Clinical Signs in
Neurology

A Compendium

Clinical Signs in
Neurology

A Compendium

William W. Campbell, MD, MSHA, COL, MC, USA (Ret)

Professor of Neurology (Emeritus)
Uniformed Services University of the Health Sciences
Bethesda, Maryland

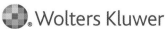
 Wolters Kluwer

Philadelphia • Baltimore • New York • London
Buenos Aires • Hong Kong • Sydney • Tokyo

Acquisitions Editor: Jamie Elfrank
Product Development Editor: Andrea Vosburgh
Marketing Manager: Stephanie Kindlick
Production Project Manager: Priscilla Crater
Design Coordinator: Elaine Kasmer
Manufacturing Coordinator: Beth Welsh
Prepress Vendor: S4Carlisle Publishing Services

9 8 7 6 5 4 3 2 1

Printed in China

Library of Congress Cataloging-in-Publication Data

Campbell, William W., Jr. (William Wesley), author.
  Clinical signs in neurology : a compendium / William W. Campbell.
    p. ; cm.
  Includes bibliographical references and index.
  ISBN 978-1-4511-9445-6
  I. Title.
  [DNLM: 1. Neurologic Manifestations—Handbooks.   2. Nervous System Diseases—diagnosis—Handbooks.   3. Neurologic Examination—Handbooks. WL 39]
  RC386.6.N48
  616.8'0475—dc23

2015021078

LWW.com

To the memory of William W. Campbell, Sr.,
Rose Campbell, and Judi Campbell Lee.
And to Rhonda, Wes, Matt, Shannon,
Will, Ella, Sara, and Mitch.

Preface

The title of this work evolved through several stages of thought and discussion. The first proposed title was *Compendium of Clinical Signs in Neurology*. The final title, *Clinical Signs in Neurology: A Compendium,* was arrived at after the recognition that the term compendium is not currently in wide circulation. It was pointed out that younger physicians might well not be familiar with it. A brief survey of medical students and house staff confirmed the validity of this point of view.

So what is a compendium? One definition is "a concise compilation of a body of knowledge." An encyclopedia is a compilation of a body of knowledge that makes little effort to remain concise. This work did not strive for encyclopedia status. *The Encyclopedia of the Neurological Sciences* runs to four volumes. This book is an attempt at a concise compilation of useful neurologic signs. There was no attempt to include every conceivable neurologic sign, as many are of marginal clinical utility, are primarily of historical interest, and are not in wide use.

This book might be viewed as a Venn diagram of three other works. The first is *DeJong's The Neurologic Examination*. The *DeJong*[1] was first published in 1950; the 7th edition was published in 2013.[2] It has been in continuous publication longer than any other major textbook in American neurology. The *DeJong* makes no attempt at conciseness. Almost every conceivable neurologic sign is at least mentioned, if not discussed in detail, and there is an accompanying discussion of the relevant neuroanatomy, neurophysiology, and clinical neurology. It is not organized in such a way that one can quickly obtain a brief discussion of a given sign. Writing books has made me acutely aware of the limitations of indexing. Even though professional indexers attempt the task, it is distressing how often entities I know are contained in my own book cannot be found in the index.

Enter another influential work: *Companion to Clinical Neurology*.[3] This book, by William Pryse-Philips, is an alphabetized listing of a host of topics of interest to the neurologist. The *Companion* might be considered a compendium, as it is at least only one volume, although it is, in its most recent edition, quite a hefty volume. The *Companion* is not limited to clinical signs and includes a vast amount of information, from the A band to Zellweger syndrome.

The objective of this compendium was to compose an alphabetized, easily accessed, richly illustrated collection limited to clinical signs, and only useful clinical signs. Although some may question whether everything in this collection is truly useful, I think the vast majority are.

The third lattice in the conceptual framework was *augenblickdiagnose*.[4] This is a German word, obviously, that roughly translates as "diagnosis in the blink of an eye." It describes a finding or phenomenon so characteristic that the differential diagnosis is essentially limited to one possibility. The diagnosis is immediately obvious and is rendered in too short a time to have permitted any amount of hypothesis generation and testing. It is familiarity with and recognition of certain physical findings that are so characteristic of a particular condition or clinical syndrome as to permit almost instantaneous diagnosis. A physician familiar with a certain condition that has a characteristic appearance can often recognize it at a glance. It does not even require medical training to recognize something such as Down's syndrome at a glance. A medical student in early clinical training could recognize neurofibromatosis type 1 at a glance. This compendium has attempted to include a large number of figures and videos to illustrate various signs and conditions.

Goethe reminded us of the proverb, "One sees only what one knows." A neurologist is unlikely to recognize Puussepp's little toe sign unless he knows of its existence. I hope readers who familiarize themselves with the contents of this book will be able to "augenblick" many more things as a result. To paraphrase Henry James, "We must know as much as possible about our art."

I have for years been giving a series of Grand Rounds on *augenblickdiagnose* that illustrates many common or classical neurologic signs and conditions. In the course of working on this book, I encountered a number of potentially useful signs not currently in my armamentarium. Another interesting talk might be titled "Neurologic Signs You Don't Know But Should."

A number of other interesting things came to light in the course of working on this book. For instance, everyone is familiar with "Babinski's sign," meaning Babinski's extensor plantar response. Some are familiar with Babinski's platysma sign and the trunk–thigh sign, but how many with the six other signs described by that prolific clinical observer, all of which might legitimately be referred to as "Babinski's sign"? Several other neurologic pioneers also described multiple signs, all of which bear their name. Robert Wartenberg is a prime example. What should a resident say when asked by an attending "what is Wartenberg's sign? The resident has at least four answers to choose from.

It has been fashionable for decades to criticize the use of eponyms. But the alternative in many instances is some verbose appellation or a convoluted acronym just as obtuse as the eponym. It is difficult to conceive of a better way to say Foster Kennedy syndrome than simply Foster Kennedy syndrome. In choosing the rubric for a certain entry, in general the name in widest current use was chosen, with Google Books and Google Scholar as the referees, with cross references to other commonly used designations. For instance, the main entry is benediction hand rather than preacher's hand, papal hand, or hand of the papal benediction.

References

1. DeJong, RN. *The Neurologic Examination, Incorporating the Fundamentals of Neuroanatomy and Neurophysiology.* New York: Hoeber; 1950.
2. Campbell, WW. *DeJong's The Neurologic Examination.* 7th ed. Baltimore, MD: Wolters Kluwer Health/Lippincott Williams & Wilkins; 2013.
3. Pryse-Phillips, W. *Companion to Clinical Neurology.* 3rd ed. Oxford: Oxford University Press; 2009.
4. Campbell, WW. Augenblickdiagnose. *Semin Neurol.* 1998;18:169–176.

Acknowledgments

I owe my gratitude to many individuals who contributed to this work. Apologies to anyone inadvertently left out. Thanks are due to Drs. Osama S. M. Amin, Jason Barton, Nabil Ebraheim, K. Figueroa, J. Goldman, J. David Karlin, J. Y. Kwan, Thomas Mathews, Ivan Paredes, John C. Pearson, Alejandro Stern, Nathan T. Tagg, S. Tazen, Niall Tubridy, and Olavo Vasconcelos, and to Mr. Alistair Hamilton.

I would like to especially acknowledge the assistance of the individuals who critiqued parts of the text. These include Drs. Francis Walker, John D. Stewart, Robert Laureno, William Pryse-Philips, John Kincaid, Stephen G. Reich, Peter Donofrio, Mark Landau, Craig Carroll, and Jason Hawley.

Ms. Shannon C. Ward provided invaluable assistance. Expert advice and support was provided by the team at Wolters Kluwer Health, including Andrea Vosburgh, Jamie Elfrank, and Julie Goolsby.

As always, I appreciate the support and forbearance of my wife, Dr. Rhonda M. Pridgeon.

Contents

Videos

 The following videos can be found in the companion eBook edition.

H

Video H-1.   Hemiballismus. The movements were unremitting and medically intractable but resolved after pallidotomy. (Courtesy of Stephen G. Reich, Department of Neurology, University of Maryland.)

Video H-2.   Two patients with hemifacial spasm. (Courtesy of Stephen G. Reich, Department of Neurology, University of Maryland.)

I

Video I-1.   A pseudo-internuclear ophthalmoplegia in a patient with myasthenia gravis. (Courtesy of Dr. Jason Barton and www.neuroophthalmology.ca.)

J

Video J-1.   Jaw winking. (Courtesy of Dr. Stephen G. Reich, Department of Neurology, University of Maryland.)

M

Video M-1.   A patient with myoclonus of the facial muscles. (Courtesy of Stephen G. Reich, Department of Neurology, University of Maryland.)

Video M-2.   Grip myotonia.

Video M-3.   Percussion myotonia.

N

Audio N-1.   An example of the voice quality of nasal speech from a popular television show. The voice does not have the characteristics of velopharyngeal insufficiency.

Video N-1.   Patient with episodic ataxia type 2 who demonstrates gaze evoked nystagmus on gaze in either direction and transient rebound nystagmus beating in the opposite direction on reassuming primary gaze. (Courtesy of Dr. Jason Barton and www.neuroophthalmology.ca.)

Video N-2.   A patient who developed upbeat nystagmus acutely after a viral infection. (Courtesy of Dr. J. David Karlin.)

Video N-3.   Downbeat nystagmus. (Courtesy of Dr. Nathan T. Tagg.)

Video N-4.   Periodic alternating nystagmus due to a Chiari II malformation. As the patient attempts to maintain fixation in primary position, initially there is a right beating nystagmus that gradually increases in amplitude and velocity, then subsides. After a period of several seconds of no nystagmus, left-beating nystagmus then gradually develops. (Courtesy of Dr. Jason Barton and www.neuroophthalmology.ca.)

Video N-5.   Bruns' nystagmus in a 71-year-old man with the recent acute onset of diplopia and nystagmus. Examination showed clumsiness of the left hand and leg, with dysdiadochokinesia of the left arm. On Romberg testing he leaned to the left with eyes closed. CT showed a left cerebellar hemorrhage with edema and mass effect upon the junction of the medulla, pons and cerebellum. (Courtesy of Dr. Jason Barton and www.neuroophthalmology.ca.)

AC	air conduction
ACTH	adrenocorticotrophic hormone
AD	Alzheimer's disease
AIM	abnormal involuntary movements
AION	anterior ischemic optic neuropathy
ALS	amyotrophic lateral sclerosis
AM	associated movement
AOS	apraxia of speech
APB	abductor pollicis brevis
APD	afferent pupillary defect
AVM	arteriovenous malformation
BC	bone conduction
BEB	benign essential blepharospasm
BP	blood pressure
BPPV	benign paroxysmal positional vertigo
BSS	bent spine syndrome
CADASIL	cerebral autosomal dominant arteriopathy with subcortical infarcts and leukomalacia
CBD	corticobasal degeneration
CDT	clock drawing test
CFP	central facial palsy
CHL	conductive hearing loss
CIDP	chronic inflammatory demyelinating polyneuropathy
CJD	Creutzfeldt-Jakob disease
CMT	Charcot-Marie-Tooth disease
CN	cranial nerve
CNS	central nervous system
CPA	cerebellopontine angle
CR	cervical radiculopathy
CRAO	central retinal artery occlusion
CSF	cerebrospinal fluid
CST	corticospinal tract
CT	computed tomography
CTS	carpal tunnel syndrome
DBP	diastolic blood pressure
DIP	distal interphalangeal
DM	dermatomyositis
DM1	myotonic dystrophy type 1
DM2	myotonic dystrophy type 2
DMD	Duchenne muscular dystrophy
DSM-5	*Diagnostic and Statistical Manual of Mental Disorders* (5th edition)
DTR	deep tendon reflex

EAST	elevated arm stress test
EDS	Ehlers-Danlos syndrome
EHL	extensor halluces longus
EMG	electromyography
EPT	enhanced physiologic tremor
ET	essential tremor
FDI	first dorsal interosseous
FEF	frontal eye fields
FLAIR	fluid-attenuated inversion recovery
FNST	femoral nerve stretch test
FOUR	full outline of responsiveness
FPA	far point of accommodation
FRS	frontal release sign
FSH	facioscapulohumeral dystrophy
FTD	frontotemporal dementia
FTN	finger-to-nose
GBS	Guillain-Barre syndrome
GEN	gaze-evoked nystagmus
GI	gastrointestinal
GTS	Gilles de la Tourette syndrome
HD	Huntington's disease
HFS	hemifacial spasm
HIV	human immunodeficiency virus
HNPP	hereditary neuropathy with liability to pressure palsies
HR	heart rate
HSP	hereditary spastic parapareis
HTLV	human T lymphocyte virus
HTS	heel-to-shin
IBM	inclusion body myositis
ICD	intercanthal distance
ICP	intracranial pressure
INO	internuclear ophthalmoplegia
IP	interphalangeal
IPD	interpupillary distance
JHS	joint hypermobility syndrome
KF	Kaiser-Fleischer
LBD	Lewy body dementia
LEMS	Lambert-Eaton myasthenic syndrome
LGMD	limb girdle muscular dystrophy
LHON	Leber's hereditary optic neuropathy
LMN	lower motor neuron
LR	likelihood ratio
LSR	lumbosacral radiculopathy
MCA	middle cerebral artery
MCP	metacarpophalangeal
MELAS	mitochondrial encephalopathy, lactic acidosis and stroke-like episodes
MERRF	mitochondrial encephalomyopathy with ragged red fibers
MG	myasthenia gravis

MLF	medial longitudinal fasciculus
MMN	multifocal motor neuropathy
MMSE	mini-mental state exam
MRC	Medical Research Council
MRI	magnetic resonance imaging
MS	multiple sclerosis
MSA	multiple system atrophy
MSE	mental status examination
MSH	melanocyte-stimulating hormone
MTP	metatarsophalangeal
NARP	neuropathy, ataxia, retinitis pigmentosa
NF1	neurofibromatosis type 1
NF2	neurofibromatosis type 2
NMS	neuroleptic malignant syndrome
NOVEL	Neuro-Ophthalmology Virtual Education Library
NOVL	nonorganic visual loss
NPA	near point of accommodation
NPH	normal pressure hydrocephalus
NPV	negative predictive value
OKN	optokinetic nystagmus
OTR	ocular tilt reaction
PD	Parkinson's disease
PEP	peak expiratory pressure
PFP	peripheral facial palsy
PIN	posterior interosseous nerve
PIP	proximal interphalangeal
PKAN	pantothenate kinase-associated neurodegeneration
PMR	palmomental reflex
POEMS	polyneuropathy, organomegaly, endocrinopathy, monoclonal gammopathy and skin changes
POTS	postural orthostatic tachycardia syndrome
PPRF	pontine paramedian reticular formation
PPV	positive predictive value
PSP	progressive supranuclear palsy
PT	parkinsonian tremor
PTO	parietotemporaloccipital
PXE	pseudoxantoma elasticum
RAM	rapid alternating movement
RAPD	relative afferent pupillary defect
ROCF	Rey-Osterreith complex figure
ROM	range of motion
RP	retinitis pigmentosa
SAH	subarachnoid hemorrhage
SBP	systolic blood pressure
SCI	spinal cord injury
SI	sacroiliac
SIC	spinal injuries center
SLE	systemic lupus erythematosus

SLR	straight leg raising
SMA	spinal muscular atrophy
SNHL	sensorineural hearing loss
SSA	Sjogren's syndrome A
SSB	Sjogren's syndrome B
SVV	subjective visual vertical
TBI	traumatic brain injury
TCA	transcortical aphasia
TD	tardive dyskinesia
TOS	thoracic outlet syndrome
TTP	thrombotic thrombocytopenic purpura
UMN	upper motor neuron
UNE	ulnar neuropathy at the elbow
UPSIT	University of Pennsylvania smell identification test
US	ultrasound
V1	the first division of the trigeminal nerve
V2	second division of the trigeminal nerve
V3	third division of the trigeminal nerve
VF	visual field
VGKC	voltage-gated K^+ channel
VOR	vestibulo-ocular reflex
WEBINO	wall-eyed bilateral internuclear ophthalmoplegia
WEMINO	wall-eyed monocular internuclear ophthalmoplegia

A pattern deviation: A strabismus pattern in which the ocular deviation varies with the vertical position of the eyes, causing **esotropia** on upgaze and **exotropia** on downgaze. See **V pattern deviation.**

Abadie's sign: The absence of pain on squeezing the Achilles tendon, which is normally quite uncomfortable, a classic sign of tabes dorsalis (see also **Biernacki's sign** and **Pitres's sign**). All these are signs of tabes dorsalis, but could result from any process causing severe sensory loss.

Abaragnosis: Loss of ability to appreciate and differentiate weight. Baresthesia is the ability to sense pressure or weight, and barognosis is the appreciation, recognition, and differentiation of weight or the ability to differentiate between weights.

Abasia: An inability to walk, presumably on a nonorganic basis, distinct from gait ataxia, gait apraxia, or other gait abnormalities; seen as part of **astasia-abasia.**

Abdominal reflexes: Reflex responses elicited from the anterior abdominal wall (Video A.1). There are two types of abdominal reflexes, superficial and deep. **Superficial reflexes** are responses to stimulation of either the skin or mucous membrane. The **superficial abdominal reflexes** consist of contraction of the abdominal muscles elicited by a light stroke or scratch of the anterior abdominal wall that pulls the umbilicus in the direction of the stimulus (Fig. A.1).[1] The umbilicus is at the level of T10. The anterior abdominal wall can be divided into four quadrants by vertical and horizontal lines through the umbilicus. Light stroking or scratching in each quadrant elicits the response, pulling the umbilicus in the direction of the stimulus. The stimulus may be directed toward, away, or parallel

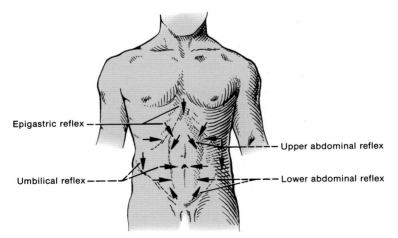

Epigastric reflex

Umbilical reflex

Upper abdominal reflex

Lower abdominal reflex

Figure A.1. Sites of stimulation employed in eliciting the various superficial abdominal reflexes. (From Campbell WW. *DeJong's the Neurologic Examination.* 7th ed. Philadelphia, PA: Wolters Kluwer Health/Lippincott Williams & Wilkins; 2013, with permission.)

to the umbilicus; stimuli directed toward the umbilicus seem more effective. The response is a quick, flicking contraction followed by immediate relaxation. The response is mediated in the upper quadrants (supraumbilical reflexes) by the intercostal nerves (T7–T10) and in the lower quadrants (infraumbilical or suprapubic reflexes) by the intercostal, iliohypogastric, and ilioinguinal nerves (T10-upper lumbar segments).

The responses are typically brisk and active in young individuals with good anterior abdominal tone. They may be sluggish or absent in normal individuals with lax abdominal tone, in the obese or in women who have borne children. Asymmetry of the abdominal reflexes is common, and in 15% of individuals the responses may be absent in all quadrants, even in adolescents and young adults.

The deep abdominal muscle stretch reflexes are obtained by brisk stretching of the muscles. These reflexes are best elicited by stretching the muscles slightly by pressing down with the fingers and then tapping with a reflex hammer. The response is contraction of the abdominal muscles and a deviation of the umbilicus toward the site of the stimulus. The innervation is by the intercostal, ilioinguinal, and iliohypogastric nerves. The abdominal muscle stretch reflexes are only minimally present in normal individuals. To elicit the symphysis pubis reflex, percussion is directed toward the site of muscle insertion.

Corticospinal tract lesions produce exaggerated **deep tendon reflexes** and decreased **superficial reflexes**. Brisk deep abdominal reflexes with absent superficial abdominal reflexes suggests a CST lesion, termed dissociation of the abdominal reflexes.

Abduction nystagmus: Nystagmus greater in the abducting eye, typical of **internuclear ophthalmoplegia**.

Abductor digiti quinti (minimi) sign: See **digiti quinti sign.**

Abductor sign: A sign used to detect nonorganic leg weakness, similar to **Hoover's sign**. It seeks to elicit a synergistic associated movement of the nonparetic leg when the patient is asked to abduct the paretic leg. In nonorganic paresis, the paretic leg demonstrates synergistic abduction when the sound leg is tested, and the sound leg does not exert normal abduction power and can be moved into a hyperadducted position when the paretic limb is tested. It may be useful when relatively preserved hip extensor strength limits the utility of Hoover's test. See **Spinal Injuries Center test.**

Abductor spasmodic dysphonia: See **spasmodic dysphonia**

Aberrant regeneration (reinnervation): Misdirection of axons in the process of repair following conditions that cause mechanical disruption of a nerve. Axons that originally innervated one muscle are mistakenly routed to a different muscle. This results from regenerating sprouts growing into the wrong Schwann cell tubes and eventually innervating some structure other than originally intended. Following a command to the original muscle to contract, the aberrantly innervated muscle contracts in addition to, or instead of, the agonist. Aberrant reinnervation may follow any type of nerve lesion and there are many examples. Aberrant reinnervation is common after Bell's palsy, causing **facial synkinesis (Video Link A.1)** and the **Marin Amat sign. Aberrant reinnervation of CN III** is common, especially after diabetic third nerve palsy.

Aberrant reinnervation of CN III: A helpful clinical feature distinguishing ischemic from mechanical, compressive lesions of CN III; also referred to as misdirection syndrome or oculomotor synkinesias **(Video Link A.2)**. Fibers originally destined to innervate the medial rectus may reinnervate the levator palpebrae and other extraocular muscles. The dual innervation of muscles causes a failure of normal reciprocal relaxation of the antagonist, resulting in co-contraction and retraction of the globe on certain movements. Attempted upgaze causes adduction and retraction because of misdirection of superior rectus fibers into the medial and inferior recti with co-contraction. The upper lid may retract on downgaze (pseudo-Graefe sign) due to inferior rectus fibers aberrantly innervating the levator. The lid retracts on adduction because of synkinesis between the medial rectus and the levator. The lid may droop on abduction because the reciprocal inhibition of the medial rectus causes the levator to relax. The dynamic lid changes with eye movement are the opposite of those seen in **Duane's syndrome**.

The common causes are aneurysm and head trauma, and less common causes are tumor and neurosyphilis; the condition can occur congenitally. Aberrant reinnervation does not occur after ischemic or idiopathic third nerve palsy.

Abnormal involuntary movements: Spontaneous movements that occur with many different neurologic disorders. There are many types of abnormal involuntary movements (AIMs), ranging from tremor to chorea to muscle fasciculations to myoclonic jerks. Common examples include tremor and dystonia. The only common characteristic is that the movements are spontaneous and, for the most part, not under volitional control. They may be rhythmic or random, fleeting or sustained, predictable or unpredictable, and may occur in isolation or accompanied by other neurologic signs **(Table A.1)**. The character of the movement depends on both the site of the lesion and the underlying pathology.

Absent muscles: Congenitally absence of a muscle. It is not uncommon for isolated muscles, such as the palmaris longus, pectoralis minor, or depressor anguli oris, to fail to develop, causing minimal deformity and no clinical deficit.

Abstraction (abstract thinking): One of the higher cerebral functions. Abstraction is often tested by asking the patient to describe similarities and differences and to interpret proverbs and aphorisms. The patient may be asked how an apple and a banana, a car and an airplane, a watch and a ruler, or a poem and a statue are alike or to tell the difference between a lie and a mistake or between a cable and a chain. Patients with impaired abstraction are said to think concretely. The patient with impaired abstraction may be unable to interpret a proverb. When interpreting "Don't cry over spilt milk," the patient thinking concretely will talk about accidents, milk, spillage, cleanup, and other things that miss the point.

Interpretation of proverbs and aphorisms are commonly used tests of abstract thinking. Frequently used proverbs include "a rolling stone gathers no moss,"

Table A.1. Abnormal Involuntary Movements as a Spectrum of Movements

Regular/Predictable	Intermediate	Fleeting/Unpredictable
Tremor	Most dystonias	Fasciculations
Hemiballism	Myokymia	Myoclonus
Palatal myoclonus	Athetosis	Chorea
	Tic	Dyskinesias
	Stereotypy	
	Myorhythmia	

From Campbell WW. *DeJong's the Neurologic Examination.* 7th ed. Philadelphia, PA: Wolters Kluwer Health/Lippincott Williams & Wilkins; 2013.

"a stitch in time saves nine," "Rome wasn't built in a day," and "people who live in glass houses shouldn't throw stones." The usefulness of proverb interpretation has been questioned because many examiners are not precisely sure themselves what some of the proverbs mean. Bizarre, peculiar proverb interpretations may be given by patients with psychiatric disease or by normal people not familiar with the idiomatic usage. A concatenated or confused proverb or saying such as "The hand that rocks the cradle shouldn't throw stones" and "don't pussyfoot around the bush" may be useful to test both the patient's abstraction ability and sense of humor. Impaired abstraction occurs in many conditions, but is particularly common with frontal lobe disorders.

Abulia: Difficulty in initiating and sustaining spontaneous movements and reduction in emotional responsiveness, spontaneous speech, and social interaction. Abulia is characteristic of frontal lobe and basal ganglia lesions. Other terms used to describe similar states include **akinetic mutism** and **apallic state**.

Acalculia: An inability to calculate; one of the components of Gerstmann's syndrome (agraphia, acalculia, finger agnosia, and right left disorientation). The acalculia may have a basis in an inability to recognize numbers, an inability to align numbers visuospatially, or a true **anarithmia**.

Accommodation: The thickening of the lens that permits clear vision of nearby objects. It occurs as contraction of the ciliary muscle relaxes the zonular fibers, permitting the lens to become more convex because of its inherent elasticity. Accommodation is measured in diopters. The **near point of accommodation** is the closest point at which an object can be seen clearly. The **far point of accommodation** is the distance at which a distant image is focused on the retina with no accommodative effort.

Accommodation reflex (near response, near reflex): Thickening of the lens, convergence of the eyes, and miosis; elicited by having the patient relax accommodation by gazing into the distance, then shifting gaze to some near object. The best near object is the patient's own finger or thumb. The pupils constrict at near to increase the depth of focus. With special techniques, each component of the response can be tested separately. Routine bedside testing elicits all three components.

Achilles reflex: See **ankle reflex**.

Achromatopsia: An inability to perceive colors. Achromatopsia is most often congenital and asymptomatic. Acquired achromatopsia may occur from ophthalmologic or neurologic processes. Achromatopsia must be differentiated from color agnosia and color anomia. It may be a very early manifestation of a focal occipital lobe lesion that later evolves into heminaopsia. Testing may be informal, as by asking the patient to recognize or point out the colors in a garment, such as a necktie, or more formally by the use of color plates, such as Ishihara or HRR plates. Achromatopsia is often an early manifestation of optic neuropathy. See **color blindness, color desaturation**.

Acopia: Difficulty copying, with or without accompanying aphasic abnormalities.

Acoustic startle reflex: Sudden spasmodic muscle contraction after a loud noise; may affect any number of muscles.

Acrocephalosyndactyly: The association of a **craniosynostosis** syndrome with fusion of the digits. Sometimes there are extra digits, creating acrocephalopolysyndactyly. These defects are characteristic of Carpenter's, Apert's, and similar syndromes. See **syndactyly**.

Acrocephaly: A **craniosynostosis** syndrome causing premature closure of the sagittal and both coronal sutures, causing **oxycephaly**, a pointed, conical skull.

Acromegaly: A condition associated with excessive secretion of growth hormone and insulin-like growth factor, most often due to an anterior pituitary adenoma. Acromegaly causes characteristic enlargement of the hands and feet and a typical facial appearance **(Fig. A.2)**. It was first described and named by Pierre Marie, the French neurologist. The facial appearance in acromegaly is due to **prognathism**,

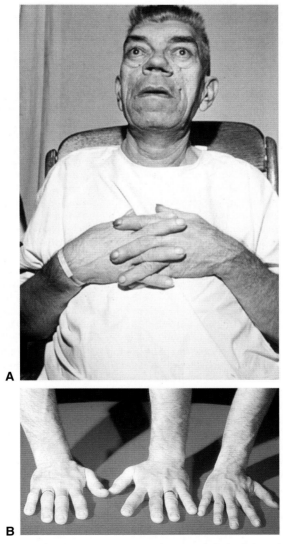

Figure A.2. Acromegaly. **A:** Note coarse facial features. **B:** Patient's large hands at left; single normal hand at right. (From McConnell TH, Paulson VA, Valasek MA. *The Nature of Disease: Pathology for the Health Professions*. 2nd ed. Baltimore, MD: Wolters Kluwer Health/Lippincott Williams & Wilkins; 2014, with permission.)

enlarged supraorbital ridges, coarse facial features and **frontal bossing.** The condition is easily recognized when these changes are advanced; recognition of early disease is more challenging. Acromegaly also causes **macroglossia**.

Acromial reflex: See **clavicle reflex**.

Action dystonia: See **dystonia**.

Action myoclonus: See **myoclonus**.

Action tremor: See **tremor.**

Adam's bend test: See **scoliosis**.

Adaptability (fatigability): Failure of the nystagmus to persist, or of the response to recur on repetition of the provocative maneuver, in patients with positional nystagmus. The **Dix-Hallpike maneuver** may elicit nystagmus by placing the patient's head into a particular position. If vertigo or nystagmus occur, the patient is held in the provoking position until the symptoms subside and then the movement is repeated to assess its recurrence. The response is transient (fatigabile) and repeating the maneuver several times consecutively provokes less of a response each time until eventually the nystagmus and vertigo are nil. After a period of 10 to 15 minutes, the response can be elicited again. This lessening of the response on repetition of the maneuver has variously been referred to as adaptability, fatigability, or habituation; these terms are used inconsistently. With positional nystagmus, latency to onset, fatigability, and adaptability all support a peripheral process. Minimal vertigo with prominent nystagmus, or lack of latency, fatigability, and adaptability suggests a central process.

Adduction lag: A sometimes subtle finding of **internuclear ophthalmoplegia** when the amplitude and velocity of the adducting saccade is reduced when compared with the abducting saccade.

Adductor reflex: The DTR elicited by tapping over the medial femoral condyle, causing the hip to adduct. A normal but usually not very active reflex, elicited with some difficulty in normal individuals. The reflex may sometimes be useful (see Table D.1). When reflexes are hyperactive, some thigh adduction may occur on eliciting the knee jerk, and bilateral thigh adduction may occur with percussion over the synthesis pubis (suprapubic reflex). See **crossed adductor reflex**.

Adductor reflex of the foot (Hirschberg's sign): A response elicited by stroking the inner aspect of the foot (not the sole) from the great toe toward the heel, causing adduction, inversion, and slight plantar flexion, seen in patients with CST disease.

Adductor spasmodic dysphonia: See **spasmodic dysphonia**.

Adenoma sebaceum: The facial skin lesions seen in tuberous sclerosis. These small papules are cutaneous hamartomas, often mistaken for acne (Fig. A.3).[2,3] See **hypomelanotic macule, periungual fibroma, poliosis, shagreen patch.**

Adiaphoresis: Absence of sweating, see **anhidrosis**.

Adie's (Holmes-Adie) syndrome: The association of **Adie's tonic pupil** with depressed or absent DTRs, particularly in the lower extremities. In Ross' syndrome, there is also involvement of sudomotor fibers, producing Adie's syndrome along with segmental **anhidrosis**, often associated with compensatory **hyperhidrosis**.

Adie's (Holmes-Adie) tonic pupil: A disorder involving the ciliary ganglion or short ciliary nerves, or both. There is **light-near dissociation** of the pupil in which the direct light reflex is impaired while pupillary constriction to near is relatively preserved (Fig. A.4). The pupillary reaction to light may appear absent, although prolonged illumination may provoke a slow constriction. The reaction to near,

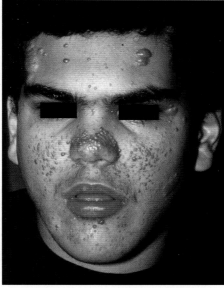

Figure A.3. Adenoma sebaceum in a patient with tuberous sclerosis. (From Wyllie E, Cascino GD, Gidal BE, et al, eds. *Wyllie's Treatment of Epilepsy: Principles and Practice.* 5th ed. Philadelphia, PA: Wolters Kluwer Health/Lippincott Williams & Wilkins; 2011, with permission.)

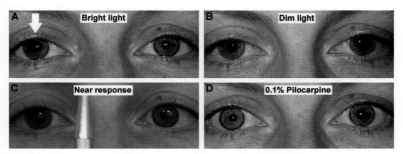

Figure A.4. Adie's pupil showing poor light reaction but prompt constriction to dilute pilocarpine, demonstrating denervation supersensitivity. There is typically better con-striction to near than shown here, although the near response may be slow and difficult to demonstrate. Impairment of the near response may be more common acutely. (From Wakerley BR, Tan MH, Turner MR. Teaching video neuroimages: acute Adie syndrome. *Neurology.* 2012;79:e97, with permission.)

although slow, is better preserved. Once constricted, the tonic pupil redilates very slowly when illumination is removed or the patient looks back at distance, often causing a transient reversal of the **anisocoria**. The abnormally slow and prolonged redilation on looking back at distance resembles the delayed relaxation seen in

myotonia. On close inspection, the constricted pupil is not perfectly round. Slit lamp examination may reveal characteristic findings. Close examination under magnification shows that what iris constriction does occur is not uniform, but involves some segments more than others, producing a slightly irregular contour to the pupil, referred to as segmental or sector palsy. Slit lamp may also show peculiar spontaneous "vermiform" movements of the iris (**Video Link A.3**). Adie's pupil is due to **aberrant regeneration** of fibers intended for the ciliary muscle innervating the pupillary sphincter muscle, usually following a presumably viral attack on the ciliary ganglion.

Tonic pupils are fairly common. The patient presenting with Adie's tonic pupil is typically a young woman who suddenly notes a unilaterally enlarged pupil, with no other symptoms. The parasympathetic denervation eventually leads to denervation supersensitivity; the pupil may then constrict to solutions of pilocarpine or methacholine too dilute to affect a normal eye. About 20% of patients develop a tonic pupil in the other eye. With the passage of time, the pupil may become smaller, and an old Adie's pupil can be a cause of unilateral miosis. The light reaction never recovers.

Examining the eyes under light and dark conditions can help greatly in sorting out asymmetric pupils (**Fig. A.5**). Recall that physiologic **anisocoria** produces about the same degree of pupillary asymmetry in the light and the dark. With **Horner's syndrome,** the small pupil dilates poorly in the dark, causing pupillary asymmetry greater in the dark than in the light. In contrast, CN III palsy and Adie's pupil cause greater asymmetry in the light because of the involved pupil's inability to constrict.

Adson's test: See **thoracic outlet syndrome provocative tests.**

Afferent pupillary defect (relative afferent pupillary defect, Marcus Gunn pupil, Gunn pupil): An abnormal pupillary response seen most often in optic nerve disease. The normal pupillary response to light is constriction. A difference in the intensity of the signal transmitted through the two optic nerves may cause an asymmetry in the light reflex. Even in normal individuals, the amplitude and velocity of the response depend on a number of factors, such as the level of

Etiologic Factor	Ambient Light		Strong Light		Dark		Conclusion
Physiologic anisocoria	•	●	•	•	●	●	Same relative asymmetry under all conditions
Right Horner syndrome	•	●	•	•	•	●	More asymmetry in the dark; abnormal pupil can not dilate
Left third cranial nerve palsy	•	•	•	●	●	●	More asymmetry in the light; abnormal pupil cannot constrict

Figure A.5. Behavior of unequal pupils in light and dark conditions. (From Campbell WW. *DeJong's the Neurologic Examination.* 7th ed. Philadelphia, PA: Wolters Kluwer Health/Lippincott Williams & Wilkins; 2013, with permission.)

ambient illumination and whether the patient is fixing at near or far. When clinical circumstances dictate careful evaluation, the amplitude of the initial pupillary constriction and the normal subsequent slight escape must be judged by comparing the two eyes.

With mild to moderate optic nerve disease, it is difficult to detect any change in pupil reactivity to the direct light stimulation as usually performed. In 1902, R. Marcus Gunn, a Scottish ophthalmologist, described an abnormal pupillary response in optic nerve disease, what he termed secondary dilatation under continued exposure, or the adapting pupillary response. This became known as a Marcus Gunn pupil, or an afferent pupillary defect (APD). In 1959, Levitan described looking for an APD by swinging a light back and forth between the two eyes (swinging flashlight test). Moving the light back and forth amplifies the asymmetry of the response. Since the finding depends on the difference between the two eyes, the state of the afferent system and activity of the light reflex in one eye relative to the other, the term relative APD (RAPD) is often used. In essence, with a unilateral optic nerve lesion the direct pupillary response is less active that the consensual response elicited by stimulating the opposite eye and the swinging flashlight exposes this imbalance. The sensitivity of an APD in detecting a unilateral optic nerve lesion exceeds 90%.[4]

The swinging flashlight test can quickly and accurately compare the light responsiveness of the two pupils (**Fig. A.6**, **Video Links A.4 and A.5**). It is a key clinical technique in the evaluation of suspected optic neuropathy and can often detect a side-to-side difference even when the lesion is mild and there is no detectable difference in the direct light reflex when testing each eye individually. An RAPD may occur even in the absence of other clinical evidence of optic nerve dysfunction.

There are two techniques for the swinging flashlight test. In the first, the light is held about one inch from the eye and just below the visual axis and rapidly alternated, pausing for about one full second on each side. The examiner only attends to the stimulated eye, comparing the amplitude and velocity of the initial constriction in the two eyes. The reaction is relatively weaker when the bad eye is illuminated. In the other technique, the light is allowed to linger a bit longer. With stimulation of the good eye, both pupils constrict smartly due to the direct reflex in the stimulated eye and the consensual reflex in the opposite eye. After 3 to 5 seconds to allow the pupil to stabilize, the light is quickly swung to the bad eye. The brain detects a relative diminution in light intensity, and the pupil may dilate a bit in response. The pupil in the other eye dilates as well because the consensual reflex constricting the pupil in the good eye is less active than its direct reflex, but this is not observed. On moving the light back to the good eye, the more active direct response causes the pupil to constrict. On moving back to the bad eye, the pupil dilates because the direct light reflex is weaker than the consensual reflex that had been holding it down. As the light passes back and forth, the pupil of the good eye constricts to direct light stimulation and the pupil of the bad eye dilates to direct light stimulation. It may require several swings to find the optimum speed to bring out the dynamic anisocoria. Over several cycles, it may be striking to see one pupil consistently dilate to the same light stimulus that causes the other to constrict (see Video Link A.5). Active hippus may cause difficulty in interpretation. Hippus is random; a true RAPD will be consistent over multiple trials. Pay attention to the

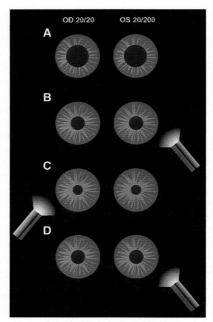

Figure A.6. Relative afferent pupillary defect. Vision on the right 20/20; vision on the left 20/200 because of optic neuropathy. **A:** The pupils in dim light are equal. **B:** Light directed into the left eye results in a partial and sluggish contraction in each eye. **C:** Light directed into the right eye results in a brisk and normal reaction in each eye. **D:** The light quickly redirected into the left eye results in a dilatation of both pupils. Swinging the light back and forth will bring out the dynamic anisocoria. (From Tasman W, Jaeger E. *The Wills Eye Hospital Atlas of Clinical Ophthalmology.* 2nd ed. Philadelphia, PA: Wolters Kluwer Health/Lippincott Williams & Wilkins; 2001, with permission.)

first movement of the pupil; if it is consistently a dilation movement, the patient has an RAPD and not hippus.

The light brightness comparison test is the subjective equivalent of the swinging flashlight test. A bright light is shone into the good eye and the patient asked to judge the intensity and then asked to compare with the symptomatic eye. The patient's estimate of the difference in intensity often correlates with the level of activity of the APD.

Afternoon ectropion: Drooping and eversion of the lower lid that occurs in patients with MG as the day wears on and the lid muscle weakens. See **ectropion**.

Age-related signs: Findings that may occur in the normal elderly. A number of neurological changes are known to occur as part of normal aging and do not indicate the presence of disease. These abnormalities are increasingly common with advancing age and are present in a substantial portion of the elderly population. Findings not attributable to major disease may include impaired olfaction, small pupils, decreased upgaze, impaired visual pursuit, high-frequency hearing loss, decreased balance, a decline in muscle bulk and power, decreased coordination, decreased vibratory sensation in the distal lower extremities, impaired ankle jerks, and changes in gait.[5,6] The ankle jerk issue may be overemphasized. Skilled examiners using good equipment find substantially less impairment than usually described.[7] **Frontal release signs**, often elicitable even in normal, younger patients, occur with even greater frequency in the normal elderly.

Ageotropic nystagmus: Nystagmus in which the upper pole beats in a direction away from the ground testing for positional nystagmus (**Video Link A.6**), as opposed to **geotropic nystagmus**. Positional nystagmus due to peripheral lesions is usually geotropic. Ageotropic nystagmus that does not convert to geotropic after positioning raises the possibility of a central lesion.

Ageusia: An inability to taste, often accompanied by anosmia. Ageusia occurs in as many as 0.5% of patients after TBI, with the incidence increasing to 5% to 6% in those who have **anosmia**. Temporary ageusia over the anterior 2/3 of the tongue occurs commonly in Bell's palsy. Perversions of taste, **dysgeusia**, are more frequent.

Agnosia: Loss or impairment of the ability to know or recognize the meaning or importance of a sensory stimulus in the absence of any impairment of perception, cognition, attention, or alertness and without any word-finding or naming limitations.

Agnosias are usually specific for a given sensory modality and can occur with any type of sensory stimulus. **Tactile agnosia** refers to the inability to recognize stimuli by feel; **visual agnosia** is the inability to recognize visually; and **auditory agnosia** is the inability to know or recognize by hearing. **Prosopagnosia** is an inability to recognize faces. **Body-image agnosia (autotopagnosia)** is loss or impairment of the ability to name and recognize body parts. **Topagnosia** is the inability to localize a tactile sensation. **Finger agnosia** is a type of **autotopagnosia** involving the fingers. Agnosias are also classified by the type of entity involved. Agnosia for physical objects (**object agnosia**) differs from agnosia for faces (**prosopagnosia**), for colors (**color agnosia**) and for letters and words (**alexia**). The most common object agnosia is visual object agnosia.

Unusual types of agnosia include time agnosia, loss of time sense without disorientation in other spheres, and visuospatial agnosia, loss or impairment in the ability to judge direction, distance, and motion and the inability to understand three-dimensional spatial relationships. Because of the impaired spatial judgment and visual disorientation, the patient with visuospatial agnosia is unable to navigate even in familiar surroundings. Multimodal agnosias may occur with dysfunction of the association areas in the parietal and temporal lobes that assimilate sensory information from more than one domain.

Two categories of agnosia are recognized. Apperceptive agnosia occurs when there is some distortion of the perception of the sensation, such as a visual agnosia due to a lesion involving the parieto-occipital region rendering an object unrecognizable. There is impairment of the more complex perceptions that allow for the synthesis of the elements necessary for object or sound recognition. Associative agnosia refers to a global inability to identify objects or sounds in the absence of sensory impairment, aphasia, or anomia. It is a defect in the association of the sensory experience with past experience and memory. Perception is intact but there is an inability to link it to the appropriate concepts in the cortical association areas, resulting in an inability to recognize it. Patients can readily identify the perception using other sensory modalities, such as by sight rather than touch. An associative agnosia is "a percept stripped of its meaning" (Teuber). Apperceptive visual agnosia lies somewhere between **cortical blindness** and associative visual agnosia.

Agrammatism (paragrammatism): An inability to use proper grammar and syntax resulting in a misuse of words and defective sentence structure. The patient knows what he wishes to say but is unable to say it or to say it correctly. Seen in patients with nonfluent **aphasia**, whose speech is parsed to the crucial, meaning-conveying nouns and verbs, omitting nonessential words (telegraphic speech).

Agraphesthesia: Inability to recognize numbers or letters by tactile stimulation, usually written on the patient's palm or fingertips. Normal individuals can recognize symbols 1 cm high on the fingertips and 6 cm high elsewhere.[8] In the presence of intact primary sensory modalities, agraphesthesia usually indicates a lesion involving the contralateral parietal lobe.

Agraphia: Loss of the ability to write not due to weakness, incoordination, or other neurologic dysfunction of the arm or hand; milder involvement may be referred to as dysgraphia. Three types are usually recognized: aphasic, constructional (due to impaired visuospatial ability), and apractic. Agraphia typically accompanies aphasia, but may occur as an isolated finding (pure agraphia). In evaluating writing ability, the patient may be asked to write spontaneously or to dictation. A spontaneous writing sample might include a few words, a sentence, or a paragraph. In aphasia, writing usually reveals the same sorts of naming difficulties and paraphasias evident in the patient's speech. Patients may be able to write elementary, overlearned things such as name, address, days of the week and months of the year, but cannot write more complex material. There may be a difference in the patient's ability to print and to write in cursive.

Akathisia: An inner restlessness and urge to move, resulting in almost constant, purposeless motion, such as rocking, pacing, and crossing and uncrossing the legs. Akathisia occurs most often as a result of treatment with dopamine-blocking agents **(Table A.2)**.

Akinesia: A paucity of movement and a slowing of movements seen in PD and related disorders. Strictly speaking, akinesia refers to an absence of movement, **bradykinesia** a slowness of movement, and **hypokinesia** a decreased amount or amplitude of movement **(Video A.2)**. All may occur to a greater or lesser degree at one time or another, although seldom is there a total absence of movement. Other conditions, such as PSP and similar parkinsonian syndromes, the effects of phenothiazines and

Table A.2. Movement Disorders Caused by Dopamine Receptor Antagonists

Acute
Drug-induced parkinsonism
Acute dystonia
Acute akathisia
Tardive
Tardive dyskinesias
Tardive dystonia
Tardive akathisia
Tardive myoclonus (rare)
Tardive tics (rare)
Tardive tremor (rare)
Neuroleptic malignant syndrome

related medications, and toxins such as MPTP and carbon monoxide, cause similar phenomena. Patients with akinesia due to PD may transiently exhibit greatly improved mobility in an emergency (paradoxical kinesia).

Akinetic mutism: A state in which the patient is mute and unmoving. The patient appears awake but is mute, immobile, and unresponsive. Akinetic mutism is a state of extreme **apathy**. It most often occurs with damage to the frontal lobes, particularly extensive, bilateral, prefrontal lesions; bilateral lesions involving the posterior intralaminar nuclei of the thalamus may also produce akinetic mutism. It has been reported with craniopharyngioma, obstructive hydrocephalus, lesions in the region of the third ventricle and lesions involving the ventral striatum, ventral globus pallidus, and anterior cingulate. Akinetic mutism is a state of persistent unresponsiveness or altered awareness similar, if not identical to, what has been termed persistent vegetative state, **abulia**, apallic state, coma vigil, and pseudocoma. Much of the nomenclature is outdated and perplexing, the distinctions vague and of marginal clinical utility. Persistent unresponsiveness and unresponsive wakefulness syndrome have been suggested as alternatives.

Akinetic-rigid gait: See **gait disorders.**

Akinetotopsia: A dissociation between the ability to see static images versus moving images in the visual field. The patient loses the ability to see objects in motion, retaining the ability to see fixed images, referred to as statokinetic dissociation or Riddoch's phenomenon.

Albert's test: See **line bisection test.**

Alcoholism, signs of: Alcohol abuse produces many neurologic complications, ranging from Wernicke's encephalopathy to cerebellar degeneration to auditory hallucinosis. There are many signs on physical examination that may provide a clue to alcohol abuse as the cause of a patient's neurological difficulties, particularly when alcoholic cirrhosis is present. Many of these in males are due to relative estrogen excess. Spider angiomas are telangiectasias that blanch on pressure, seen most often on the anterior chest wall. Other findings include palmar erythema, gynecomastia, testicular atrophy, glossitis, parotid enlargement, splenomegaly, and pseudo-Cushing syndrome. Some of these changes may also occur with cirrhosis due to other conditions, such as hepatitis C or primary biliary cirrhosis. The presence of spider angiomas along with either splenomegaly or thrombocytopenia is a strong indicator of cirrhosis.[4] Patients in liver failure obviously also have jaundice and other abnormalities.

Alexia: Loss of the ability to read in the absence of actual loss of vision (word blindness, visual receptive aphasia, visual sensory aphasia). Alexia is distinct from illiteracy, where the ability to read is never acquired. Alexia is usually related to a lesion of the dominant angular or supramarginal gyrus or its connections to the visual cortex. There is loss of the ability to recognize, interpret, and recall the meaning of visual language symbols; printed words simply have no meaning.[9]

Reading aloud is a different task from reading comprehension. Oral reading (visual input–oral output) is comparable to copying (visual input–manual output), repetition (auditory input–oral output), and transcribing dictation (auditory input–manual output), and may be preserved despite impaired reading comprehension.

Types of alexia commonly recognized include **alexia with agraphia, alexia without agraphia,** frontal alexia, deep alexia, and pure alexia. Patients with pure alexia may suffer from a specific word form processing deficit; they see "wrods with trasnpsoed letters." Alexia with agraphia is classically associated with a lesion involving the dominant angular gyrus and adjacent inferior parietal lobule; commonly associated deficits include right hemianopia and elements of Gerstmann's syndrome. Aexia without agraphia usually results from a left occipitotemporal lesion with involvement of the splenium causing disconnection between the visual cortex and the angular gyrus.

Alexia with agraphia: Loss of the ability to read and write. **See alexia.**

Alexia without agraphia: Loss of the ability to read with preservation of the ability to write. Alexia without agraphia is one of the cerebral disconnection syndromes, due to a lesion involving the left occipital lobe and the splenium of the corpus callosum, impairing the transfer of visual information from the intact right occipital lobe to the reading centers in the region of the opposite angular gyrus in the left hemisphere. The patient may write spontaneously or to dictation and then be unable to read the words just written. The syndrome was elegantly described by Dejerine. See **alexia.**

Alien hand (limb): Spontaneous, involuntary, wandering movements and bizarre behavior of an extremity. In alien hand syndrome, there is interruption of the cortical connections that control smooth bimanual operations. The hands no longer work as a team. The affected hand begins to function autonomously and loses the ability to cooperate with its fellow. There may be outright intermanual conflict. There are at least two forms: callosal and frontal.[10] Intermanual conflict is typical with lesions in the anterior corpus callosum. With a lesion of the medial frontal lobe, the alien hand is uncooperative but not contentious. It may display reflex grasping (alien grasp) and other autonomous behavior, but there is little or no intermanual conflict. A sensory alien hand syndrome has also been described following right posterior cerebral distribution stroke. There are typically parietal sensory deficits and hemineglect involving the left side of the body, which resemble anosognosia. The right arm may then involuntarily attack the left side of the body. For a video of a patient with an alien hand after callosal section for epilepsy that repeatedly slapped her in the face, see **Video Link A.7.** In Dr. Strangelove, Peter Sellers was repeatedly attacked by his alien hand.

Allen's sign: See **minor extensor toe signs.**

Allesthesia (alloesthesia): Perception of a sensory stimulus at a site other than where it was delivered. Tactile allesthesia is feeling something other than at the site of the stimulus; visual allesthesia is seeing something other than where it actually is. See **allochiria.**

Allochiria: Displacement of images or stimuli from one place to another, usually from the left to the right, often seen in association with **anosagnosia** and other manifestations of hemispatial neglect. The Greek *allo* meaning "other" or "different" is a combining form that occurs frequently in neurology. *Alias* is a related term. Rather than complete inattentiveness or neglect of a stimulus or image on the left, it is projected to the right or to a different location on the same side.

Allodynia: Pain felt following a stimulus that is not normally painful or an exaggerated response to a stimulus that should be only minimally painful. The terms hyperalgesia and hyperpathia convey the same concept but are less frequently used. Allodynia often occurs after a peripheral nerve injury in the setting of a complex regional pain syndrome in which there is sensory loss, but once the sensory threshold is exceeded the response is excessive. Such patients may also have a painful response to any stimulus, even a puff of air. Patients with migraine often develop allodynia of the scalp once a headache has persisted past a certain point.

Allographia: A transposition of letters when writing, similar to dyslexia, but more severe, with transposing letters, changing cases, and other lexical aberrations seen as part of agraphia or dysgraphia syndromes due to parietal lobe lesions.

Alopecia: Premature hair loss or thinning. Alopecia, or balding, occurs in several disorders with neurologic features or complications, including myotonic dystrophy, hypothyroidism, Leigh's disease, sarcoidosis, secondary syphilis, and SLE.

Alternating hemiplegia: Conditions in which there is paralysis on one side of the body and dysfunction of one or more cranial nerves on the opposite side due to a lesion of the brainstem, usually a stroke.

Alternating sensory loss: A pattern of sensory loss that involves one side of the head or face and the opposite side of the body, typical of lateral medullary syndrome.

Alternating sequences tests: Tests first developed by the Russian Neuropsychologist Aleksandr Luria to assess frontal lobe and executive function. These tests require concentration, planning, and resistance to distraction. The patient may be asked to write a series of alternating M's and W's or draw alternating squares and triangles or perform the **fist-edge-palm test**. **Perseveration** may cause the patient to write the same letter several times in a row or draw the same shape repetitively or have difficulty with the fist-edge-palm test.

Alternating skew deviation (paroxysmal skew, periodic alternating skew): See **skew deviation**.

Altitudinal visual field defect: A visual field defect that involves either the upper or the lower portion of the visual hemifield, respecting the horizontal meridian. An altitudinal defect is most commonly associated with retinal emboli causing amaurosis fugax, in which the patient briefly loses either the upper or lower half of the visual field in one eye due to a transient retinal artery branch occlusion involving either the superior or inferior arterial supply. More permanent altitudinal defects may accompany frank branch artery occlusions. Rarely, homonymous altitudinal defects occur with occipital lobe lesions that involve either the upper or lower bank of the calcarine cortex bilaterally, as from TBI. A monocular altitudinal defect may also be a symptom of retinal detachment.

Amaurotic pupil: The pupil of a blind eye. There is no reaction to light, but the pupil constricts to consensual stimulation and to near. The consensual response is absent in the fellow eye. An amaurotic pupil causes the most extreme example of an **afferent pupillary defect**.

Amblyopia: Loss of vision. The term is often used synonymously with **amblyopia ex anopsia**, a very common condition, but there are other important causes. Tobacco-alcohol (alcoholic, nutritional) amblyopia is an optic neuropathy usually seen in malnourished, chronic alcoholics who develop insidious, progressive visual loss. The disease has been attributed to nutritional deficiency, but some individuals with the tobacco-alcohol amblyopia phenotype have the genetic mutation of LHON.[11]

Amblyopia ex anopsia: Loss of vision in an otherwise healthy eye due to cortical suppression of vision because of conflicting images from the two eyes in patients with strabismus or refractive error. The brain picks an eye to use and suppresses the vision in the other eye. Also called strabismic or anisometropic amblyopia.

Amimia: Inability to mimic gestures.

Amnesia: Loss of memory or inability to acquire new memories. The term is primarily used in one of two ways. One is to describe any severe memory impairment, whatever the cause. The other is to describe memory impairment in the absence of other substantial cognitive difficulty. In the latter disorders, referred to as amnesic or amnestic disorders, memory impairment is the main feature.[12] Amnesia may occur in the setting of TBI, stroke, epilepsy, limbic encephalitis, herpetic encephalitis, thiamine deficiency, and medication and substance use and abuse. Zolpidem and related drugs are as particularly risky (the Ambien zombie). Typically, left hemisphere lesions cause verbal memory deficits and right hemisphere lesions nonverbal memory deficits. Transient global amnesia and transient epileptic amnesia are disorders that cause temporary memory dysfunction. **Confabulation** is a common feature in some amnestic disorders.

Psychogenic, dissociative or functional amnesia is a psychiatric disorder characterized by an inability to recall personal information.[13] Characteristically, autobiographical memory is much more severely affected than memory in general (semantic memory). The patient cannot remember his name but recalls the winner of the Super Bowl and the score. Patients with psychogenic amnesia have often experienced some severely stressful life event. The memory loss may be global, causing a fugue state, or situation specific, resulting in an inability to recall a certain event, such as committing a crime. Feigned amnesia occurs in malingering.

Neuropsychological testing is indispensable in providing an objective assessment of the nature and severity of memory impairment.

Amoss' sign: See **tripod sign.**

Amusia: Loss of musical ability, either production or comprehension. Amusia may occur in patients with aphasia or agnosia, or develop independently. Melody and rhythm may be affected separately. The centers that control musical ability are largely undefined, and different features of musical ability appear to be distributed between the two hemispheres.

Amyotrophy: A term synonymous with muscle atrophy and implying a decrease in muscle volume or bulk, usually accompanied by changes in shape or contour. Neurologic conditions likely to cause muscle atrophy are primarily those that affect the anterior horn cell, the nerve root(s), the peripheral nerve, or the muscle. The term amyotrophy is generally restricted by convention to amyotropic lateral sclerosis and related conditions and to certain conditions involving the brachial and lumbosacral plexuses.

Analgesia: Loss of pain sensation. Many terms have been used, not always consistently, to describe sensory abnormalities. Algesia refers to the sense of pain (Gr. *algos* "pain"). Hypalgesia is a decrease, and analgesia (or analgesthesia) an absence, of pain sensation. The combining form "algia" refers to any painful condition. This term is seldom used currently except to refer to the effectiveness of a local anesthetic.

Anal reflex: Contraction of the anal musculature to external stimulation. There are two components to the anal reflex: the superficial or cutaneous anal reflex (anal wink) and the internal anal sphincter reflex. The anal wink consists of contraction of the external sphincter in response to stroking or pricking the skin or mucous membrane in the perianal region. The internal anal sphincter reflex is contraction of the internal sphincter on insertion of a gloved finger into the anus. If the reflex is impaired there is decreased sphincter tone and the anus does not close immediately after withdrawal. Assessment of the anal reflexes is particularly important when a spinal cord, cauda equina, or conus medullaris lesion is suspected.

Anal wink: See **anal reflex.**

Anarchic hand: Alien hand syndrome with pronounced intermanual conflict.

Anarithmia (anarithmetria): A primary disturbance of calculating ability, when not part of an aphasic syndrome. See **acalculia**.

Anarthria: A total inability to articulate because of a defect in the control of the peripheral speech musculature.

Anesthesia: Absence of sensation. The definition of esthesia is perception, feeling, or sensation (Gr. *aesthesis* "sensation"), hypesthesia a decrease, and anesthesia an absence, of all sensation.

Anesthesia dolorosa: Pain in an area of sensory loss. Seen primarily in disorders of cranial and peripheral nerves, where, despite dramatic loss of sensation, a chronic pain syndrome develops. Classically a complication of trigeminal rhizotomy done for tic doloreux in which the patient develops severe facial pain in the distribution of the rootlets that were operated upon.

Angioid streaks: Long dehiscences in Bruch's membrane that resemble blood vessels, associated with degeneration of the retinal pigment epithelium. They appear as jagged, irregular lines that radiate from the peripapillary retina toward the periphery. Angioid streaks occur in pseudoxanthoma elasticum, sickle-cell anemia, diabetes, Ehlers-Danlos, acromegaly, neurofibromatosis, Paget's disease, and in normals. The appearance can be striking (Fig. A.7). Nearly 50% of patients with angioid streaks have some underlying disease.[4]

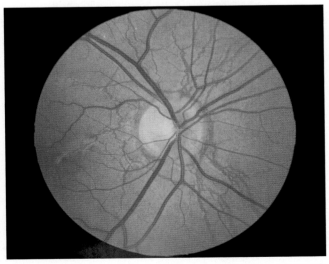

Figure A.7. Angioid streaks radiating from the optic nerve. (From Chern KC, Saidel MA. *Ophthalmology Review Manual.* 2nd ed. Philadelphia, PA: Wolters Kluwer Health/Lippincott Williams & Wilkins; 2012, with permission.)

Angiokeratoma: The skin lesion seen in Fabry's disease, which consist of reddish-purplish papules that often occur in a "bathing trunks" distribution, particularly on the scrotum (Fig. A.8).

Anhidrosis: Lack of sweating, seen primarily as a manifestation of sympathetic dysfunction in **Horner's syndrome,** spinal cord injury, MSA, PD, or peripheral neuropathy with autonomic failure. Ross' syndrome is segmental anhidrosis with **Adie's pupil** and **areflexia.** The anhidrosis is usually asymmetric and often accompanied by compensatory hyperhidrosis nearby.

A simple bedside test to demonstrate the distribution of abnormal skin dryness related to loss of sweating is to note the resistance to stroking of the skin with a finger or an object such as the barrel of a pen or a spoon (spoon test). When a spoon is drawn over the skin, it pulls smoothly over dry (sympathectomized) skin but irregularly and unevenly over moist, perspiring skin.

Anismus: Involuntary contraction or spasm of the anal sphincter. On examination, anismus manifests as an inability to relax the sphincter for digital rectal examination. Some instances are due to a focal dystonia, and anismus can occur as a manifestation of PD. It may cause constipation.

Anisocoria: A difference in pupillary size. The pupils are generally of equal size. A difference of 0.25 mm in pupil size is noticeable, and a difference of 2 mm is considered significant. Physiologic anisocoria, mild degrees of inequality with less

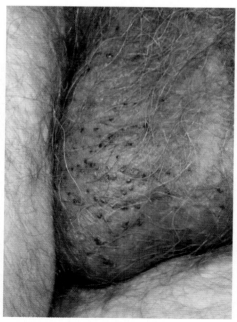

Figure A.8. Angiokeratomas. These small red-purple papules are most often found on the scrotum and usually first noticed in young adulthood. (From Elder DE, Miller J, Miller OF, et al. *Altas and Synopsis of Lever's Histopathology of the Skin.* 3rd ed. Philadelphia, PA: Wolters Kluwer Health/Lippincott Williams & Wilkins; 2013, with permission.)

than 1 mm of difference between the two sides, occurs in 15% to 20% of normal individuals. Rarely does the difference exceed 0.6 mm. With physiologic anisocoria the degree of inequality remains about the same in light and dark, and the pupils react normally to all stimuli (see Fig. A.5).[14]

Ankle reflex: The DTR obtained by striking the Achilles tendon just above its insertion on the calcaneus **(Video A.3)**. The resulting contraction of the posterior crural muscles, the gastrocnemius, soleus, and plantaris causes plantar flexion of the foot at the ankle. The reflex is mediated by the tibial nerve and the S1 root. If the ankle jerk is hyperactive, it may be elicited by tapping other areas of the sole of the foot or by tapping the anterior aspect of the ankle, the paradoxical ankle reflex. A hyperactive reflex may also result in extra beats or even clonus when the tendon is percussed. The ankle reflex is frequently impaired bilaterally in peripheral neuropathy and unilaterally in S1 radiculopathy. For the diagnosis of S1 radiculopathy, a decreased ankle jerk has an LR of 2.7, a PPV of 67% to 84%, and an NPV of 79% to 84%.[8] Although the ankle reflex, when carefully elicited, should be present in normal individuals, it tends to diminish with age and its bilateral absence in elderly individuals is not necessarily of clinical significance (see **age-related signs**). How to elicit the ankle reflex is nicely demonstrated at the website for Stanford Medicine 25, An Initiative to Revive the Culture of Bedside Medicine (http://stanfordmedicine25.stanford.edu/the25/tendon.html).

Anomia: Difficulty naming. Anomia occurs as a feature in most aphasias and as the primary manifestation of **anomic aphasia.** Patients have word-finding pauses and circumlocutions because of the inability to retrieve names and often use descriptive phrases instead of single words. They are able to recognize and point out or describe an object yet not able to name it. See **naming.**

Anomic aphasia: An type of **aphasia** that causes a deficit in naming ability with preservation of other language functions. Anomic aphasia is the most common, but least specific, type of aphasia. Anomia occurs with every type of aphasia. Patients with any aphasia type as it develops or recovers may pass through a stage in which anomia is the primary finding, and it may be the most persistent deficit. Only when anomia occurs as an isolated deficit throughout the course of the illness is the designation anomic aphasia appropriate. Dysnomia is sometimes used to refer to mild difficulty with naming. Anomic aphasia is regarded as a nonlocalizing syndrome; the lesion cannot be readily localized to any particular cortical area. See **naming.**

Anosmia: Loss or impairment of the sense of smell. There are many etiologies. Common causes of impaired smell are sinonasal disease, trauma, and normal aging. Persistent olfactory loss following a URI is the most common etiology, accounting for 15% to 25% of cases. Anosmia complicates 5% to 20% of major head injuries. Anosmia may accompany some degenerative dementias, especially Alzheimer's disease, and olfactory dysfunction has been recognized as a common finding in patients with PD. In these conditions, testing can detect anosmia in most patients even early in the course of the disease. Anosmia is a common, and often the first, manifestation of olfactory groove meningioma. See **olfaction testing.**

Anosodiaphoria: A term, coined by Babinski, to refer to a condition in the spectrum of **anosognosia**. At the far end of the spectrum is the denial of the existence of one's own limbs (**asomatognosia**). Less severe is acknowledgment of the limbs, but denying that there is anything wrong with them, that is, denial of disability. Yet less severe is anosodiaphoria, acknowledgement of the disability with failure to be concerned about it, such as adopting a *la belle indifference* attitude toward a hemiplegia. The patient concedes the deficit is present, but is not worried or troubled about it. See **attentional deficit.**

Anosognosia (anosagnosia): A spectrum of disorders seen particularly in patients with nondominant parietal lesions. **Kortte anosognosia** is a type of **attentional deficit,** which ranges from the denial of the existence of one's own limbs, to acknowledging ownership of the limbs but denying any disability, to acknowledging the disability with failure to be concerned about it (**anosodiaphoria**).

Most common is a patient with severe left hemiplegia denying there is anything wrong with the involved limbs. Even when the examiner dangles the patient's paralyzed left hand before her face and asks if there is anything wrong with this hand, the patient may deny it. The most severe form of anosognosia is when the patient denies owning the hand (**asomatognosia**). Occasionally, patients become belligerent in denying that the hand dangling before them is theirs. They commonly say the hand belongs to the examiner. One patient stated it was, "Queen Elizabeth's hand." When asked where Queen Elizabeth was, the patient replied, "behind the curtain." Patients with severe anosognosia may refuse to remain in the bed with this "other person." One patient thought her left arm was her grandbaby lying beside her. Another patient, convinced her left arm was not her own, threw it over the side rail of the bed, fracturing the humerus. In **misoplegia**, also seen with right hemisphere lesions, patients hate and may reject their paralyzed limbs.

Patients with persistent anosognosia typically have large right hemisphere strokes causing severe left hemisensory loss and left hemispatial neglect. Anosognosia for hemiplegia has also been reported with pontine lesions. Using special techniques to compensate for aphasia, it may be detected more often in dominant hemisphere lesions than previously suspected. Patients may deny or neglect other neurologic deficits as well, particularly loss of vision due to bilateral occipital lobe lesions (**cortical blindness, Anton's syndrome**).

Anserina (cutis anserina): Goose flesh, **piloerection.** Anserina means "of the goose."

Antalgic gait: See **gait disorders.**

Anterior tibial sign (Strümpell's sign): An **associated movement** sign unmasked with CST disease. Normally, vigorous flexion of the hip and knee are accompanied by plantar flexion of the foot. In lower extremity weakness due to a CST lesion, voluntary flexion of the hip is accompanied by involuntary dorsiflexion and inversion of the paretic foot; there may also be dorsiflexion of the great toe or of all the toes. The patient is unable to flex the hip without dorsiflexing the foot (Fig. A.9). The response is accentuated if the movement is carried out against resistance. The sign may also be elicited by flexing the knee with the patient lying prone (Fig. A.10).

Anterocollis: One of the abnormal head positions that can be caused by cervical dystonia in which there is primarily forward flexion of the neck with the chin pulled down; see **cervical dystonia.** Other conditions, such as the **dropped head** syndrome and **bent spine syndrome** (camptocormia), can produce this head position.

Antisaccade task: A test of the ability to inhibit automatic responses. Antisaccades are voluntary saccades away from a target. The dorsolateral prefrontal cortical area is involved in mechanisms responsible for inhibiting unwanted saccades. Patients with frontal lobe disease, such as PSP, PD, or AD, when asked to look away from a visual stimulus may be unable to inhibit a saccade toward the target (prosaccade)

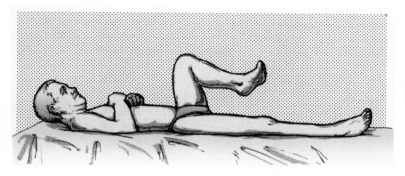

Figure A.9. Anterior tibial sign in a patient with left hemiparesis. (From Campbell WW. *DeJong's the Neurologic Examination.* 7th ed. Philadelphia, PA: Wolters Kluwer Health/ Lippincott Williams & Wilkins; 2013, with permission.)

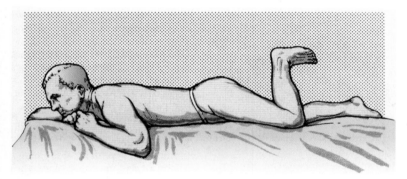

Figure A.10. Anterior tibial sign elicited with the patient in the prone patient. (From Campbell WW. *DeJong's the Neurologic Examination.* 7th ed. Philadelphia, PA: Wolters Kluwer Health/Lippincott Williams & Wilkins; 2013, with permission.)

and are therefore unable to make an antisaccade or make it only after a prosaccade. Inability to inhibit saccades toward the target has been termed the visual grasp reflex. One way to perform the antisaccade test is for the examiner to hold up the index finger of each hand on either side of the patient, who is then instructed to look at the finger that does not wiggle. The patient who repeatedly looks at the moving finger has an impairment of the ability to inhibit unwanted saccades.

The antisaccade test falls in the category of tests designed to detect **defective response inhibition.** See **applause sign, automatic responses, Stroop test, Go/ No-Go, alternating sequences tests,** and **imitation and utilization behavior.**

Apallesthesia (pallanesthesia): Absence of vibratory sensation.

Apallic state: See **abulia.**

Apathy: A lack of emotion, feeling, motivation, interest, or concern. In neurologic patients, it occurs primarily as a manifestation of frontal lobe disorders and lesions involving the anterior cingulate gyrus, but may also occur with subcortical lesions.

Patients say little, move little, and think little. **Akinetic mutism** is an extreme form of apathy. See **abulia**.

Aphasia: An acquired disorder of language, including various combinations of impairment in the ability to spontaneously produce, understand, and repeat speech, as well as defects in the ability to read and write.[15] Six separate components of language function are typically tested at the bedside: spontaneous (conversational) speech, auditory comprehension, naming, reading (aloud and for comprehension), writing (spontaneous, to dictation and copying), and the ability to repeat. Speech and language pathologists do much more comprehensive testing. Using bedside testing, the aphasias may be categorized into numerous types: expressive–receptive, fluent–nonfluent, motor–sensory, anterior–posterior, **Broca's, Wernicke's, conduction, crossed, global, transcortical** (motor, sensory, and mixed), **anomic, subcortical,** and others.

A key distinguishing feature is fluency, the volume of speech output. Normal speech is 100 to 115 words per minute, which are uttered effortlessly. Nonfluent speech is laborious, with single words, short phrases, pauses, and hesitation. Speech output is often as low as 10 to 15 words per minute, sometimes less. If the maximum sentence length is fewer than seven words, then the patient is nonfluent. Patients are usually aware of nonfluency and frustrated by it. Their speech may tend toward the laconic, answering questions but trying to speak no more than necessary. Aphasic patients may use pantomime or gesture, shaking or nodding the head, shrugging the shoulders, or demonstrating visible emotional reactions. In severe aphasia, the patient may be unable to utter a single word or endlessly repeat a **monophasia**.

Instruments such as the Boston Diagnostic Aphasia Examination, Western Aphasia Battery, and the Boston Naming Test provide a more formal evaluation.

See **agrammatism, agraphia, alexia, apraxia of speech, circumlocution, jargon aphasia, isolation of the speech area, naming, neologisms, paraphasia, sympathetic apraxia.**

Aphemia: See **pure word mutism.**

Aphonia: Complete voice loss in which the patient must resort to mouthing or whispering words. Laryngeal disorders may alter the volume, quality, or pitch of the voice (dysphonia), or, when severe, produce aphonia. Laryngitis causes dysphonia. The most common nonorganic voice disorders are dysphonia and aphonia. In functional, nonorganic aphonia, there is profound speech difficulty but no disturbance of coughing or respiration. Aphonia is distinct from mutism, in which the patient makes no effort to speak, and anarthria, in which the patient is able to make sounds but is not able to articulate.

Aphthongia: A type of dysarthria, even anarthria, due to spasm of the speech muscles; it is possibly a dystonia.

Apley scratch test: A method to assess shoulder range of motion; see **shoulder examination tests.**

Apneustic breathing: One of the abnormal respiratory patterns that may be seen in patients with neurologic disease and depressed consciousness. Apneustic (Gr, *a pneusis,* not breathing) breathing, which is rare, causes a prolonged inspiratory gasp and a pause at full inspiration with erratic and incomplete expiration. It occurs in pontine lesions just rostral to the trigeminal motor nuclei, or with cervicomedullary compression. Other patterns include **ataxic breathing, central neurogenic hyperventilation, Biot breathing, and Cheyne-Stokes respirations.**

Appendicular ataxia: **Ataxia** involving the limbs, as opposed to **truncal ataxia** or gait ataxia (**see gait disorders**).

Apperceptive agnosia: See **agnosia.**

Applause sign (three clap test): An inability to stop clapping after being asked to clap three times. The applause sign was initially touted as a way to distinguish PSP from PD and FTD.[16] Later studies found the applause sign was a nonspecific sign of frontal lobe dysfunction.

Apraxia: A deficit involving the inability to carry out motor acts. Apraxia (Gr. *praxis* "action") is defined in several ways. Common to all definitions is the inability to carry out on request a motor act in the absence of any weakness, sensory loss, or other deficit involving the affected part in a patient who has intact comprehension and is cooperative and attentive to the task.[17] One definition requires the task be high level, familiar, and purposeful, such as saluting or using an implement. But the term is also used to refer to loss of the ability to execute some very elemental functions, such as opening or closing the eyes (eyelid apraxia), glancing to the side (**oculomotor apraxia**), walking (gait apraxia), talking (apraxia of speech), or a behavior as basic as smacking the lips (**buccofacial apraxia**). Another definition of apraxia is the inability to perform an act on command that the patient is able to perform spontaneously. But the patient with gait apraxia cannot walk spontaneously any better than to command (see **gait disorders**). So all the definitions and applications of the term suffer in one respect or another. See **constructional apraxia, dressing apraxia, ideational apraxia, ideomotor apraxia, limb kinetic apraxia, sympathetic apraxia.**

Apraxia of eyelid closure: Inability to close the eyes on command with preserved ability to close the eyes and keep them closed at other times, such as when blinking. Much less common than **apraxia of eyelid opening**, it is also seen in extrapyramidal disorders, especially PSP.

Apraxia of eyelid opening: A nonparalytic inability to open the eyes at will, or to keep the eyes open, in the absence of visible contraction of the orbicularis oculi. The condition is often associated with extrapyramidal disorders, particularly PSP, and with essential **blepharospasm**, with which it is easily confused.[18]

Apraxia of gait: See **gait disorders.**

Apraxia of gaze: See **gaze apraxia.**

Apraxia of speech (AOS): A condition causing difficulty with speech, which differs from **aphasia** because comprehension is perfect and writing is not affected.[19] Patients with AOS have more of a speech problem than a language problem. AOS may or may not be accompanied by buccofacial apraxia. This condition has also been called verbal apraxia, cortical dysarthria, acquired apraxia of speech, Broca's area aphasia, mini-Broca, or baby-Broca. Patients with AOS appear to have forgotten how to make the sounds of speech. There is speech sound distortion as their articulatory muscles grope for the right position. Prosody may be impaired, and speech may have a stuttering quality. The speech pattern may change so that the patient sounds as though he has developed a **foreign accent.**

There is greater difficulty with polysyllabic words and complex phrases than with simple words. Transposition is common ("pasghetti"). The speech resembles the hesitant nonfluency seen in Broca's aphasia, but the patient speaks in correct English sentences, using proper grammar and syntax. The lesion in these cases may be confined to Broca's area and seems to affect areas of the brain that control speech but not language, while in the more typical case of Broca's aphasia the lesion is usually more extensive, involving Broca's area as well as the subjacent white matter. AOS is often the first symptom of neurodegenerative diseases such as primary progressive aphasia and corticobasal degeneration.

Aprosodia: Impairment of prosody, or the melodic aspects of speech. Prosody refers to the modulation of pitch, volume, rhythm, intonation, and inflection that convey nuances of meaning and emotional content. Dysprosody, typically hypoprosody or aprosody, may occur with right hemisphere lesions. Patients lose the ability to convey emotion in speech (motor aprosodia) or to detect the emotion expressed by others (sensory aprosodia or "affective agnosia"). Dysprosodic speech lacks inflections, accents, modulation, or emotion; it is flat and monotonous. The patient speaks in a monotone and is unable to say the same neutral phrase (e.g., "I am going to the store") in an angry or happy way. Patients with right hemisphere lesions also often lose the capacity to understand metaphors and to appreciate sarcasm, irony, and humorous remarks in discourse.

Arachnodactyly: Long, slender fingers (Fig. A.11). Some of the conditions with neurologic features or complications associated with arachnodactyly include Marfan's syndrome, Ehlers-Danlos syndrome, Schwartz-Jampel syndrome, sickle cell disease and osteogenesis imperfecta.[20]

Archimedes spiral: A figure frequently used to assess tremor (Fig. A.12).

Arcuate scotoma: See **scotoma.**

Arcus senilis: The grayish-white discoloration around the limbus that occurs in normal aging and prematurely in hyperlipidemia. When asymmetric or unilateral, it may indicate carotid stenosis on the side of the eye less affected.

Areflexia: Loss of **deep tendon reflexes.** The significance depends entirely on the distribution and the circumstances. Loss of one ankle jerk in a patient with back pain

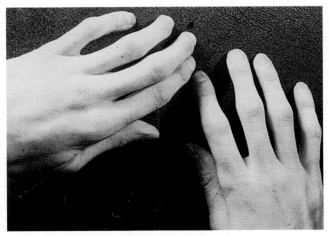

Figure A.11. Arachnodactyly in a patient with Marfan's syndrome. (From Rubin E, Gorstein F, Rubin R, et al. *Rubin's Pathology: Clinicopathologic Foundations of Medicine.* 4th ed. Philadelphia, PA: Wolters Kluwer Health/Lippincott Williams & Wilkins; 2005: 244, with permission.)

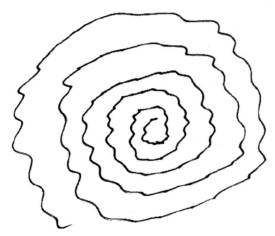

Figure A.12. Archimedes spiral drawn by a patient with essential tremor.

suggests radiculopathy, loss of both knee jerks in a young woman with unreactive pupils is consistent with **Adie's syndrome,** and loss of all reflexes in a patient with subacute generalized weakness suggests Guillain-Barré syndrome. Reflexes may be lost acutely in CNS disorders, such as below the level of a traumatic spinal cord lesion (spinal shock) or contralateral to an acute hemispheric lesion.

Argyll Robertson (AR) pupil: Small (1 to 2 mm) pupils, irregular in outline, with **light near dissociation** (Fig. A.13). They react poorly or not at all to light, but very well to near. AR pupils are generally bilateral and asymmetric. They are the classic eye finding of neurosyphilis. The lesion lies in the periaqueductal region, pretectal area and rostral midbrain dorsal to the Edinger-Westphal nuclei. Other conditions may cause an AR-like pupil, and with the declining incidence of neurosyphilis, AR-like pupils with light near dissociation are increasingly likely to be of some other etiology. **Adie's pupil** is a much more common cause of **light near dissociation** than AR pupils. The near response in AR pupils is brisk and immediate; in **Adie's pupil** it is slow and prolonged. Other causes of **light near dissociation** include lesions involving the dorsal rostral midbrain (**tectal pupils**), diabetic autonomic neuropathy (tabes diabetica), Lyme disease, chronic alcoholism, chiasmal lesions (tabes pituitaria), myotonic muscular dystrophy, amyloidosis, **aberrant regeneration of CN III**, sarcoidosis, multiple sclerosis, and severe retinal or optic nerve disease.[21]

Arm–diaphragm synkinesia: A co-contraction between the diaphragm and proximal arm muscles, usually most evident in the biceps, due to **aberrant regeneration** following a brachial plexus lesion. The muscle twitches with each inspiration; best appreciated by EMG.

Arm dropping test: A method for testing muscle tone. The patient's arms are briskly raised to shoulder level, then dropped. In spasticity, there is a delay in the downward movement of the affected arm, causing it to hang up briefly on the affected side (**Bechterew's sign**); with hypotonicity, the dropping is more abrupt than normal. A similar maneuver may be carried out by lifting, then dropping the extended legs of the recumbent patient.

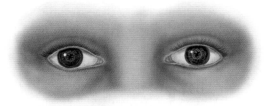

Figure A.13. Argyll Robertson pupils are small, irregular pupils that do not react to light but do react to near, usually but not always caused by neurosyphilis. (From Bickley LS, Szilagyi P. *Bates' Guide to Physical Examination and History Taking.* 8th ed. Philadelphia, PA: Wolters Kluwer Health/Lippincott Williams & Wilkins; 2003, with permission.)

Arm (hand) drop sign: The tendency of a patient in nonorganic coma to avoid hitting himself in the face when one hand is held above the head and dropped. In a patient with organic coma, the hand and arm will plummet down and strike the patient in the face, whereas the patient with nonorganic alteration of consciousness will avert the arm at the last instant. This should be done only in the absence of sensitive observers who might misinterpret the proceedings. This is also used as a test of nonorganic weakness; when letting an arm with functional weakness drop, the descent is slower and jerkier than would be expected for the degree of weakness. The **drop arm sign** is unrelated and occurs in rotator cuff disease.

Arthrogryposis: Joint contractures. When these occur in utero, from a variety of orthopedic and neurological conditions, the child is born with severely deformed limbs; this is congenital arthrogryposis, where the term is most often applied. For acquired arthrogryposis, the term *contracture* is preferred.

Aschner's cardiac phenomenon: See **oculocardiac reflex.**

Ash leaf spots: See **hypomelanotic macule.**

Asomatognosia: The most severe form of **anosognosia.** The patient fails to recognize a body part, most often the left arm. It occurs with contralateral parietal lobe lesions and is in the spectrum of **attentional deficit** disorders.

Associative agnosia: See **agnosia.**

Associated movements and associated movement signs: An associated movement (AM) is an unintentional, involuntary, spontaneous, automatic movement that accompanies some other movement. The AM is often one that serves to fix a part of the body as another part is voluntarily activated. Common examples of normal AMs include swinging of the arms when walking; facial contortions or grimaces with extreme exertion; movements of the head and neck with movements of the eyes; contraction of the frontalis muscle with elevation of the eyes; and extension of the wrist on making a fist.

AMs often occur because of activation of synergistic and fixation muscles involved in a particular motion. AMs may occur under normal circumstances or in neurologic disease. When a normal motor engram is activated, spread of activation to nearby motor neuron pools is normally suppressed by the descending motor pathways. In the face of disease, this overflow activation may become apparent.

The corticospinal pathways are concerned primarily with fine, fractionated distal extremity movements. Disease in the corticospinal pathways may eliminate discrete distal movement while preserving the synergistic mass movements of the proximal muscles that play a secondary, supportive role, particularly in fixation of the part to be moved. When the distal muscles are paralyzed, the primary movement left may be the associated mass movement. Normal AMs are difficult to suppress and their presence in the face of apparent weakness may be a sign of nonorganicity, as in **Hoover's sign**, where the patient is unable to control the normal AM of hip extension when trying to feign leg paralysis.

In the presence of disease, abnormal AMs may make an appearance or normal ones may disappear or be exaggerated. Loss of normal AMs is characteristic of extrapyramidal disorders, especially in **parkinsonism**, where masking of facial expression and absence of arm swing when walking are prominent manifestations. **Babinski's platysma sign** is another example of the loss of a normal AM.

Abnormal or pathologic AMs are usually activity in paretic muscle groups brought out by active movement of other groups and seen predominantly in disease of the corticospinal pathways. They usually accompany vigorous voluntary movements of another part and occur on the hemiplegic side. AMs are slow, forceful movements of the already spastic parts. The greater the spasticity, the greater the extent and duration of the AMs. An involuntary, automatic movement such as a yawn or cough may cause the affected arm to extend at the elbow, wrist, and fingers. In CST disease, abnormal AMs may occur in the paretic limb when the normal contralateral limb is forcefully moved. When squeezing the examiner's hand with the healthy hand, the paretic hand may flex. Any forceful movement on the normal side may be followed by a similar but slow tonic duplication of the movement on the paretic side. With all the associated movement-related signs, a paradoxical situation exists: the presence of movement signifies organic disease, and the absence of movement indicates nonorganic disease.

Familiar examples of abnormal AMs include the Wartenberg thumb adduction sign (see **Wartenberg signs**), the **Babinski trunk-thigh sign,** and the **anterior tibial sign**. Many other AM signs have been described that are not of major clinical importance. See **mirror movements**.

Astasia: An inability to stand; classically a nonorganic sign, but may occur with lesions in some parts of the brain. Patients with unilateral thalamic lesions may have an inability to stand or sit out of proportion to weakness or sensory loss, with a tendency to fall backward or to the side contralateral to the lesion (**thalamic astasia**).

Astasia-abasia: A gait abnormality usually of a nonorganic basis; see **gait disorders**.

Astereognosis (stereoanesthesia): Loss of the ability to recognize and identify an object by touch despite intact primary sensory modalities. There is no loss of perceptual ability. The patient can feel the object, sensing its dimensions, texture, and other relevant information. But there is an inability to synthesize this information and correlate it with past experience and stored information about similar objects in order to recognize and identify it.

Stereognosis is tested by asking the patient to identify, with eyes closed, common objects placed into the hand (e.g., coin, key, button). Normal individuals can identify 90% of objects in five seconds or less.[8] The most convincing deficit is when the patient is able to identify with the other hand an object she was unable to identify with the tested hand. Astereognosis usually indicates a lesion involving the contralateral parietal lobe. If there is hand weakness, the examiner may hold and move the object between the patient's fingers. It is striking to see a patient with a paralyzed hand from a pure motor capsular stroke demonstrate exquisitely intact stereognosis when tested in this fashion.

Asterixis: A sign seen primarily in metabolic encephalopathy, particularly hepatic and renal encephalopathy. Asterixis is an inability to sustain normal muscle tone.[22] Other causes include cardiac and respiratory disease, electrolyte abnormalities, and drug intoxication. With the arms outstretched and wrists extended, "like stopping traffic," the lapse in postural tone may cause the hands to suddenly flop downward and then quickly recover, causing a slow and irregular flapping motion (Video A.4). When severe, the entire arm may drop. Asterixis may affect other muscles as well (Video A.5). In unresponsive patients, asterixis can sometimes be brought out by passively flexing and abducting the hips and placing the feet together so that the thighs form a "V." In this position, the periodic loss of adductor tone may cause the knees to flap up and down. Asterixis is usually bilateral. The presence of asterixis due to metabolic encephalopathy indicates serious disease and is often a poor prognostic sign. In alcoholic liver disease, asterixis is the only physical finding that has a statistically significant predictive value for mortality.[23]

Asterixis may occasionally occur with structural CNS lesions, when it is typically unilateral. The most common structural cause of asterixis is ischaemia or haemorrhage in the CNS, most frequently involving the genu and anterior portion of the internal capsule or ventrolateral thalamus. The exact mechanism underlying asterixis remains elusive, despite many proposed explanations.

Pseudoasterixis refers to brief, rapid, voluntary action tremors of the hands and fingers, elicited by slow flexion and extension movements of the hands at the wrists, while keeping the fingers in full hyperextension.[24] Subtle movements can trigger pseudoasterixis, and it may mimic asterixis, but in pseudoasterixis the patient is aware of the hand twitching in contrast to asterixis, which is involuntary.

Asynergia: See **dyssynergia.**

Ataxia: Disordered movement that may arise from any number of causes, roughly from the Greek *taxis* for order. The common forms are **cerebellar ataxia** and **sensory ataxia**; less common are **frontal ataxia** (Bruns ataxia), **optic ataxia**, episodic ataxia, and the hereditary ataxias.

Ataxic breathing: One of the abnormal respiratory patterns that may be seen in patients with neurologic disease and depressed consciousness. In respiratory ataxia, the pattern of breathing is completely irregular, with erratic shallow and deep respiratory movements, erratic pauses, and increasing periods of apnea. Ataxic breathing occurs with dysfunction of the medullary respiratory centers and may signify impending agonal respirations and apnea. See **apneustic breathing, central neurogenic hyperventilation, Biot breathing, Cheyne-Stokes respirations.**

Ataxic hemiparesis: A lacunar syndrome causing homolateral ataxia with accompanying CST impairment, most often due to a small deep infarction in the basis pons or internal capsule.[25] The presence of sensory loss is highly associated with a capsular localization. The syndrome is defined by ipsilateral ataxia and pyramidal signs, ataxia out of proportion to weakness, and absent or minimal cortical signs.

Weakness is often worse in the leg, particularly the foot; the original designation was homolateral ataxia and crural paresis.[26] The ataxia may be equal in the arm and leg or worse in the arm, but is always out of proportion to any weakness.

Ataxic respirations: See **ataxic breathing.**

Athetosis: A hyperkinetic movement disorder in which the movements are slower, more sustained, and larger in amplitude than those in **chorea.** They are involuntary, irregular, coarse, somewhat rhythmic, and writhing or squirming in character. Athetotic movements may involve the extremities, face, neck, and trunk. In the extremities, they affect mainly the distal portions, the fingers, hands, and toes **(Video Link A.8).** The movements are characterized by any combination of flexion, extension, adduction, abduction, pronation, and supination, often alternating and in varying degrees. They flow randomly from one body part to another, and the direction of movement changes randomly. The affected limbs are in constant motion (Gr. *athetos* "without fixed position"). Hyperextension of the fingers and wrist and pronation of the forearm may alternate with full flexion of the fingers and wrist and supination of the forearm. The movements can often be brought out or intensified by voluntary activity of another body part (overflow phenomenon). They disappear in sleep. Athetosis is usually unilateral; bilateral involvement is called double athetosis.

Athetotic dystonia: See **dystonia.**

Atrophy: A decrease in muscle volume or bulk, usually accompanied by changes in shape or contour **(Fig. A.14).** Neurologic conditions likely to cause muscle atrophy are primarily those that affect the anterior horn cell, the nerve root(s), the peripheral nerve, or the muscle. Loss of trophic influence from the LMN leads to breakdown of actin and myosin and myofibrillar degeneration. Atrophy may also result from such things as disuse or inactivity, immobilization, tendonotomy, muscle

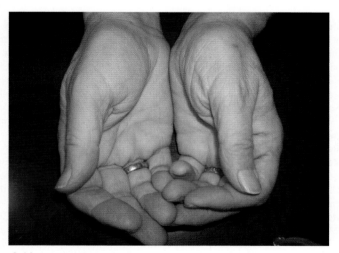

Figure A.14. Atrophy of the left APB.

ischemia, malnutrition, endocrine disorders, and normal aging. CST lesions do not cause the sort of severe, early focal muscle atrophy seen in LMN lesions, but there may be some mild, late atrophy of the involved part due to disuse. As a generalization, when weakness and wasting are comparable the process is more likely to be neurogenic; when the weakness is disproportionately greater than the wasting the process is more likely to be myopathic. When a muscle appears wasted but is not weak, the cause is likely to be nonneurologic, such as disuse. See **amyotrophy.**

Attentional deficits: Selective defects of attention that occur in patients with focal cerebral lesions, primarily in right-handed patients with right (nondominant) hemisphere lesions, especially those that involve the temporoparietal junction and inferior parietal lobule. A variety of terms have been used to describe the phenomenon, including extinction, neglect, hemineglect, hemispatial neglect, visuospatial neglect, hemi-inattention, denial, and spatial inattention. Thalamic lesions, especially those involving the medial thalamus, may produce similar findings, often accompanied by a tendency not to use the involved limbs without any weakness (thalamic neglect). In a series of 140 consecutively admitted patients with right hemisphere strokes, 56% had an attentional deficit.[27]

The mildest manifestation is extinction of the contralateral stimulus with double simultaneous stimulation on visual field or somatosensory testing. Patients with multimodal hemineglect may extinguish all types of contralesional stimuli and may completely ignore the left side of space. On the **line bisection test,** they fail to see the left half of the line or fail to bisect any of the lines on the left. When presented with a complex drawing, the patient fails to notice what is occurring on the left. The most fully developed form is **asomatognosia,** a severe form of **anosognosia** in which the patient fails to recognize his own paralyzed limbs.

Motor neglect refers to bradykinesia of the limbs contralateral to a nondominant brain lesion despite normal strength, reflexes, and sensation. It has been reported with lesions involving the parietal and frontal cortex, internal capsule, lenticulostriate nuclei, thalamus and cingulum.[28]

Auditory agnosia: The loss of recognition of sounds in the absence of any hearing impairment; may involve either verbal or nonverbal sounds. Verbal auditory agnosia has been called pure word deafness. Patients have difficulty in the comprehension of spoken language not due to aphasia or explicable on the basis of any defect in generalized auditory processing. Reading is normal, and comprehension of nonverbal sounds is not affected. Patients with nonverbal auditory agnosia may be unable to recognize music or the sound of traffic, a dog barking, or the crying of a baby. Vocal agnosia is the inability to recognize a known human voice. See **agnosia.**

Auditory Go/No-Go test: See **Go/No-Go test.**

Auditory reflexes: Responses to a loud, sudden noise, such as blink or reflex eye closure, pupillary dilation, or eye deviation or jerking of the body. These responses are occasionally useful in evaluating hearing in children, patients with altered mental status, and hysteria or malingering.

Auditory-palpebral (auro- or acousticopalpebral) reflex: Reflex contraction of the orbicularis oculi causing eye closure, usually bilateral but more marked on the ipsilateral side, in response to a sudden loud noise. See **acoustic startle reflex, auditory reflexes.**

Automatic obedience: A disorder in which a command is unquestioningly obeyed. The response is involuntary, or unvoluntary, usually seen in association with an excessive startle response in conditions such as latah, miryachit, and the jumping Frenchmen of Maine. See **hyperekplexia.**

Automatic responses: A type of **defective response inhibition**, a common manifestation of frontal lobe dysfunction. A useful response inhibition task is to have the patient respond oppositely to the examiner, e.g., asking the patient to tap once if the examiner taps twice and vice versa, or telling the patient to point to his chin as the examiner points to her nose. The ability to inhibit automatic responses can be measured in several ways, such as the **Stroop test, antisaccade task, alternating sequences test, applause sign,** and the **Go/No-Go test.** See **imitation behavior** and **utilization behavior.**

Automatic-voluntary dissociation: The difference between voluntary activation of the bulbar musculature and the preservation of automatic and reflex movements seen in the bilateral anterior opercular syndrome. Patients with the Foix-Chavany-Marie (bilateral anterior opercular) syndrome have loss of voluntary bulbar movements, with preservation of involuntary movements and reflexes, due to a lesion involving the frontal opercular regions bilaterally.

Automatic writing behavior: A form of **hypergraphia** related to **utilization behavior** that may occur in frontal lobe disease.

Automatism: An activity done by a patient during or after an absence or complex partial seizure when there is altered awareness but not unconsciousness. Automatisms are simple, primitive motor activities that are not done purposefully, but reflect the activity of some elementary motor engram that emerges during the seizure. Common examples include chewing, swallowing, lip smacking, scratching, and idly picking at the clothing with one hand. De novo automatisms arise spontaneously, reactive automatisms are reactions to external stimuli, and perseverative automatisms are continuations of acts in progress at seizure onset.

Autonomic function testing: Maneuvers for quantifying autonomic nervous system function.[29] More sophisticated testing requires laboratory testing, but some testing can be done at the bedside.[30] Tests of parasympathetic cardiovagal regulation include heart rate analysis during standing (the 30:15 ratio), heart rate variation with deep breathing, and the Valsalva ratio. Tests of sympathetic adrenergic vascular regulation include blood pressure analysis while standing, the Valsalva maneuver, sustained handgrip, mental stress, and cold water immersion. Tests of sympathetic cholinergic sudomotor function include the sympathetic skin response, quantitative sudomotor axon reflex test, sweat box testing, and quantification of sweat imprints. The available tests have various sensitivities and ease of administration. They are typically administered in a battery of multiple tests, which improves sensitivity and reliability, and allows probing of various autonomic functions. See **orthostatic hypotension.**

Autoprosopagnosia: See **prosopagnosia**

Autotopagnosia: Loss or impairment of the ability to name and recognize body parts. Finger agnosia is a type of autotopagnosia (body-image agnosia) involving the fingers. See **agnosia.**

axial dystonia: A **dystonia** primarily affecting the paravertebral muscles of the trunk, causing scoliosis, lordosis, and other deformities; a common manifestation of dystonia musculorum deformans.

Video Links

A.1. Facial synkinesias. (From Dr. Joshy EV, MBBS, MD, DM(NIMHANS), Neuromuscular dis., Fellowship (USA), Chief of Neurology, SSSIHMS, Bangalore, India.) Available at: http://www.doctor shangout.com/video/facial-synkinesis

A.2. Third nerve synkinesias due to midbrain injury. (From Taieb G, Renard D, Jeanjean L, et al. Unusual third nerve synkinesis due to midbrain injury. *Arch Neurol.* 2011;68(7):948–949.) Available at: http://archneur.jamanetwork.com/multimediaPlayer.aspx?mediaid=2522009

A.3. Acute Adie's syndrome. Paralysis of the iris results in characteristic segmental vermiform movements, which are visible superolaterally acutely and inferomedially. (From Wakerley BR, Tan MH, Turner MR. Teaching video neuroimages: acute Adie syndrome. *Neurology.* 2012;79:e97.) Available at: http://www.ncbi.nlm.nih.gov/pmc/articles/PMC3525299/bin/supp_79_11_e97__index.html

A.4. Relative afferent pupillary defect. A video that demonstrates pupillary response testing and how to assess and grade relative afferent pupillary defects with an overview of the general anatomic pathways. (From Reinholt M, Indiana University School of Optometry.) Available at: http://www.youtube.com/watch?v=soiKbngQxgw

A.5. A relative afferent pupillary defect in the left eye. (From the Helmut Wilhelm collection, Neuro-ophthalmology Virtual Education Library [NOVEL], University of Utah.) Available at: http://stream.utah.edu/m/dp/frame.php?f=510a475d2cc7f749093

A.6. Ageotropic nystagmus. Head-turning to either side while supine induces ageotropic nystagmus that lasts more than five minutes. (From Nam J, Kim S, Huh Y, et al. Ageotropic central positional nystagmus in nodular infarction. *Neurology.* 2009;73:1163.) Available at: http://www.neurology.org/content/suppl/2009/10/04/73.14.1163.DC1/Video.mov

A.7. A patient with an alien hand after callosal section for epilepsy that repeatedly slapped her in the face. (From Mosley M. Alien hand syndrome sees woman attacked by her own hand. *BBC News*; 2011.) Available at: http://www.bbc.co.uk/news/uk-12225166

A.8. Athetosis of the fingers due to a contralateral basal ganglia tumor. (From Dr. Osama SM Amin., Sulaimaniya General Teaching Hospital, Sulaimaniya College of Medicine, Iraq.) Available at: https://www.youtube.com/watch?v=ZF1uTCf4ZIg

References

1. Dick JP. The deep tendon and the abdominal reflexes. *J Neurol Neurosurg Psychiatry.* 2003;74: 150–153.
2. Staley BA, Vail EA, Thiele EA. Tuberous sclerosis complex: diagnostic challenges, presenting symptoms, and commonly missed signs. *Pediatrics.* 2011;127:e117–e125.
3. Ghosh SK, Bandyopadhyay D, Chatterjee G, et al. Mucocutaneous changes in tuberous sclerosis complex: a clinical profile of 27 Indian patients. *Indian J Dermatol.* 2009;54:255–257.
4. Dennis M, Bowen WT, Cho L. *Mechanisms of Clinical Signs.* Sydney, New South Wales, Australia: Churchill Livingstone; 2012.
5. Kaye JA, Oken BS, Howieson DB, et al. Neurologic evaluation of the optimally healthy oldest old. *Arch Neurol.* 1994;51:1205–1211.
6. Odenheimer G, Funkenstein HH, Beckett L, et al. Comparison of neurologic changes in 'successfully aging' persons vs the total aging population. *Arch Neurol.* 1994;51:573–580.
7. Impallomeni M, Kenny RA, Flynn MD, et al. The elderly and their ankle jerks. *Lancet.* 1984;1: 670–672.
8. McGee, S. *Evidence Based Physical Diagnosis.* 3rd ed. Philadelphia, PA: Elsevier/Saunders; 2012.
9. Bub D. Alexia and related reading disorders. *Neurol Clin.* 2003;21:549–568.
10. Feinberg TE, Schindler RJ, Flanagan NG, et al. Two alien hand syndromes. *Neurology.* 1992;42:19–24.
11. Korkiamaki P, Kervinen M, Karjalainen K, et al. Prevalence of the primary LHON mutations in Northern Finland associated with bilateral optic atrophy and tobacco-alcohol amblyopia. *Acta Ophthalmol.* 2013;91:630–634.
12. Markowitsch HJ, Staniloiu A. Amnesic disorders. *Lancet.* 2012;380:1429–1440.
13. Brandt J, Van Gorp WG. Functional ("psychogenic") amnesia. *Semin Neurol.* 2006;26:331–340.
14. Martin TJ. Horner's syndrome, Pseudo-Horner's syndrome, and simple anisocoria. *Curr Neurol Neurosci Rep.* 2007;7:397–406.
15. de Freitas, GR. Aphasia and other language disorders. *Front Neurol Neurosci.* 2012;30:41–45.
16. Dubois B, Slachevsky A, Pillon B, et al. "Applause sign" helps to discriminate PSP from FTD and PD. *Neurology.* 2005;64:2132–2133.
17. Dovern A, Fink GR, Weiss PH. Diagnosis and treatment of upper limb apraxia. *J Neurol.* 2012;259: 1269–1283.
18. Boghen, D. Apraxia of lid opening: a review. *Neurology.* 1997;48:1491–1494.

19. Ogar J, Slama H, Dronkers N, et al. Apraxia of speech: an overview. *Neurocase.* 2005;11:427–432.
20. Grahame R, Hakim AJ. Arachnodactyly—a key to diagnosing heritable disorders of connective tissue. *Nat Rev Rheumatol.* 2013;9:358–364.
21. Thompson HS, Kardon RH. The Argyll Robertson pupil. *J Neuroophthalmol.* 2006;26:134–138.
22. Pal G, Lin MM, Laureno R. Asterixis: a study of 103 patients. *Metab Brain Dis.* 2014;29:813–824.
23. Hardison WG, Lee FI. Prognosis in acute liver disease of the alcoholic patient. *N Engl J Med.* 1966;275:61–66.
24. Jacome DE. Blepharoclonus, pseudoasterixis, and restless feet. *Am J Med Sci.* 2001;322:137–140.
25. Gorman MJ, Dafer R, Levine SR. Ataxic hemiparesis: critical appraisal of a lacunar syndrome. *Stroke.* 1998;29:2549–2555.
26. Fisher CM, Cole M. Homolateral ataxia and crural paresis: a vascular syndrome. *J Neurol Neurosurg Psychiatry.* 1965;28:48–55.
27. Karnath HO, Fruhmann BM, Kuker W, et al. The anatomy of spatial neglect based on voxelwise statistical analysis: a study of 140 patients. *Cereb Cortex.* 2004;14:1164–1172.
28. Migliaccio R, Bouhali F, Rastelli F, et al. Damage to the medial motor system in stroke patients with motor neglect. *Front Hum Neurosci.* 2014;8:408.
29. Ravits JM. AAEM minimonograph # 48: autonomic nervous system testing. *Muscle & Nerve.* 1997;20:919–937.
30. Weimer LH. Autonomic testing: common techniques and clinical applications. *Neurologist.* 2010; 16:215–222.

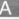

Babcock sentence: A test of memory. Ask the patient to recall this after 5 minutes: "One thing a nation must have to be rich and great is a large, secure supply of wood." Normal patients can do this in three attempts.

Babinski signs: Babinski was a prolific clinical observer, and several signs bear his name, the major ones are as follows. See **pathologic reflexes.**

Babinski's ankle sign: Loss of the ankle reflex in sciatica.

Babinski's brow lift sign: See **brow lift sign.**

Babinski's plantar sign: Normally, plantar stimulation produces plantar flexion of the toes. In disease of the corticospinal system, there may instead be extension (dorsiflexion) of the toes, especially the great toe, with variable separation or fanning of the lateral four toes: the Babinski sign or extensor plantar response (Fig. B.1). The Babinski sign has been called the most important sign in clinical neurology. It is one of the most significant indications of disease of the CST at any level from the motor cortex through the descending pathways.

A small but provocative study questioned whether the Babinski sign should be part of the routine neurologic examination, contending that its validity and interobserver reliability was limited, and suggested that slowed foot tapping was a more useful clinical sign (see **finger tapping test**).[1] A subsequent study documented moderate interobserver reliability with a kappa of 0.5491 (see below). Studies of the foot tapping test have shown a sensitivity of 11% to 23%, a specificity of 89% to 94%, and insignificant LRs in the detection of contralateral hemispheric disease.[2] Studies of the Babinski's sign have shown a sensitivity of 9% to 45%, a specificity of 98%, and a positive LR of 8.5.[2] Given these results, replacing the Babinski sign with foot tapping does not seem prudent.

The Babinski sign is obtained by stimulating the plantar surface of the foot with a blunt point, such as an applicator stick, handle of a reflex hammer, a broken tongue blade, the thumbnail, or the tip of a key. Strength of stimulus is an important variable. It is not true that the stimulus must necessarily be deliberately "noxious," although most patients find it at least somewhat uncomfortable even if the examiner is trying to be considerate. The stimulus should be firm enough to elicit a consistent response, but as light as will suffice. Some patients are very sensitive to plantar stimulation, and only a slight stimulus will elicit a consistent response; stronger stimuli may produce confusing withdrawal. When the response is strongly extensor, only minimal stimulation is required. Merely a fingertip stimulus may elicit a response when the toe is briskly upgoing. If no response is obtained, progressively sharper objects and firmer applications are necessary. Although some patients require a very firm stimulus, it is not necessary to aggressively rake the sole as the opening gambit. Both tickling, which may cause voluntary withdrawal, and pain, which may bring about flexion as a nociceptive response, should be avoided.

Plantar stimulation must be carried out far laterally, in the S1 root/sural nerve sensory distribution. More medial plantar stimulation may not only fail to elicit a positive response when one is present, but may actually elicit a plantar grasp

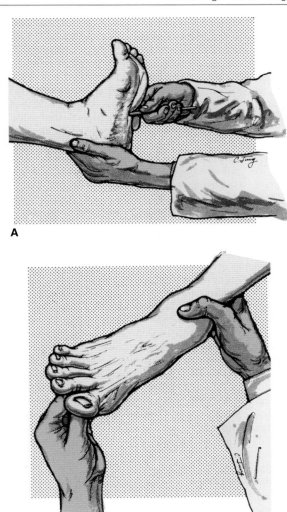

A

B

Figure B.1. Method of eliciting Babinski's sign, **(A)** with a sharp instrument and **(B)** with the thumb. (From Campbell WW. *DeJong's the Neurologic Examination.* 7th ed. Philadelphia, PA: Wolters Kluwer Health/Lippincott Williams & Wilkins; 2013, with permission.)

response and obscure an extensor response. The only movements of significance are those of the great toe. Fanning of the lateral toes without an abnormal movement of the great toe is seldom of any clinical significance, and an absence of fanning does not negate the significance of great toe extension. The knee must be extended, even if the patient is sitting; an upgoing toe may be abolished by flexion of the knee. Usually, the upward movement of the great toe is a quick, flicking motion sometimes mistaken for withdrawal by the inexperienced. The response may sometimes be a slow, tonic, sometimes clonic, dorsiflexion of the great toe with fanning, or separation, of the other toes **(Video B.1)**. Babinski's sign is a part of a primitive flexion reflex. One of the most common mistakes is to misinterpret the hip and knee flexion that sometimes accompany an upgoing toe as voluntary withdrawal when in fact they are part of a **triple flexion reflex**.

There are many other CST responses in the lower extremities characterized by dorsiflexion of the toes. With severe CST disease, the threshold for eliciting an upgoing toe is lower, the reflexogenic zone is wider, and more and more of the other components of the primitive flexion reflex appear as part of the response. This led to a profusion of variations on the Babinski method of eliciting the extensor plantar response. The years around the turn of the 20th century were referred to as "open season for the hunting of the reflex" and the "assault on the great toe" as clinicians sought eponymic immortality by describing different ways of making the toe go up, other components of the reflex, and other variations on the theme. The most useful variation by far is **Chaddock's sign**; the **Oppenheim** sign is also sometimes useful. Other responses may occasionally be useful in cases where, for some reason, the plantar surface of the foot cannot be stimulated.

A study of 34 patients examined by six neurologists compared the inter- and intraobserver consistency of the Babinski, Gordon, Chaddock, and Oppenheim reflexes.[3] The Babinski reflex had the highest interobserver consistency with a kappa value of 0.5491. The Chaddock, Oppenheim, and Gordon reflexes had kappa values of 0.4065, 0.3739, and 0.3515, respectively. For intraobserver consistency, Gordon was the most consistent with a kappa value of 0.6731, but the small sample size limits conclusions regarding this calculation. When reflexes were combined in pairs, the Babinski and Chaddock reflexes together were the most reliable.

See **minor extensor toe signs, Bing's sign, Cornell's sign, Gonda's sign, Gordon's sign, Moniz's sign, Schaefer's sign, Stransky's sign, Strümpell's phenomenon**.

Babinski's platysma sign: Decreased contraction of the platysma on facial grimace on the side of a hemiparesis, due to the loss of the normal **associated movement (Fig. B.2)**.[4]

Babinski's pronator sign: See **pronator sign**.

Babinski's reinforcement sign: A coordinated **associated movement** seen on the side of a hemiparesis. With the patient seated and legs hanging free, the **Jendrassik maneuver** causes knee extension on the paretic side.

Babinski's tonus test: With the arms abducted at the shoulders, the forearms are passively flexed at the elbows. With hypotonicity, there is increased flexibility and mobility, and the elbows can be bent to an angle more acute than normal. With hypertonicity, there is reduced flexibility, and passive flexion cannot be carried out beyond an obtuse angle.

Babinski's trunk–thigh sign (combined flexion of the trunk and thigh): The patient, lying supine with legs abducted, attempts to sit up while holding the arms crossed on the chest. Normally, the legs remain motionless and the heels down. In corticospinal hemiparesis, the hip flexes as the trunk flexes, and there is an involuntary elevation of the paretic limb off the bed **(Fig. B.3)**. The normal limb remains on the bed or rises slightly, but not as high as the paretic one. In paraparesis, both

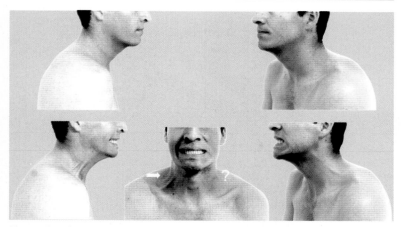

Figure B.2. On the patient's right side, there is a clear difference between the appearance of the platysma muscle at rest **(view at upper left in composite photograph)** and during voluntary effort to retract both corners of the mouth **(view at lower left)**. On the patient's left side, there is only a minimal contraction **(views at upper and lower right)**. In the frontal view, the fully contracting right platysma (*arrow*) can be directly compared with the paretic muscle on the left (*question mark*). Note also the incomplete retraction of the left corner of the mouth. (From Leon-Sarmiento FE, Prada LJ, Torres-Hillera M. The first sign of Babinski. *Neurology.* 2002;59:1067, with permission.)

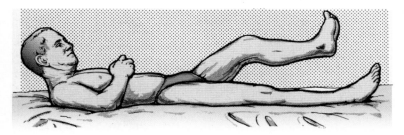

Figure B.3. Trunk–thigh sign in patient with left hemiparesis. (From Campbell WW. *DeJong's the Neurologic Examination.* 7th ed. Philadelphia, PA: Wolters Kluwer Health/ Lippincott Williams & Wilkins; 2013, with permission.)

legs rise equally. In nonorganic weakness, the normal leg rises, and the paretic one does not, or neither leg rises. The same phenomenon occurs if the standing patient bends over **(Fig. B.4)**.

Babinski–Weil test: See **star walking, Unterberger–Fukuda stepping test.**

Bachtiarow's sign: An upper extremity pathologic reflex seen with corticospinal tract disease; stroking downward along the radius with thumb and index finger causes extension and slight adduction of thumb.

Back handing: A maneuver done by the patient with pelvic girdle weakness, who will often begin the movement to rise from the floor by placing one hand behind. Backhanding is typically the first movement in **Gower's maneuver.**

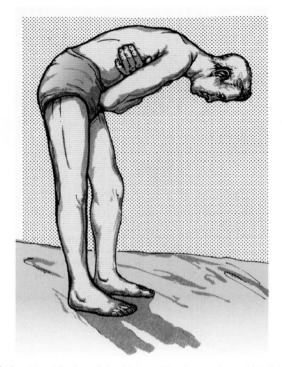

Figure B.4. Combined flexion of the thigh and leg in a patient with left hemiparesis. (From Campbell WW. *DeJong's the Neurologic Examination.* 7th ed. Philadelphia, PA: Wolters Kluwer Health/Lippincott Williams & Wilkins; 2013, with permission.)

Back kneeing: See **genu recurvatum.**

Bajonet posture: Tonic extension of the great toe along with hyperflexion and hyperpronation of the hands and feet seen in some basal ganglia disorders. See **striatal toe.**

Bakody's sign (shoulder abduction relief sign, hand-on-head sign): Relief of pain in cervical radiculopathy by placing the hand on top of the head (Video B.2), see **cervical radiculopathy signs, cervical distraction test, Naffziger's sign, Viets' sign, upper limb tension test.**

Balaclava helmet sensory loss: A pattern of facial sensory loss that may occur with intrinsic brainstem and cervical spinal cord lesions, especially syringomyelia and syringobulbia (Fig. B.5). The nucleus of the spinal tract of CN V is somatotopically organized so that the face is represented as concentric rings from the perioral region to the preauricular region. Fibers from the foreface (lips, mouth, and tip of the nose) synapse most rostrally, and those from the hindface synapse more caudally, adjacent to the sensory input from C2 and C3. Because of this onionskin organization, there is occasionally sparing, less frequently selective involvement, of the perioral region compared with the posterior face. The pattern of the sensory

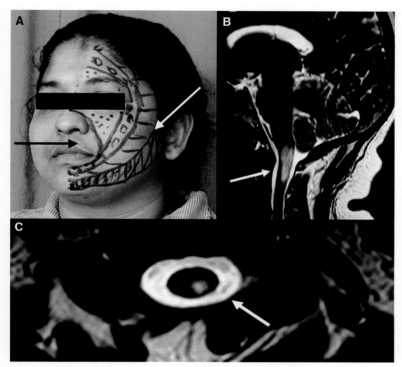

Figure B.5. Onion skin sensory loss in a patient with an acute demyelinating lesion involving the lower brainstem and upper cervical cord. **A:** Different patterns showing gradation of loss. White arrow, maximal loss peripherally; black arrow, spared central part of face. **B:** Sagittal T2 MRI shows a hyperintense lesion in the brainstem and spinal cord extending from the lower medulla to C2 level. **C:** Axial T2 MRI at the level of the upper cervical cord shows a hyperintense lesion in the left posterior-lateral cervical cord. (From Das A, Shinde PD, Kesavadas C, et al. Teaching neuroimages: onion-skin pattern facial sensory loss. *Neurology.* 2011;77(8):e45–e46, with permission.)

loss resembles that of a balaclava or ski mask; it is also referred to as an onion skin or onion peel pattern.

Balding: See **alopecia.**

Balduzzi's sign: Striking the sole of the foot causes adduction of the opposite leg in patients with CST disease.

Ballet's sign: The absence of internal ophthalmoplegia despite external ophthalmoplegia in thyroid eye disease.

Ballet dancer's foot: An occupational dystonia of the foot.

Ballism: See **hemiballismus.**

Band atrophy: A pattern of optic atrophy characterized by a transverse pattern of pallor of the disc contralateral to a lesion of the optic tract. It is due to retrograde axonal degeneration that affects the retinal nerve fiber layers, particularly the papillomacular bundle, as they enter the nasal and temporal portions of the disc. The pattern has also been referred to as "bowtie" or hemianopic atrophy. The disc ipsilateral to the lesion may show disproportionate atrophy of the superior and inferior poles. There is sometimes an RAPD on the side of the transverse band atrophy (Fig. B.6).

Band keratopathy: A transverse band of corneal calcium deposits (Fig. B.7). It may develop in patients with hypercalcemia, hyperuricemia, chronic kidney disease, or chronic uveitis.

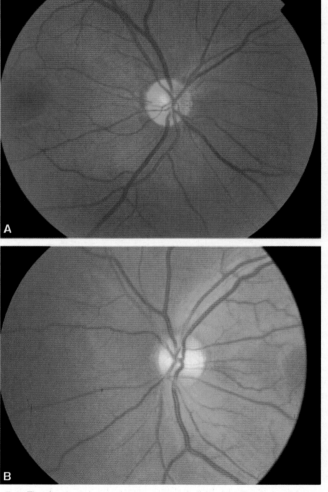

Figure B.6. The fundus above shows a normal disc, the disc below demonstrates optic atrophy in a transverse band across the disc. (From Gálvez-Ruiz A, Arishi N. Band atrophy of the optic nerve: a report on different anatomical locations in three patients. *Saudi J Ophthalmol.* 2013;27:65–69, with permission.)

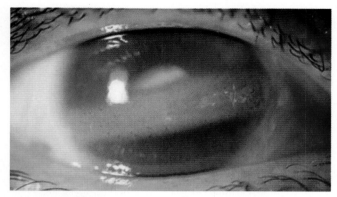

Figure B.7. Band keratopathy.

Bárány's sign: Reduced vestibular response to caloric stimulation.

Bárány's test: See **caloric tests.**

Barré's sign: See **pronator drift.**

Barré's leg sign (leg drift, leg sign of Barré): One of the **subtle signs of hemiparesis,** elicited in the lower extremity by having the patient lie prone and attempt to maintain both knees flexed at about 45° from horizontal with the feet slightly apart. When the knee flexors are weak on one side, as in a CST lesion, the involved leg will sink, gradually or rapidly, similar to the way the upper extremity drifts and pronates.

Barré-Liéou test: One of several maneuvers sometimes performed by practitioners contemplating therapeutic spinal manipulation. These movements are designed to assess the patency of the vascular system, particularly the vertebrobasilar system, by rotating or bending the neck. The primary change that may occur is occlusion of the contralateral vertebral artery with rotation of the head. Depending on individual vascular anatomy, if the vertebral artery is stenotic or atretic, vertebrobasilar ischemia may occur. The patient may experience vertigo, nausea, diplopia, or other symptoms of vertebrobasilar insufficiency or may develop nystagmus or other clinical manifestations. Should any of these occur, the prudent practitioner then avoids spinal manipulation. Depending on the individual and the particular motion performed, occlusion of the ipsilateral vertebral may occur. Variants include lateral bending rather than rotation and performing these movements with the neck extended or flexed.

Bartender's sign: On testing the biceps, the patient with elbow flexion weakness may use a compensatory trick movement of pulling the elbow backward. The movement resembles the one bartenders make when drawing a draft beer.

Bathmocephaly: A craniosynostosis syndrome with prominence of the occiput.

Battle's sign: Discoloration over the mastoid seen in basilar skull fracture (Fig. B.8). See **hemotympanum.**

Beatty maneuver: A maneuver used in the diagnosis of piriformis syndrome; see **piriformis syndrome provocative tests.**

Bechterew's (Bekhterew's) sign: (1) the **arm dropping test.** With spasticity, there is a delay or catch in the descent of the affected arm, causing it to hang up briefly on

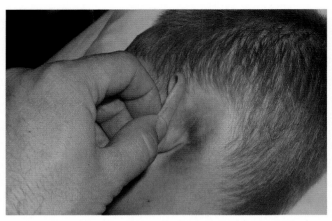

Figure B.8. Battle's sign: Superficial ecchymosis over the mastoid process. (From van Dijk GW. The bare essentials: head injury. *Pract Neurol.* 2011;11:50–55, with permission.)

the involved side; (2) extending the knee in the sitting position in the patient with low back pain, the seated **straight leg raising sign (Video B.3)**. The maneuver is known as Bechterew's test. See **Waddell signs.**

Beevor's sign: Movement of the umbilicus on raising the head. Normally, when the supine patient raises the head or attempts a sit-up, the abdominal muscles contract equally in all four quadrants, and the umbilicus does not move. If the lower abdominal muscles are paralyzed, as in a T10 myelopathy, the upper abdominal muscles will pull the umbilicus cephalad **(Video B.4).**[5]

Behr's pupil: Slightly dilated pupil contralateral to optic tract lesion, existence dubious.

Bekhterew's sign: See **Bechterew's sign.**

Bell's phenomenon (palpebro-oculogyric reflex): Reflex upgaze with forceful eyelid closure. Tight eye closure causes the eyeballs to turn upward, a normal response but obvious only when eye closure is weak, as in peripheral facial palsy, when the rolling of the eyes is seen through the incompletely closed lids. The iris may completely disappear upwardly. Testing for the reflex is a method for testing reflex upgaze in patients with upgaze deficits. In some conditions, such as PSP, reflex upgaze may be preserved when upgaze is otherwise paralyzed. Other conditions, such as chronic progressive external ophthalmoplegia, cause loss of both voluntary and reflex eye movements, and Bell's phenomenon is absent.

Belly dancers dyskinesia (dystonia): Focal **dyskinesia** of the abdominal musculature; may occur as a side effect of psychotropic medications or after abdominal surgery. Some instances may be a form of spinal **myoclonus.**

Bending reflex: An upper extremity reflex seen in frontal lobe disease. Forced passive flexion of the wrist is accompanied by flexion of the elbow in normal subjects (**Leri's sign**). In the bending reflex, attempted passive extension of the elbow during its phase of flexion reinforces the bending reflex and causes it to spread to the shoulder muscles. With frontal lobe lesions, the associated contraction of the

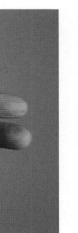

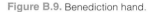

Figure B.9. Benediction hand.

proximal muscles is greatly increased and can be obtained even with passive radial flexion of the wrist. See **pathologic reflexes.**

Benediction hand (preacher's hand, papal hand, hand of the papal benediction): A hand posture with flexion of the ring and small fingers and extension of the index and middle fingers. The literature is contradictory regarding whether this is indicative of an ulnar or a median neuropathy. There are two possibilities: (1) an **ulnar griffe** with the hand at rest or (2) a high median neuropathy or anterior interosseous nerve palsy with the patient attempting to make a fist (Fig. B.9). The hand posture is somewhat similar, and usage is inconsistent. As a broad sweep, the neurology and neurosurgery literature uses the benediction hand designation to refer to median neuropathy, and the rest of medicine uses it to refer to ulnar neuropathy.

Bent knee pulling: See **reverse straight leg raising, femoral nerve stretch test.**

Bent spine syndrome (BSS, camptocormia): An abnormal flexion posture of the trunk that is present when standing, increases with walking, and abates in the supine position (Fig. B.10).[6] BSS was initially considered as a psychogenic disorder, but it is now recognized that many cases are related to a number of musculoskeletal or neurological disorders. Some cases are due to a primary late onset progressive axial myopathy that appears in elderly patients and is associated with massive fatty infiltration of paravertebral muscles. Paravertebral muscle weakness causing BSS or the **dropped head syndrome**, due to involvement of the cervical paraspinal musculature, can occur with a number of neuromuscular conditions, including ALS, myasthenia gravis, metabolic myopathies, especially acid maltase deficiency, polymyositis, and some forms of muscular dystrophy.[7] BSS may also occur with Parkinson's disease (PD) and related disorders, long noted for their tendency to produce an abnormal flexion posture.[8] It is now recognized that some of the abnormal flexion is due to an axial dystonia. Inflammatory spondyloarthropathies such as ankylosing spondylitis can of course produce a similar posture, but the deformity does not reduce when supine.

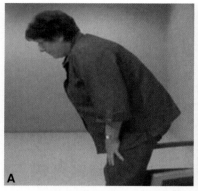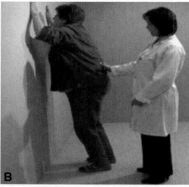

Figure B.10. Patient with a generalized inflammatory myopathy who presented with camptocormia. The patient demonstrated a flexed posture while standing **(A)**, but was able to correct the posture by "climbing up" the wall with her hands **(B)**. (From Kuo SH, Vullaganti M, Jimenez-Shahed J, et al. Camptocormia as a presentation of generalized inflammatory myopathy. *Muscle Nerve*. 2009;40:1059–1063, with permission.)

Bergara–Wartenberg sign: Loss of the normal fine vibrations palpable with the thumbs or fingertips resting lightly on the eyelids as the patient tries to close the eyes as tightly as possible; a sensitive sign of facial weakness.

Biceps reflex: The DTR elicited by percussion of the biceps tendon, causing contraction of the biceps muscle and flexion of the elbow (C5,6) **(Fig. B.11, Video B.5).** Pressure on the tendon should be light; too much pressure against the tendon makes the reflex much harder to obtain. If the reflex is exaggerated, the reflexogenic zone is increased, and there may be abnormal spread with accompanying flexion of the wrist and fingers and adduction of the thumb. The most common cause of reflex depression is cervical radiculopathy. A decreased biceps jerk has an LR of 14.2 for the diagnosis of C6 radiculopathy.[2] How to elicit the biceps reflex is nicely demonstrated at the website for Stanford Medicine 25, An Initiative to Revive the Culture of Bedside Medicine (http://stanfordmedicine25.stanford.edu/the25/tendon.html).

Biceps femoris reflex: See **hamstring reflexes.**

Biceps tendonopathy tests: See **shoulder examination tests** and **Video S.1 shoulder signs.**

Bielschowsky's head tilt test: A maneuver used in the evaluation of vertical diplopia and suspected fourth nerve palsy that consists of tilting the head to each side and noting the changes in diplopia that result.[9] The superior oblique functions primarily as an intorter, and forcing the involved eye to intort worsens the diplopia. If the diplopia improves with head tilt to the left and worsens with tilt to the right, the patient has a right fourth nerve palsy; the right superior oblique fails to intort the eye on tilting to the right, and the diplopia worsens.

The three-step test for vertical diplopia includes the head tilt test. Using objective cover tests or one of the subjective tests (see **diplopia rules**), three determinations are made. Step 1 is to determine the higher (hypertropic) eye, repositioning to remove any head tilt if necessary. If the hypertropia is on the right, the involved

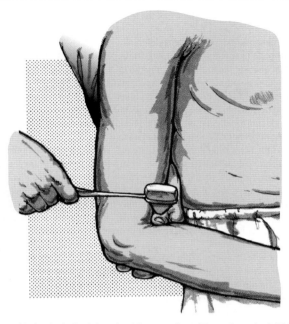

B

Figure B.11. Method of obtaining the biceps reflex. (From Campbell WW. *DeJong's the Neurologic Examination.* 7th ed. Philadelphia, PA: Wolters Kluwer Health/Lippincott Williams & Wilkins; 2013, with permission.)

muscle is either one of the depressors of the right eye (inferior rectus or superior oblique) or one of the elevators of the left eye (superior rectus or inferior oblique). In step 2, the patient gazes to the right and left. If the diplopia worsens on the left gaze, the involved muscle is either the left elevator, the superior rectus, which works best in abduction, or the right depressor, the superior oblique, which works best in adduction. Step 3 is to perform the Bielschowsky's head tilt test.[9]

Biernacki's sign: The absence of pain on pressure on the ulnar nerve, a classic sign of tabes dorsalis (see also **Abadie's** and **Pitres's signs**).

Bikele's sign: A sign of meningeal inflammation (see **meningeal signs**). With the elbow flexed, and the shoulder abducted, elevated, and externally rotated, the examiner attempts to passively extend the elbow. There is abnormal resistance to elbow extension, similar to Kernig's sign in that it stretches irritated nerve roots; also reported to occur in brachial plexitis. See **brachial plexus tests**.

Bing's sign: A pathologic reflex; pricking the dorsum of the foot or great toe with a pin causes toe extension. Bing's sign is an alternate method for eliciting great toe dorsiflexion in lesions of the corticospinal tract. The normal response is toe flexion as an avoidance response. In Bing's sign, the toe pulls upward toward the noxious stimulus rather than downward and away from it. Considered a **minor extensor toe sign**.

Bing's test: A tuning fork hearing test similar to the **Rinne test**. Normally and with sensorineural hearing loss, a tuning fork vibrating on the mastoid becomes louder when the tragus is occluded. Failure of the fork to sound louder suggests conductive hearing loss.

Binasal hemianopia: See **visual field defects.**

Biot breathing: One of the abnormal breathing patterns seen in patients with acute neurological disease. Various definitions can be found, but Plum and Posner[10] use it synonymously with **ataxic breathing**, a completely irregular breathing pattern with erratic pauses and increasing periods of apnea merging with agonal respirations. Many of the definitions given of Biot breathing are inaccurate, and it is often confused with cluster breathing. Wijdicks[11] provided a succinct review.

Bitemporal hemianopia: See **visual field defects.**

Blepharospasm: Involuntary closure of the eye(s) due to contraction of the orbicularis oculi, usually bilateral, repetitive, transient, and involuntary, as in benign essential blepharospasm (BEB). In BEB, patients suffer repetitive attacks of involuntary, bilateral eye closure multiple times daily that become more frequent and more sustained with the passage of time, may interfere with vision, and are often treated with botulinum toxin **(Video Link B.1)**. The condition is classified as a focal dystonia. In Meige's or Brueghel syndrome, blepharospasm is accompanied by oromandibular dystonia.

Similar movements sometimes occur as a **tic**, habit spasm, or **stereotypy**, especially in adolescents. Blepharospasm may be confused with **apraxia of eyelid opening**. Rarely, the movements in **hemifacial spasm** are more prominent in the upper face and appear to cause unilateral blepharospasm, but subtle lower facial movements are always present in addition. **Facial synkinesis**, as after Bell's palsy, may cause similar confusion (see **Marin Amat sign**). Related phenomena are blepharoclonus (repetitive blinking) and blepharismus (winking).

Blind spot: A scotoma corresponding to the optic nerve head. The physiologic blind spot (Mariotte's spot) is located 15° lateral to and just below the center of fixation because the disc lies nasal to the macula and the blind spot is projected into the temporal field. Elliptical in shape, it averages about 7° vertically and 5° horizontally. On a tangent screen with the patient 1 m away using a 1-mm white object, the average measurements for the blind spot are from 9 to 12 cm horizontally and 15 to 18 cm vertically. The blind spot is enlarged in papilledema and optic neuritis.

Blink reflex: The clinical blink reflex is eye closure following sudden unexpected visual stimulation or tactile stimulation around the eyes. There is also an electrophysiologic blink reflex. See **orbicularis oculi reflex.**

Blue rubber bleb: A rare skin lesion occurring in a neurocutaneous disorder, the blue rubber bleb syndrome, characterized by vascular malformations involving the skin and other organs, particularly the brain and the GI tract.[12] The skin lesions are bluish, nipple-like, and easily compressible **(Fig. B.12)**. MRI typically shows venous malformations.

Blue sclera: A condition, usually congenital, producing a bluish or grayish discoloration of the sclera because of scleral thinning and the resultant visibility of choroidal pigment **(Fig. B.13)**. Blue sclera are a classical manifestation of osteogenesis imperfecta. Other conditions associated with this finding include: Ehlers–Danlos syndrome, Marfan's syndrome, Crouzon's syndrome, Paget's disease, pseudoxanthoma elasticum, relapsing polychondritis, and phenylketonuria.

Body part as object: A phenomenon seen in apraxia when patients are asked to pantomime the use of an object. For example, when asked to demonstrate how to

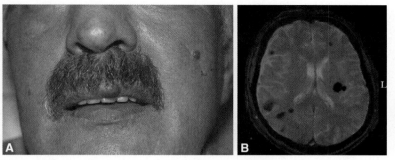

Figure B.12. Patient with blue rubber bleb syndrome who presented after a seizure. **A:** The cutaneous lesions were bluish, nipple-like, and easily compressible and present on the face and trunk. **B:** MRI showed multiple venous angiomas. (From den Heijer T, Boon AJ. Blue rubber bleb nevus syndrome. *Neurology.* 2007;68(13):1075, with permission.)

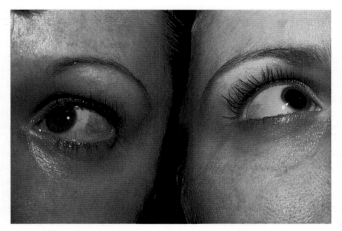

Figure B.13. Characteristic blue sclera in a patient with Ehlers–Danlos syndrome (normal patient on right for comparison). Thinning of the sclera allows the underlying choroid to cast a blue hue on the sclera. (From Gold DH, Weingeist TA. *Color Atlas of the Eye in Systemic Disease.* Baltimore, MD: Lippincott Williams & Wilkins; 2001, with permission.)

use a comb, the patient may rake the fingers through the hair rather than showing how to properly hold and use the actual implement.

Bodybuilder sign: A posture of abduction of the shoulders and flexion of the elbows described in acute traumatic central cord syndrome **(Fig. B.14).**[13] The bodybuilder sign is likely the same as the **Bradborn's sign and Thorburn's signs,** the authors reporting it being apparently unaware of these previous reports. See **Jolly's sign.**

Bon bon sign: A dystonic or dyskinetic movement of the tongue characterized by protrusion or lateral tongue movements within the mouth producing a bulge in

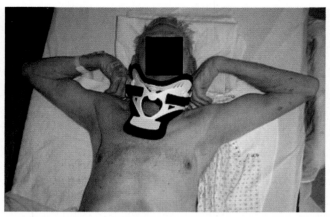

Figure B.14. Patient with acute traumatic central cord syndrome and the bodybuilder posture, abduction of the shoulders, flexion of the elbows, and bilateral wrist drops. This is the identical posture described by Bradborn and Thorburn years ago in patients with spinal cord injury. (From Espinosa PS, Berger, JR. Acute central cord syndrome with bodybuilder sign. *Clin Neurol Neurosurg.* 2007;109:354–356, with permission.)

the cheek as if the patient were storing a piece of candy there. Reportedly helpful in distinguishing tardive dyskinesias, where it is present, from chorea, where it is not. See **dyskinesias, tardive dyskinesias, orofacial dyskinesias, rabbit syndrome.**

Bonnet's sign: A modification of the **straight leg raising test**. The pain is more severe, or elicited sooner, if the test is carried out with the thigh and leg in a position of adduction and internal rotation (see also **Bragard's sign, Sicard's sign, Spurling's sign, bowstring sign**).

Bouche de tapir: A facial expression commonly seen in myopathies causing facial weakness, especially FSH. Because of the weakness, the lips move little, but droop tonelessly, leaving an involuntary protrusion of the upper lip, thought to resemble the mouth of the tapir with its overhanging upper lip. When the patient with FSH laughs, the lower face does not move; mirth shows in the eyes but not in the mouth. The appearance is characteristic and instantly recognizable.

Bovine cough: A cough without a glottal coup, seen in vocal cord palsy or conditions causing bulbar weakness. The cough is soft, feeble, and lacks the explosive quality of a normal cough.

Bowed-head sign: Tucking the chin to compensate for an inferior altitudinal hemianopia.

Bowstring sign (popliteal compression test): A **root stretch sign** seen in lumbosacral radiculopathy. A quick push on the sciatic nerve in the popliteal fossa just as stretch begins to cause pain during the **straight leg raising test** causes pain in the lumbar region, in the affected buttock, or along the course of the sciatic nerve (Video B.6).

Bowtie atrophy: See **band atrophy.**

Bowtie nystagmus: Oblique upbeat nystagmus with horizontal quick phases that alternate from right to left, the pattern of jerks thought to resemble neckwear. It has been reported in association with cerebellar disease and brainstem anomalies.[14]

Brachial diplegia: Weakness of both arms, with relative sparing of the legs and bulbar musculature (dangling arms), a pattern of weakness that occurs in several conditions. One of the most common etiologies is motor neuron disease. It may also occur with the man-in-the-barrel syndrome due to bilateral watershed cerebral infarctions, in central cord syndrome due to cervical spine trauma or ischemia, due to a lesion at the foramen magnum involving the rostral portion of the pyramidal decussation, and after sequential attacks of neuralgic amyotrophy or due to other causes of bilateral brachial plexopathy.

Brachial plexus stretch and tension tests: Maneuvers designed to elicit pain by stretching the brachial plexus in patients with brachial plexopathy. There is no information on the sensitivity, specificity, or reliability of these tests. The tests are similar to the **upper limb tension test,** which is said to be capable of eliciting pain in patients with brachial plexus "irritation" or cervical radiculopathy. The brachial plexus stretch test and brachial plexus tension test both involve having the patient place the arm in abduction and extend the arm down and back while depressing the shoulder and bending or rotating the head to the opposite side.

Brachioradialis (radial periosteal, supinator) reflex: The DTR elicited by tapping just above the styloid process of the radius with the forearm in semiflexion and semipronation, causing flexion of the elbow with variable supination (**Fig. B.15,** Video B.5). How to elicit the brachioradialis reflex is nicely demonstrated at the website for Stanford Medicine 25, An Initiative to Revive the Culture of Bedside Medicine (http://stanfordmedicine25.stanford.edu/the25/tendon.html). The most common cause of reflex impairment is cervical radiculopathy. A decreased brachioradialis

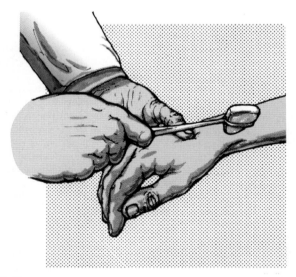

Figure B.15. Method of obtaining the brachioradialis reflex. (From Campbell WW. *DeJong's the Neurologic Examination.* 7th ed. Philadelphia, PA: Wolters Kluwer Health/ Lippincott Williams & Wilkins; 2013, with permission.)

reflex has an LR of 14.2 for the diagnosis of C6 radiculopathy.[2] It is normal for percussion of the brachioradialis tendon to also cause slight finger flexion. In the presence of spasticity and hyperreflexia, contraction of the brachioradialis may be accompanied by pronounced flexion of the fingers and adduction of the thumb. When the afferent limb of the reflex is impaired, there may be a twitch of the flexors of the hand and fingers without flexion and supination of the elbow; this is termed inversion of the reflex. The brachioradialis reflex is occasionally referred to as the radial periosteal or radioperiosteal reflex, an unfortunate misnomer as the periosteum has nothing to do with triggering the reflex. See **inverted reflexes.**

Brachycephaly: See **craniosynostosis.**

Bradborn's sign: See **Jolly's sign** and **bodybuilder sign.**

Bradykinesia: Slowness of movement, a cardinal manifestation of PD and other related hypokinetic movement disorders. These conditions are characterized by a paucity of movement and a slowing of movements (see Video A.2). Strictly speaking, **akinesia** means an absence of movement, bradykinesia a slowness of movement, and **hypokinesia** a decreased amount or amplitude of movement, but the term bradykinesia is often used to encompass all three. If bradykinesia, rigidity, and tremor are all present with asymmetry and no atypical features, there is a positive LR of 4.1 and a negative LR of 0.4 for the diagnosis of PD.[2]

Current models of basal ganglia function include a direct and an indirect loop or pathway for the connection between the striatum and thalamus. The direct pathway serves to facilitate cortical excitation and carry out voluntary movement. The indirect pathway serves to inhibit cortical excitation and prevent unwanted movement. Dysfunction of the direct pathway, as from a lack of dopamine, produces hypokinesia, e.g., parkinsonism; disease of the indirect pathway produces hyperkinesias, e.g., **chorea** or **hemiballismus.**[15]

Bradylalia: Slowness of speech, seen in hypokinetic movement disorders, especially PD.

Bradyphrenia: Slowness of thinking, typically seen in subcortical disorders causing cognitive impairment, such as PSP and HD. The patient may answer a question correctly, but with a prolonged response time.

Bragard's sign: An enhancement of the **straight leg raising test**; passively dorsiflexing the patient's foot, or great toe (Sicard's sign), just at the elevation angle at which the increased root tension begins to produce pain causes a further increase in pain (see Video B.6). The term **Spurling's sign** is also used for the same maneuver. See also **bowstring sign, Bonnet's sign.**

Breathing arm/hand: Aberrant regeneration of diaphragm axons into upper extremity muscles producing contraction synchronous with respiration; see **arm-diaphragm synkinesia.**

Brissaud reflex: Contraction of the tensor fascia lata on scratching the sole of the foot, seen in CST disease, part of the **triple flexion reflex.**

Brissaud–Sicard sign: Hemifacial spasm with contralateral hemiparesis, due to a lesion in the pons.

Broca's aphasia: A nonfluent type of **aphasia** due to a lesion involving the anterior perisylvian speech areas in the posterior inferior frontal region, also frequently called expressive aphasia. Patients have labored, uninflected, nonfluent spontaneous speech with a decreased amount of linguistic output: few words, short sentences, and poor grammar. In severe Broca's aphasia, the speech consists of nouns and substantive verbs produced with great effort. There is a tendency to leave out nonessential words such as adjectives, adverbs, and functor words (telegraphic speech). Speech comprehension is relatively unimpaired. Because of the severe nonfluency, patients are unable to repeat what they hear and unable to read aloud. The patient can identify objects but not name them. There may be preservation of emotional and automatic speech, and the patient may be able to sing. Patients with Broca's aphasia classically have a contralateral hemiparesis or faciobrachial paresis but no **visual field defect** (**Audio B.1**). See **agrammatism**.

Brow lift sign: A sign seen in **hemifacial spasm.** Cocontraction of the frontalis and orbicularis oculi causes simultaneous eye closure and paradoxical elevation of the eyebrow during a spasm (**Fig. B.16**). The sign was described by Babinski (see **Babinski signs**). This movement is impossible to execute voluntarily, and does not occur in blepharospasm. It seems very specific for HFS.[16]

Brown's superior oblique tendon syndrome: Limitation of the free movement of the superior oblique tendon through the trochlea. The restriction of movement is analogous to trigger finger and causes an impairment of upgaze in adduction simulating inferior oblique palsy (**Video B.7**). The disorder is most often congenital.

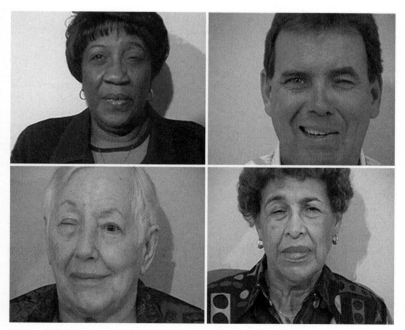

Figure B.16. Patients with hemifacial spasm (HFS) demonstrating the "other Babinski sign" manifested by elevation of the eyebrow caused by contraction of the frontalis muscle ipsilateral to the facial spasm. (From Stamey W, Jankovic J. The other Babinski sign in hemifacial spasm. *Neurology.* 2007;69:402–404, with permission.)

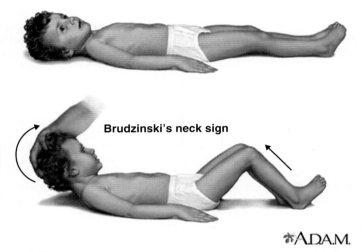

Figure B.17. Flexing the neck causes the knees to flex. (From Campbell WW. *DeJong's the Neurologic Examination.* 7th ed. Philadelphia, PA: Wolters Kluwer Health/Lippincott Williams & Wilkins; 2013, with permission.)

Brudzinski's neck sign: One of the **meningeal signs.** Placing one hand under the patient's head and flexing the neck while holding down the chest with the other hand causes flexion of the hips and knees bilaterally, often accompanied by extensor plantar responses **(Fig. B.17)**. With severe meningismus, it may prove impossible to hold the chest down, and the patient may be pulled into a sitting position with only the examiner's hand behind the head. Brudzinski described this as a sign of meningitis, but it is also sometimes listed as a method for reproducing pain in lumbosacral radiculopathy; in this context, it is essentially identical to **Lindner's sign** or the **Soto-Hall test** (see **straight leg raising test**).

Brudzinski's cheek sign: Pressure against the cheeks on or just below the zygoma causes flexion at the elbows with an upward jerking of the arms; a sign of meningeal irritation (see **meningeal signs**).

Brudzinski's contralateral leg sign: Passive flexion of one hip, especially with the knee extended, or passive knee extension after the hip has been flexed to a right angle, causes flexion of the opposite hip and knee; a sign of meningeal irritation (see **meningeal signs**).

Brudzinski's reciprocal contralateral leg sign: One knee and hip are flexed with the other leg extended; when the flexed limb is lowered, the contralateral extended leg goes into flexion; a sign of meningeal irritation (see **meningeal signs**).

Brudzinski's symphysis sign: Pressure on the symphysis pubis causes flexion of both lower extremities; a sign of meningeal irritation (see **meningeal signs**).

Bruit: The swishing sound created by turbulent arterial blood flow. The turbulence is often due to an obstruction, but bruits may occur in the absence of any demonstrable pathology, particularly in children. Any rapidly moving fluid produces noise, especially when the volume is high; no better example in medicine than the churning roar of a dialysis fistula. By convention, noises arising from arteries are called bruits, those from the heart murmurs, and those from veins are called hums, but the acoustics are the same. A focal bruit over the carotid bifurcation in a patient with acute symptoms of ipsilateral cerebral or ocular ischemia is particularly ominous, but in high-grade, malignant stenosis the bruit may soften or disappear because of low flow. In some instances, carotid occlusion on one side increases collateral flow and causes a bruit on the opposite side. As many as 1% of the normal population has a benign, insignificant bruit. The presence or absence of a bruit is of limited value in patient management except as a marker of atherosclerotic vascular disease in the appropriate clinical setting.[17] However, in the face of a known carotid stenosis, the presence of a bruit triples stroke risk. The ability of a bruit to pick up high-grade carotid stenosis has been found to have a sensitivity ranging from 30% to 75%, with a specificity ranging from 60% to 95% and a positive LR of 1.6-5.7.[18] Bruits may be heard over the cranium, particularly over the temporal regions, the eyeballs, and the mastoids, in patients with large aneurysms and arteriovenous malformations, and in the presence of intracranial occlusive cerebrovascular disease.

A carotid bruit is often transmitted to the mastoid, and this may be helpful in distinguishing a bruit from a transmitted murmur. About 10% of bruits arise from the external carotid. Internal carotid bruits are said to increase and external carotid bruits to decrease with breath holding or compression of the ipsilateral superficial temporal artery, but the reliability of these maneuvers is debatable and certainly less useful than ultrasonography.[19]

Venous hums are common and often confused with carotid bruits. With a hum, the sound is softer and more continuous, is less pulsatile, is located lower in the neck, and disappears with light finger pressure just above the location of the hum.

Bruns' ataxia: One of the **gait disorders** seen in conditions affecting the frontal lobe or its connections. In general, these conditions lead to a flexed posture with short, shuffling steps on a widened base and particular difficulty with gait initiation, so-called magnetic gait. Many terms have been used to refer to what is more or less the same disorder, one of which is Bruns' ataxia or apraxia; others are gait apraxia, frontal disequilibrium or ataxia, lower half/body parkinsonism, and marche à petits pas.

Bruns' nystagmus: An unusual direction-changing nystagmus that is coarse and slow on gaze toward the side of the lesion, and fine and rapid on gaze away from the lesion, characteristic of large tumors of the CPA (**Video Link B.2**). The coarse ipsilateral nystagmus is gaze paretic, and the fine contralateral nystagmus is vestibular in origin.[20]

Brushfield spots: Light-colored specks arranged in a ring near the outer margin of the iris (**Fig. B.18**). These are seen in 90% of patients with Down's syndrome who have light irises and in 25% of the normal population; difficult to see in dark irises.

Buccal apraxia: See **buccofacial apraxia.**

Buccal reflex: See **snout reflex.**

Buccofacial (oral) apraxia: An inability to execute on request complex acts involving the lips, mouth, and face. Buccofacial (orofacial, orobuccal) apraxia may include such activities as whistling, coughing, pursing the lips, sticking out the tongue, blowing a kiss, pretending to blow out a match, or sniffing a flower. There is no weakness of the mouth, lips, or face, but the patient is unable to make the requested movement. The patient may spontaneously lick the lips or stick out the tongue, but is not able to do so on command. Apraxia of such midline functions is common

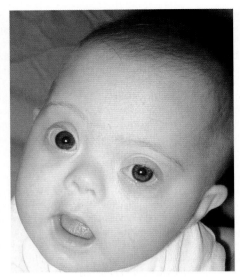

Figure B.18. A child with Down's syndrome showing Brushfield spots and heterochromia. (From Ryan E. Wikimedia Commons.)

in patients with lesions involving either hemisphere. Failure to execute such acts should not necessarily be construed as evidence of impaired comprehension in aphasic patients. Buccofacial apraxia usually occurs in association with **aphasia** or **apraxia of speech,** but may occur in isolation.[21] See **apraxia, ideomotor apraxia, ideational apraxia, constructional apraxia, dressing apraxia.**

Buccolingual dyskinesias: See **orofacial dyskinesias.**

Buckling sign: Knee flexion during straight leg raising to avoid sciatic nerve tension, evidence of lumbosacral radiculopathy. See **straight leg raising test.**

Bulbocavernosus reflex: A reflex elicited by stimulating the glans penis or clitoris (clitoroanal reflex), which causes contraction of the anal sphincter. The reflex is primarily useful in assessing the integrity of the cauda equina, lower sacral roots, and conus medullaris.[22]

Bulldog reflex: A **frontal release sign** causing involuntary clenching of the teeth in response to an object, usually a tongue blade, inserted between them.

Butt first maneuver: See **Gower's sign.**

Buzzard reflex: A method for facilitating the knee jerk by having the patient press the toes against the floor.

Video Links

B.1. A patient with benign essential blepharospasm. (From the Shirley H. Wray, Neuro-ophthalmology Collection, Neuro-ophthalmology Virtual Education Library (NOVEL), University of Utah.) Available at: http://stream.utah.edu/m/dp/frame.php?f=f46da46aa9a47c55037

B.2. Bruns' nystagmus due to a left cerebellar hemorrhage with edema and mass effect upon the junction of the medulla, pons, and cerebellum. (From Jason Barton, Canadian Neuro-ophthalmology Group.) Available at: http://www.neuroophthalmology.ca/case-of-the-month/eye-movements/diplopia-and-an-unusual-nystagmus

References

1. Miller TM, Johnston SC. Should the Babinski sign be part of the routine neurologic examination? *Neurology.* 2005;65:1165–1168.
2. McGee S. *Evidence Based Physical Diagnosis.* 3rd ed. Philadelphia, PA: Elsevier/Saunders; 2012.
3. Singerman J, Lee L. Consistency of the Babinski reflex and its variants. *Eur J Neurol.* 2008;15:960–964.
4. Leon-Sarmiento FE, Prada LJ, Torres-Hillera M. The first sign of Babinski. *Neurology.* 2002;59:1067.
5. Hilton-Jones D. Beevor's sign. *Pract Neurol.* 2004;4:176–177.
6. Lenoir T, Guedj N, Boulu P, et al. Camptocormia: the bent spine syndrome, an update. *Eur Spine J.* 2010;19:1229–1237.
7. Lawson VH, King WM, Arnold WD. Bent spine syndrome as an early manifestation of myotonic dystrophy type 1. *J Clin Neuromuscul Dis.* 2013;15:58–62.
8. Revuelta GJ. Anterocollis and camptocormia in parkinsonism: a current assessment. *Curr Neurol Neurosci Rep.* 2012;12:386–391.
9. Muthusamy B, Irsch K, Peggy Chang HY, et al. The sensitivity of the Bielschowsky head-tilt test in diagnosing acquired bilateral superior oblique paresis. *Am J Ophthalmol.* 2014;157:901–907.
10. Posner JB, Plum F. *Plum and Posner's Diagnosis of Stupor and Coma.* 4th ed. Oxford, NY: Oxford University Press; 2007.
11. Wijdicks EF. Biot's breathing. *J Neurol Neurosurg Psychiatry.* 2007;78:512–513.
12. den Heijer T, Boon AJ. Blue rubber bleb nevus syndrome. *Neurology.* 2007;68:1075.
13. Espinosa PS, Berger JR. Acute central cord syndrome with bodybuilder sign. *Clin Neurol Neurosurg.* 2007;109:354–356.
14. Choi KD, Jung DS, Park KP, et al. Bowtie and upbeat nystagmus evolving into hemi-seesaw nystagmus in medial medullary infarction: possible anatomic mechanisms. *Neurology.* 2004;62:663–665.
15. Campbell WW. *DeJong's the Neurologic Examination.* 7th ed. Baltimore, MD: Wolters Kluwer Health/Lippincott Williams & Wilkins; 2012.
16. Stamey W, Jankovic J. The other Babinski sign in hemifacial spasm. *Neurology.* 2007;69:402–404.
17. Nemeth J. Physical exam myths: listening for carotid artery bruits in stroke patients. *CJEM.* 2007;9: 368–370.
18. Sauve JS, Laupacis A, Ostbye T, et al. The rational clinical examination: does this patient have a clinically important carotid bruit? *JAMA.* 1993;270:2843–2845.
19. Orient JM, Sapira JD. *Sapira's Art & Science of Bedside Diagnosis.* 4th ed. Philadelphia, PA: Wolters Kluwer Health/Lippincott Williams & Wilkins; 2010.
20. Venkateswaran R, Gupta R, Swaminathan RP. Bruns nystagmus in cerebellopontine angle tumor. *JAMA Neurol.* 2013;70:646–647.
21. Kwon M, Lee JH, Oh JS, et al. Isolated buccofacial apraxia subsequent to a left ventral premotor cortex infarction. *Neurology.* 2013;80:2166–2167.
22. Wester C, FitzGerald MP, Brubaker L, et al. Validation of the clinical bulbocavernosus reflex. *Neurourol Urodyn.* 2003;22(6):589–591.

Café-au-lait spot: Hyperpigmented macules sometimes present in normals, but which when present in abundance suggest NF1. The macules are tan in color against white skin, but much more difficult to see against dark skin (Fig. C.1). The spots usually develop in the first year of life, but may be present at birth and are often the first apparent feature of NF1. The presence of six or more with a diameter of 0.5 cm before puberty or 1.5 cm after puberty is diagnostic (see Table N-1).[1]

Calcinosis (calcinosis cutis): See **dermatomyositis skin changes.**

Calf enlargement: An increase in the size of the calf that may result from various conditions. Both true muscle hypertrophy and **pseudohypertrophy**, symmetric and asymmetric, occur as a frequent and nonspecific clinical feature of many neuromuscular diseases. Calf pseudohypertrophy is a classic and consistent finding in Duchenne's and Becker's muscular dystrophy (Fig. C.2). Calf enlargement, either from true hypertrophy or pseudohypertrophy, may also be seen in juvenile proximal spinal muscular atrophy (Kugelberg-Welander disease), Kennedy's disease, central core disease, centronuclear myopathy, LGMD, acid maltase deficiency, polymyositis, granulomatous myositis, FSH, and IBM.[2] Neurogenic hypertrophy of the calf happens rarely, most often due to S1 radiculopathy (Fig. C.3).[3]

Caloric tests: Responses frequently used to check for brainstem integrity in comatose patients or to evaluate patients with vertigo. Ice water instilled into one ear canal will abruptly decrease the tonic activity from the labyrinth on the irrigated side.

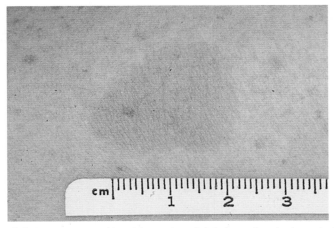

Figure C.1. The common café-au-lait spot is a slightly but uniformly pigmented macule or patch with a somewhat irregular border. Most of these spots are 0.5 to 1.5 cm in diameter and are of no consequence. After puberty, six or more such spots with a diameter of >1.5 cm suggests NF1. (From Bickley LS, Szilagyi, P. *Bates' Guide to Physical Examination and History Taking.* 8th ed. Philadelphia, PA: Wolters Kluwer Health/Lippincott Williams & Wilkins; 2003, with permission.)

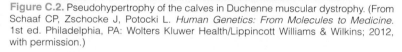

Figure C.2. Pseudohypertrophy of the calves in Duchenne muscular dystrophy. (From Schaaf CP, Zschocke J, Potocki L. *Human Genetics: From Molecules to Medicine.* 1st ed. Philadelphia, PA: Wolters Kluwer Health/Lippincott Williams & Wilkins; 2012, with permission.)

In a comatose patient with an intact brainstem, this causes tonic deviation of the eyes toward the side of irrigation as the normally active labyrinth pushes the eyes toward the hypoactive, irrigated labyrinth. In an awake patient, ice water calorics cause nystagmus with the fast component away from the irrigated side because the cerebral cortex produces a compensatory saccade that jerks in the direction opposite the tonic deviation. The familiar mnemonic "COWS" (cold opposite, warm same) refers to the fast phase of the nystagmus, not to the tonic gaze deviation. Nystagmus is seen only when the cortex is functioning normally. Warm water irrigation produces opposite effects.

In comatose patients, large volumes of ice water, 30 to 50 cc, are commonly used since it is imperative to elicit the response if it is present. Calorics can also be done to assess vestibular function in dizzy patients, either using much smaller volumes, 2 to 10 cc of an ice and water slush (minicalorics), or larger volumes of water less cold. The latency to onset and the duration of the nystagmus elicited is compared on the two sides. A difference of more than 20% in nystagmus duration suggests a lesion on the side of the decreased response, a condition termed *canal paresis.*

Camptocormia: See **bent spine syndrome.**

Camptodactyly: A congenital malformation of the fingers, predominantly the small finger, which causes flexion at the PIP joint. It occurs often as an isolated abnormality of no clinical significance, but is also associated with many hereditary disorders, some of which, such as Zellweger's cerebrohepatorenal syndrome and Marfan's

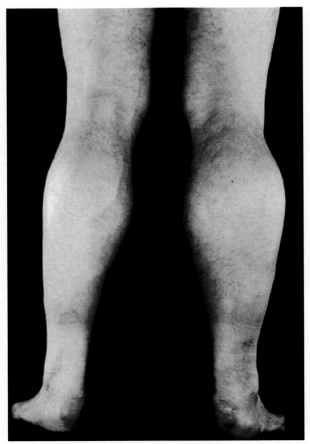

Figure C.3. Hypertrophy of the calf due to S1 radiculopathy. (From Coles A, Dick D. Unilateral calf hypertrophy. *J Neurol Neurosurg Psychiatry*. 2004;75:1606, with permission.)

syndrome, have neurologic features or complications. Clinodactyly is similar but causes primarily an incurvation of the small finger.

Carp mouth: A disparaging term used to describe the small oral aperture and tented upper lip that may be seen in myotonic dystrophy, especially in the congenital form.

Carpal compression (Durkan's) test: A test used in the evaluation of suspected CTS; see **carpal tunnel syndrome provocative tests.**

Carpal tunnel syndrome provocative tests: Maneuvers used to reproduce symptoms in patients with suspected CTS, such as Phalen's test, carpal compression test, pressure provocative test, the Elevated Arm Stress Test (EAST), the hand elevation test, the tourniquet test, percussing for Tinel's sign, and attempting to elicit the flick sign while taking the history (**Videos C.1** and **C.2**). When objectively studied, these provocative tests have proven disappointing, with high proportions of false positives and false negatives and are of limited value in the diagnosis of CTS.[4,5] They may be more sensitive and specific for the diagnosis of tenosynovitis of the flexor tendons than for CTS.[6] The EAST has been touted as useful in both thoracic outlet syndrome and CTS but has a high incidence of false positives in both; see **thoracic outlet syndrome provocative tests.**

D'Arcy and McGee, in a meta-analysis of 12 articles, concluded that several traditional tests for CTS have little or no diagnostic value, including Phalen's and Tinel's signs, thenar atrophy, and 2-point, vibratory, and monofilament sensory testing.[7] Findings that best distinguished between patients with electrodiagnostic evidence of CTS and patients without it were hypalgesia in the median nerve territory (LR 3.1), classic or probable Katz hand diagram results (LR 2.4), and weak thumb abduction strength (LR 1.8). Summarizing several studies, the calculated positive LRs were poor: 1.5 for Tinel's sign, 1.4 for Phalen's sign, and not significant for the pressure provocative test or flick sign.[8] The negative LR was 0.7 for Phalen's sign and not significant for Tinel's, the flick sign, or the pressure provocative test.

To perform Phalen's test, the wrists are flexed to 90° and held for 1 minute. The test is considered positive if the patient develops median distribution paresthesias. If the traditional Phalen's is negative, a "reverse Phalen's" may be performed with the wrists hyperextended and the patient holding the hands together in a position of prayer. Studies indicate that Phalen's test has only limited utility in the diagnosis of CTS. There is a wide range of sensitivities (10% to 91%) and specificities (33% to 76%), positive LRs of 1.1 to 2.1, and negative LRs of 0.3 to 1.0.[9]

Tinel's sign is paresthesias produced by percussion over a peripheral nerve that may indicate focal nerve pathology. It is a classical and commonly used test for CTS. Studies have shown sensitivities for CTS in the range of 25% to 60%, specificities in the range of 65% to 80%, positive LRs of 0.7 to 2.7, and negative LRs of 0.5 to 1.1.[9] The rare "reverse Tinel's sign" with paresthesias radiating retrograde up the forearm may be more specific for CTS.

In the carpal compression (Durkan's) test, the examiner applies firm thumb pressure over the transverse carpal ligament just distal to the wrist crease for 30 seconds, seeking to reproduce symptoms. Despite initial reports of high sensitivity and specificity, when studied more rigorously the carpal compression test performs no better than other carpal tunnel syndrome provocative tests.[5] The pressure provocative test (median nerve compression test) is a maneuver similar to the carpal compression test except that pressure is applied just proximal to the wrist crease over the median nerve between the flexor carpi radialis and palmaris longus tendons at the proximal margin of the transverse carpal ligament. The test is considered positive if numbness or paresthesias occur within 30 seconds. Despite initial reports of high sensitivity and specificity, when studied more rigorously the test also performs no better than other provocative tests.[5]

The Elevated Arm Stress Test (EAST, Roos, "hands up" test) is a maneuver first described as helpful in the diagnosis of TOS. The patient hold the arms horizontally and externally rotated with the elbows flexed to 90° in the "90-90" or "surrender" position, then opens and closes the hand for 3 minutes. The development of pain, heaviness, numbness, and tingling is abnormal. Subsequent studies showed the EAST maneuver was positive in 77% of patients with CTS and in 47% of normal controls.[10] In the hand elevation test, the patient raises the arm overhead for 1 minute, seeking to reproduce symptoms.[11] Some clinicians combine wrist flexion, creating an overhead Phalen's maneuver. There is some similarity to the elevated arm stress test but no exercise is involved. Studies indicate it may be slightly more useful than the other provocative tests but experience is not yet sufficient to judge its utility.

In the tourniquet test, inflation of a blood pressure cuff attempts to precipitate symptoms. Studies have shown low sensitivity and specificity, and it is of little practical use. To elicit the flick sign, the patient is asked to demonstrate what they do to "restore the circulation" when awakened with hand numbness (see Video C.1). The sign is considered positive if the patient flicks or shakes the wrist. Studies have shown the sensitivity and specificity is no better than the traditional carpal tunnel syndrome provocative tests.[12]

Carphology: An involuntary tugging at the sheets and picking of imaginary objects from the bedclothes that may be seen in acute disease, fever, and delirium, often along with a tossing to and fro on the bed.

Carpometacarpal (carpophalangeal) reflex of (von) Bechterew: Flexion of the wrist and fingers on tapping the dorsum of the wrist (carpometacarpal area). A variant of the finger flexor reflex, presumably due to spread of the reflexogenic zone that may occur with a CST lesion.

Carpopedal spasm: A contraction of the muscles of the fingers and hand with the thumb strongly adducted and the fingers stiffened, slightly flexed at the metacarpophalangeal joints, and forming a cone clustered about the thumb (see Fig. T-10). Carpopedal spasm is a common manifestation of hypocalcemia, **tetany,** and hyperventilation. See **Chvostek's sign** and **Trousseau's sign.**

Cataract: A corneal opacity, sometimes grossly visible on inspection and sometimes apparent on direct ophthalmoscopy as attenuation of the red reflex, haziness, or a frank media opacity. Mild or early cataracts are seen only on slit lamp examination. Early cataract formation is a feature of many neurologic conditions, such as myotonic dystrophy, Wilson's disease, lysosomal storage disorders, Refsum's disease, Down's syndrome, cerebrotendinous xanthomatosis, and Marinesco-Sjögren syndrome. Cataracts may develop as an adverse effect of some medications, most notably corticosteroids.

In myotonic dystrophy, the cataracts typically appear on slit lamp examination as bright, colorful spots, known as the "Christmas tree" cataract (Fig. C.4).

Catatonia: A complex neuropsychiatric syndrome that occurs primarily in psychiatric disorders, especially schizophrenia, but also in general medical and neurologic conditions and in drug-induced states such as NMS. It may occur without precedent psychiatric illness.[13] Catatonia is a movement disorder as well as a neuropsychiatric syndrome and may respond dramatically to benzodiazepines. Patients typically display a combination of immobility, **mutism,** and withdrawal with negativism, posturing, grimacing, and rigidity. More unusual are so-called waxy flexibility, **stereotypy, echolalia, echopraxia,** and episodic verbigeration. The abnormal muscle tone in catatonia is in many respects similar to extrapyramidal rigidity and may be physiologically related. There is a lead-pipe type of resistance to passive movement that may be accompanied by posturing and bizarre mannerisms. It may be possible to mold the extremities into any position, in which they remain indefinitely. Patients often appear frozen in an immobile, mute, withdrawn state and refuse to eat or drink. There is some overlap with neuroleptic malignant and serotonin syndromes as patients may have received medications known to precipitate these conditions.

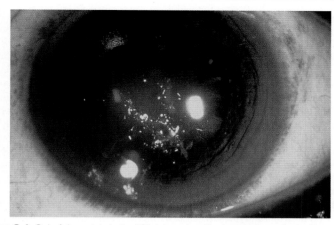

Figure C.4. Colorful crystals in the "Christmas tree" cataract of a patient with myotonic dystrophy. (From Chern KC, Saidel MA. *Ophthalmology Review Manual.* 2nd ed. Philadelphia, PA: Wolters Kluwer Health/Lippincott Williams & Wilkins; 2012, with permission.)

Catch-up saccade: A compensatory eye movement. During the **head impulse test**, when the vestibulo-ocular reflex is impaired the compensatory eye movement velocity is less than the head movement velocity and the eyes lag behind the head movement. A corrective "catch-up" saccade is required to resume fixation in the eccentric position. Also seen when the smooth pursuit eye movement system is impaired, the eyes lose the ability to track a moving target and corrective, catch-up saccades are necessary to maintain foveation, producing the phenomenon of **saccadic pursuit**.

Category (semantic) fluency: The ability to name as many items as possible in 1 minute from a particular category, such as animals or furniture. **Letter (phonemic) fluency** is the ability to name as many words as possible in 1 minute beginning with a particular letter. Commonly used letters are F, A, and S. Category fluency has been found to rely on lateral and inferior temporal lobe regions known to be involved in object perception, recognition, and naming. In contrast, letter fluency tests the ability to use phonemic and/or graphemic cues to guide retrieval. Letter fluency requires greater effort and a more active search strategy and poses more executive demands than category fluency and correlates better with prefrontal lobe functioning. The two tests of fluency may be affected differently in various disease processes. Decreased category fluency with relatively preserved letter fluency is often found in AD; the reverse pattern occurs in frontotemporal dementia and vascular dementia.

Cautious gait: See gait disorders.

Cecocentral (centrocecal) scotoma: See scotoma.

Central neurogenic hyperventilation: One of the abnormal respiratory patterns sometimes seen in patients with neurologic disease and depressed consciousness. It refers to sustained, rapid, and regular hyperpnea and is primarily associated with disease affecting the paramedian reticular formation in the low midbrain and upper pons, but may also occur with lesions in other brainstem locations, either intra-axial or extra-axial. See **apneustic breathing, Biot breathing, ataxic breathing, and Cheyne-Stokes respirations.**

Central nystagmus: Nystagmus due to a lesion of the CNS, usually involving the brainstem or cerebellum, as opposed to nystagmus due to a lesion of the peripheral vestibular apparatus or disease of the eyes. Central nystagmus has some differences in characteristics that allow for its differentiation from peripheral nystagmus, especially on electronystagmography. Central nystagmus tends to change directions whereas peripheral nystagmus does not.[14] Visual fixation suppresses peripheral nystagmus but has no effect on central nystagmus. Central nystagmus has a variable pattern; peripheral nystagmus is usually mixed horizontal-torsional. Peripheral nystagmus tends to attenuate rapidly after an acute illness, but central nystagmus may persist for weeks or months.

Central scotoma: See **scotoma.**

Centripetal rash: A rash that spreads from the extremities to the trunk. Most rashes begin on the trunk and spread to the extremities (centrifugal). Rarely a rash begins on the extremities, usually the palms and soles, and spreads centrally (centripetal). Important diseases that cause a centripetal rash include secondary syphilis, Rocky Mountain spotted fever, and Coxsackie virus infection.

Cerebellar ataxia: The cardinal sign of cerebellar disease (see **cerebellar signs**). Cerebellar **ataxia** consists of varying degrees of dyssynergia, dysmetria, lack of agonist–antagonist coordination, and tremor. One of the major elements of ataxia is dyssynergia. Loss of coordination between the component parts of a motor act produces a breakdown into its individual elements and causes execution in a disorganized, jerky erratic fashion. **Dysmetria** disrupts smooth movements because of misjudgments of the distance and speed of movement. A loss of normal coordination between agonist and antagonist causes **dysdiadochokinesia,** an inability to execute **rapid alternating movements**. Cerebellar ataxia produces a characteristic **intention tremor** on **finger-to-nose** and toe-to-finger testing. **Heel-to-shin** testing produces an erratic oscillation back and forth across the shin.

Cerebellar ataxia may affect the limbs, causing **appendicular ataxia**, the trunk, causing **truncal ataxia**, or the gait, causing **gait ataxia**. It is important not to confuse cerebellar ataxia with **sensory ataxia** (see **gait disorders**).

Cerebellar drift: Drift of the outstretched arm with the eyes closed, occasionally seen with ipsilateral cerebellar hemispheric disease. Typically the arm moves laterally, rising or sinking slightly, without the pronation or elbow flexion that accompany **pronator drift.**

Cerebellar signs: The clinical manifestations of cerebellar disease (Video C.3). **Ataxia** is the cardinal sign of cerebellar disease; it consists of varying degrees of **dyssynergia, dysmetria,** and **tremor**. Ataxia may affect the limbs, the trunk, or the gait. Patients with cerebellar dysfunction also suffer from various combinations of **dysdiadochokinesia, decomposition of movement, dysarthria,** and **nystagmus**. Cerebellar disease may also cause **hypotonia,** asthenia or slowness of movement, deviation or drift of the outstretched limbs (**cerebellar drift**), and pendular knee jerks (see **knee reflex**). Lack of agonist–antagonist coordination produces loss of the **rebound phenomenon** and impairment of the **checking reflex.**

Cerebellar disease may affect all or only a specific part of the cerebellum (Table C.1). The primary clinical manifestation of dysfunction of the

Table C.1. Clinical Manifestations of Disorders of the Cerebellum Related to the Different Zones of the Cerebellum

Zone of Cerebellum	Clinical Manifestation	Possible Disorder
Flocculonodular lobe (archicerebellum)	Nystagmus; extraocular movement abnormalities	Drug intoxication
Vermis	Gait ataxia	Alcoholic degeneration
Hemisphere (neocerebellum)	Appendicular ataxia	Tumor, stroke
Pancerebellar	All of the above	Paraneoplastic

flocculonodular lobe (archicerebellum) is **nystagmus** and other abnormalities of extraocular movement. Dysfunction of the vermis (paleocerebellum) produces **gait ataxia**, and when severe **titubation.** Disease of the cerebellar hemispheres (neocerebellum) produces **appendicular ataxia.** Disease involving the cerebellar connections in the brainstem causes abnormalities indistinguishable from disease of the cerebellum itself.

Cerebellar hemispheric deficits occur ipsilateral to the lesion, as the pathways are uncrossed (or, more correctly, double crossed). The occurrence of cerebellar ataxia in a "hemi-" distribution usually signals a unilateral, ipsilateral lesion of the cerebellum or cerebellar connections (e.g., cerebellar astrocytoma, multiple sclerosis, lateral medullary stroke).

Cerebellar outflow tremor: See **rubral tremor.**

Cerebellar tremor: The types of tremor seen in disease of the cerebellum. The most common type of cerebellar tremor is an **intention tremor.** A **postural tremor** of the outstretched limbs may also occur, without the patient reaching for a target. The heel resting on the opposite knee may tremble even before beginning to slide down the shin. Cerebellar tremor often involves the proximal muscles. When severe, cerebellar tremor may involve not only the extremities, but also the head or even the entire body (**titubation**). Severe cerebellar tremor may at times take on an almost myoclonic character.

The tremors and other movements probably result from disease involving the cerebellar efferent pathways or their connections with the red nucleus and thalamus (dentorubral and dentothalamic pathways, or superior cerebellar peduncle).

Cerebral ptosis: Bilateral, usually asymmetrical, ptosis in patients with cerebral lesions in the absence of any evidence of oculomotor or sympathetic dysfunction and without evidence of blepharospasm or lid apraxia. Cerebral ptosis was initially reported with right hemisphere lesions and accompanied by gaze palsies, but later reported to occur with left hemisphere lesions as well.[15]

Cerebrospinal fluid otorrhea: Leakage of CSF from the ear, classified as spontaneous or acquired. Trauma to the temporal bone is the most common cause of acquired CSF otorrhea, but it may also develop because of neoplasms, infections, or occasionally due to increased ICP in patients with idiopathic intracranial hypertension (Fig. C.5). The CSF leak increases the risk of meningitis. Detection of beta-2 transferrin in the secretions confirms the presence of CSF. The presence of glucose is not specific, and beta-2 transferrin is the preferred biochemical marker for the presence of CSF. See **cerebrospinal fluid rhinorrhea.**

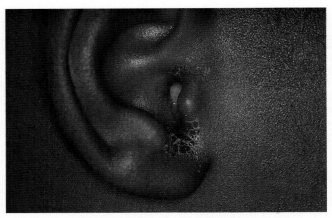

Figure C.5. CSF otorrhea associated with a cholesteatoma. (From Chung EK, Atkinson-McEvoy LR, Lai N et al. *Visual Diagnosis and Treatment in Pediatrics*. 3rd ed. Philadelphia, PA: Wolters Kluwer Health/Lippincott Williams & Wilkins; 2015, with permission.)

Cerebrospinal fluid rhinorrhea: Leakage of CSF from the nose. CSF rhinorrhea is classified as traumatic (>90%) or nontraumatic (<10%). About 80% of traumatic leaks are due to accidental trauma; the rest follow surgical procedures.[16] Idiopathic nontraumatic CSF rhinorrhea may occur in patients with idiopathic intracranial hypertension and empty sella syndrome. A typical clinical presentation of CSF rhinorrhea is a unilateral watery nasal discharge with a characteristic metallic or salty taste. The discharge characteristically occurs when the head is lowered, as when leaning over to tie the shoes **(Video Link C.1)**.[17] Sometimes the discharge can be provoked by having the patient lean forward. A "halo sign" is a clear ring around a central bloody spot after a bloody nasal discharge is dropped on a handkerchief or paper towel; it is suggestive but not diagnostic of CSF rhinorrhea. The differential diagnosis can be difficult because watery nasal discharges due to allergic and vasomotor rhinitis are much more common and may even coexist. Detection of beta-2 transferrin in nasal secretions confirms the presence of CSF. The presence of glucose is not specific, and beta-2 transferrin is the preferred biochemical marker for the presence of CSF. The leak increases the risk of meningitis. See **cerebrospinal fluid otorrhea.**

Cervical distraction test: See **cervical radiculopathy signs.**

Cervical dystonia (spasmodic torticollis): A relatively common form of focal dystonia that affects the neck, and sometimes the shoulder, muscles producing either a sustained or jerky turning of the head to one side, often with some element of head tilt **(Fig. C.6, Video Link C.2)**. Less common variants include retrocollis (extension movement), laterocollis (lateral bending), and **anterocollis** (flexion movement). In the beginning, the twisting and turning may be intermittent or present only in paroxysms (spasmodic), but later in the course there is persistent contraction of the involved muscles with resulting deviation of the head. Many, if not most, patients with cervical dystonia learn they can straighten the head by placing

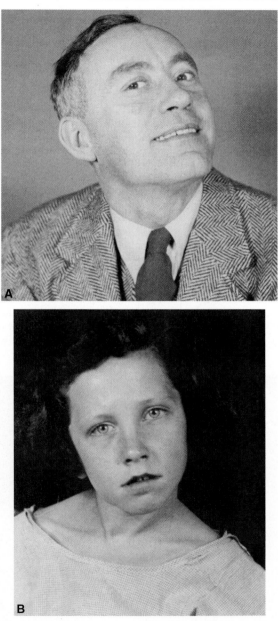

Figure C.6. Two examples (**A, B**) of cervical dystonia. (From Campbell WW. *DeJong's the Neurologic Examination.* 7th ed. Philadelphia, PA: Wolters Kluwer Health/Lippincott Williams & Wilkins; 2013, with permission.)

a hand or finger somewhere on the face or performing some other maneuver to provide sensory stimulation or light counterpressure (geste antagoniste, sensory trick, counterpressure sign).

Cervical radiculopathy signs: Maneuvers that may either exacerbate or relieve the radicular pain in patients with cervical radiculopathy (CR). The cervical spine range of motion is highly informative **(Video C.4)**. Patients should be asked to put chin to chest and to either shoulder, put each ear to shoulder, and to hold the head in full extension; these maneuvers all affect the size of the intervertebral foramen. Pain produced by movements that narrow the foramen suggests CR. Pain on the symptomatic side on putting the ipsilateral ear to the shoulder suggests radiculopathy, but increased pain on leaning or turning away from the symptomatic side suggests a myofascial origin.

Spurling's sign is a maneuver to reproduce symptoms of CR by narrowing the neural foramina.[18] The development of radicular symptoms, such as unilateral shoulder, arm, pectoral, or periscapular pain or radiating paresthesias into the arm or hand with the head in extension and tilted slightly to the symptomatic side, is highly suggestive of radiculopathy **(Fig. C.7**, Video C.4). Brief breath holding or gentle Valsalva in this position will sometimes elicit the pain if positioning alone is not provocative. Occasionally, Valsalva alone will elicit symptoms even with the neck in a neutral position (Valsalva test). The addition of axial compression by pressing down on the crown of the head does not seem to add much. There is a very prevalent misconception that Spurling's sign must involve downward pressure on the head; that is not what Spurling described, and this author has found it singularly uninformative, especially the variant that involves pounding on the patient's head. Some contend downward pressure may elicit pain from diseased

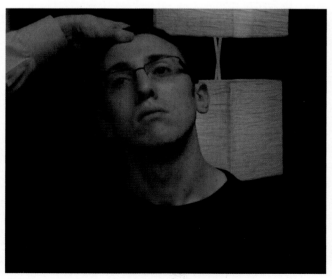

Figure C.7. Elicitation of Spurling's sign for cervical radiculopathy.

apophyseal joints; Spurling did not address that point and there is scant evidence to support this contention. Jackson's compression test is essentially the same as Spurling's maneuver.

The Spurling's test is specific, but not very sensitive. In a study of 255 patients, the Spurling test had a sensitivity of 30% and a specificity of 93%.[19] Viikari-Juntura et al[20] found a sensitivity of 40% to 60% and a specificity of 92% to 100%. McGee calculated a positive LR of 4.2.[8] In a study of the variations on Spurling's sign, Anekstein[21] et al suggested extension and lateral bending first, followed by axial compression only in cases with inconclusive results, exactly what Spurling described.

In Naffziger's sign, occlusion of the jugular veins causes an increase in radicular symptoms in compressive radiculopathy (**Fig. C.8**, Video C.4). Naffziger did this by placing a blood pressure cuff around the patient's neck; now it is done with light digital pressure. As the face becomes suffused, radicular pain or paresthesias in a nerve root distribution develop. Also known as Viets' sign, the two eponyms are often used interchangeably. Jugular compression is thought to engorge epidural veins or the CSF reservoirs, which in the normal individual is harmless. But when some element of foraminal narrowing and nerve root pressure exists, the additional compression causes the acute development of symptoms. The same mechanism likely underlies the exacerbation of root pain by coughing, sneezing, and straining (Dejerine's sign). The Viets'/Naffziger's sign is highly specific, but has low sensitivity, and is less useful in lumbosacral than in cervical radiculopathy. The upper limb tension test is a convoluted maneuver that attempts to stretch the involved

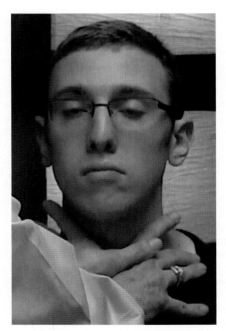

Figure C.8. Elicitation of Naffziger's (Viets' sign) for cervical radiculopathy.

structures and reproduce the pain in both CR and brachial plexopathy. It has not been validated, and there is limited evidence supporting it.[22]

Other maneuvers aid in the diagnosis of CR by producing a decrease in the pain. **Bakody's sign** (shoulder abduction relief sign, hand-on-head sign) is relief of arm and shoulder pain by resting the hand on top of the head (see Video B.1).[23,24] In one study, this sign had a sensitivity of 43% to 50% and a specificity of 80% to 100%.[20] Bakody's sign is reportedly pathognomonic for CR and more likely to be present with soft disc herniation, but occurred in at least one case with a Pancoast tumor. Patients with lesions of the brachial plexus have been reported to obtain relief from holding the elbow flexed and the shoulder adducted, the opposite from putting the hand on the head (**flexion-adduction sign**). The cervical distraction test produces relief of pain with manual upward neck traction, particularly with the neck in slight flexion (see Video B.1). In a study using 10 to 15 kg of traction in the supine position, this sign had a sensitivity of 40% to 43% and a specificity of 100%.[20] An increase in pain with cervical distraction suggests musculoskeletal or myofascial pain.

The shoulder depression test is the opposite of Bakody's sign and seeks to reproduce pain by having the patient flex the neck laterally while the examiner depresses the opposite shoulder. It is said to elicit pain due to root stretch in the presence of CR, but may also elicit myofascial pain.

A review of the literature regarding the various tests for cervical radiculopathy concluded the evidence indicated high specificity, low sensitivity, and good to fair interexaminer reliability for Spurling's test, the cervical distraction test, and Bakody's sign.[25] Flexion of the neck may provoke **Lhermitte's sign** in patients with cervical spondylosis or large disc herniations. The differentiation of CR from primary shoulder disease (e.g., bursitis, capsulitis, tendonitis, impingement syndrome) can be particularly difficult (see **shoulder examination tests**).

Chaddock's sign: An extensor toe sign seen with disease of the CST, elicited by stimulating the lateral aspect of the foot, beginning about under the lateral malleolus near the junction of the dorsal and plantar skin, drawing the stimulus from the heel forward to the small toe. The response of the toes is the same as with the Babinski. The reflex was described first by Yoshimura, but since it was described in Japanese, the observation was lost.[26] In the reverse Chaddock, the stimulus moves from the small toe toward the heel. See **pathologic reflexes.**

Chaddock's wrist sign: An upper-extremity pathologic reflex seen with CST disease. Pressure or scratching in the depression at the ulnar side of the flexor carpi radialis and palmaris longus tendons at wrist, or pressure on the palmaris longus tendon, and at times stimulation almost anywhere on ulnar side of volar forearm as high as the elbow, causes flexion of the wrist and simultaneous extension and separation of digits.

Chameleon tongue: See **trombone tongue.**

Charcot joint (neuropathic arthropathy): The arthropathy that occurs when a joint is deafferented, classically seen in neurosyphilis but now more common with sensory neuropathies, especially diabetic neuropathy, syringomyelia, or other conditions (Fig. C.9).[27] The acute Charcot foot in a diabetic is characterized by erythema, edema and warmth that can mimic cellulitis, injury, or acute arthritis such as gout. Neuropathic arthopathy due to syringomyelia tends to involve the larger joints of the upper extremity and may present as painless shoulder enlargement.[28]

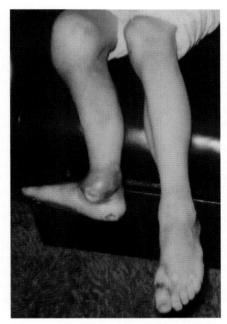

Figure C.9. Charcot joints in a patient with HSAN IV or congenital insensitivity to pain with anhidrosis. The left knee and left ankle are enlarged and distorted. The skin over the medial aspect of the ankle is darkened with a draining wound secondary to super-imposed osteomyelitis. There are other areas of trauma and ulcers including a site on the left heel. (From Axelrod FB, Gold-von Simson G. Hereditary sensory and autonomic neuropathies: types II, III, and IV. *Orphanet J Rare Dis.* 2007;2:39, with permission.)

Charcot's triad: The combination of **nystagmus, intention tremor,** and scanning speech (see **dysarthria**), once thought to be diagnostic of MS. This combination of findings can be seen in other conditions, and when it occurs in MS it is a late feature and of little use in the diagnosis early in the course.

Checking reflex (response): Contraction of the antagonist after a load is unexpect-edly removed during strong contraction of the agonist. The agonists must immedi-ately relax, and the antagonists must contract to provide braking after the sudden release of resistance. Impairment of checking is seen in cerebellar disease because of disruption of the smooth reciprocal relationship between agonist and antagonist. The checking reflex is tested with the **Holmes rebound test**, in which the examiner pulls on the wrist and attempts to extend the elbow as the patient strongly resists, with the arm adducted at the shoulder and flexed at the elbow and the fist firmly clenched. The examiner then suddenly releases his grip. Normally, with the sudden unloading the elbow flexors immediately relax and the elbow extensors contract to arrest the sudden flexion movement and stop the patient from hitting himself. The normal patient is able to control the unexpected flexion movement of the elbow, and there is a slight extension movement as the elbow extensors overcompensate, referred to as the **rebound phenomenon**. Rebound is a normal response that is reduced in disorders of the cerebellum and sometimes enhanced in spasticity. In cerebellar disease, when the strongly flexed extremity is suddenly released the patient cannot stop the flexor contraction and engage the extensors to stop the elbow movement. Because of loss of the checking response, the fist flies up to the shoulder or mouth, often with considerable force. Both the impaired checking response and the loss of rebound occur in cerebellar disease. Impaired checking and loss of rebound are both manifestations of the loss of agonist–antagonist coordination and are often confused with one another.

In the arm-stopping test, the patient holds both arms overhead or by his sides, the examiner holds his arms outstretched horizontally, and then the patient tries to quickly bring his arms up or down so that his fingertips are at the exact same level as the examiner's. With a unilateral hemispheric lesion, the good arm will stop on target, the affected arm often overshoots and then corrects in the opposite direction, oscillating around the target before eventually coming to rest. This technique allows for comparison of the checking movements on the two sides.

Chemosis: Edema of the conjunctiva. Swelling can become marked, causing difficulty with eye closure. Chemosis is a nonspecific sign that occurs in many conditions. It is often associated with **proptosis** in cavernous sinus thrombosis or carotid-cavernous fistula **(Fig. C.10)**. The classical triad of carotid-cavernous fistula is pulsatile proptosis, an ocular bruit and chemosis. See **corkscrew vessels.**

Cherry red spot: The appearance of the macula in a variety of storage diseases and in central **retinal artery occlusion (Fig. C.11)**. In storage disorders, the appearance is due to the accumulation of abnormal material within the cell layers of the retina. Because the macula is relatively devoid of cellular layers and comparatively transparent, the underlying red choroid is visible. In the younger patient, the presence of a cherry red spot indicates a condition such as gangliosidosis. The cherry red spot was originally described in Tay-Sachs disease (Tay's sign). A cherry red spot may also occur in lipid storage disease, mucopolysaccharidosis, lysosomal storage

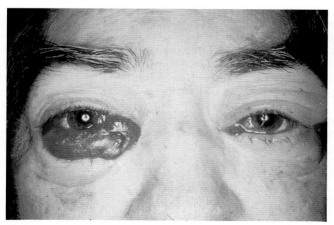

Figure C.10. Proptosis and chemosis in a direct, high-flow, right carotid cavernous fistula following trauma. (From Gold DH, Weingeist TA. *Color Atlas of the Eye in Systemic Disease.* Baltimore: Lippincott Williams & Wilkins; 2001, with permission.)

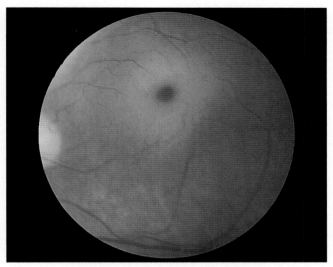

Figure C.11. Cherry-red spot in the macula of a patient with Tay-Sachs disease. (From Tasman W, Jaeger E. *The Wills Eye Hospital Atlas of Clinical Ophthalmology.* 2nd ed. Wolters Kluwer Health/Lippincott Williams & Wilkins; 2001, with permission.)

disease, and multiple sulfatase deficiency. In central retinal artery occlusion, the preservation of blood supply to the macula from the choroidal circulation makes it stand out against the retina made pale by ischemia.

Cheyne-Stokes respirations: One of the abnormal respiratory patterns that may be seen in patients with neurologic disease and depressed consciousness. Periods of hyperpnea alternate with periods of apnea **(Video Link C.3)**. Respirations increase in depth and volume up to a peak and then decline until there is a period of apnea, after which the cycle repeats. Cheyne-Stokes respirations may be due to bilateral hemisphere lesions or bilateral thalamic lesions, as well as to increased ICP. In Cheyne-Stokes variant breathing, there is hypopnea but not frank apnea. The other patterns that may be seen include **apneustic breathing, Biot breathing, ataxic breathing, and central neurogenic hyperventilation.**

Cholesteatoma: A cystic structure lined with squamous epithelium in the middle ear cavity that may occur congenitally or develop as a consequence of chronic otitis media. On examination, a grayish white mass may appear in the ear canal, frequently accompanied by a foul-smelling discharge **(Fig. C.12)**. Cholesteatomas usually arise in the attic and eventually invade the mastoid. They grow slowly due to the accumulation of epithelial debris and may erode bone to extend intracranially. They may penetrate into the CPA and produce a CPA syndrome. Central extension may also lead to meningitis and other complications. Erosion into the labyrinth may cause a perilymphatic fistula.

Chorea: Abnormal, involuntary, hyperkinetic movements that are irregular, purposeless, random, and nonrhythmic. Choreic movements are abrupt, brief, rapid, jerky, and unsustained. Individual movements are discrete, but they vary in type and

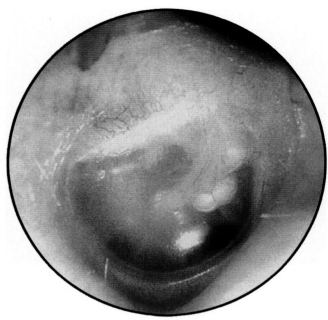

Figure C.12. A cholesteatoma. (From Chung EK, Atkinson-McEvoy LR, Lai N, et al. *Visual Diagnosis and Treatment in Pediatrics*. 3rd ed. Philadelphia, PA: Wolters Kluwer Health/Lippincott Williams & Wilkins; 2015, with permission.)

location, causing an irregular pattern of chaotic, multiform, constantly changing movements that seem to flow from one body part to another. The movements may at times appear purposeful to a casual observer, but they are actually random and aimless **(Video C.5)**.

The distribution of the movements is variable. They may involve one extremity or one half of the body (hemichorea) or be generalized. They occur most characteristically in the distal parts of the upper extremities, but may also involve the proximal parts, lower extremities, trunk, face, tongue, lips, and pharynx. Repeated twitching and grimacing movements of the face change constantly in character and location. The abnormal movements interfere with and distort voluntary movements, and the latter are frequently short, jerky, and unsustained. Constant unwanted movements of the hands may interfere with activities of daily living. When asked to hold the hands outstretched, characteristic constant random movements of individual fingers keep the fingers in perpetual motion (**piano-playing movements**). If the patient holds the examiner's finger in her fist, constant twitches of individual fingers cause variations in grip strength as individual fingers grip and relax randomly (**milkmaid grip**). When chorea is generalized, the patient is in a constant state of motion with continual adventitial movements randomly scattered.

The patient may try to incorporate a spontaneous, involuntary movement into a semipurposeful movement in order to mask the chorea (parakinesia). If a choreic movement suddenly makes a hand fly upward, the patient may continue the movement and reach up and scratch her nose. Motor **impersistence,** the inability to sustain a contraction, frequently accompanies chorea. The patient is frequently unable to hold the tongue out for any length of time; when asked to do so, the tongue shoots out, then jerks back quickly (snake, darting, flycatcher, or **trombone tongue,** Video C.5).

Choreic gait: The gait abnormality in chorea. There is often abundant extraneous movement and a dancing or prancing quality that may appear histrionic or nonorganic but is all too real **(Video Link C.4).**

Choreic hand: See **spooning.**

Choreoathetosis: a movement disorder with elements of both **chorea** and **athetosis**. There is a combination of quick, flicking, primarily distal movements and slower, more sustained, writhing, primarily proximal movements.

Chvostek's (Chvostek-Weiss) sign: A spasm or tetanic, cramp-like contraction, of the ipsilateral facial muscles on tapping just below the zygomatic process of the temporal bone, in front of the ear, in patients with nerve hyperexcitability **(Video C.6).**[29] This is the location of the pes anserinus, so Chvostek's sign is essentially a **motor Tinel's sign**. It is classically a sign of **tetany** due to hypocalcemia of any cause. When very active, the response may be elicited merely by stroking the skin in front of the ear. The sign is minimal if only a slight twitch of the upper lip or the angle of the mouth results; moderate if there is movement of the ala nasi and the entire corner of the mouth; maximal if the muscles of the forehead, eyelid, and cheek also contract. A minimal Chvostek is common in normal individuals.[30] See **Trousseau's sign.**

Ciliospinal reflex: Dilation of the pupil on stimulation of the skin of the ipsilateral neck. Local cutaneous stimulation activates sympathetics through connections with the ciliospinal center at C8–T2 that cause the ipsilateral pupil to dilate. An intact ciliospinal reflex is evidence of brainstem integrity when evaluating a comatose patient. Efferent impulses are relayed through the cervical ciliospinal center and the sympathetic nervous system. The response is minimal and often difficult to see even when normal.

Circumduction gait: The gait abnormality typical of hemiparesis. Because of foot dorsiflexion weakness, the patient tends to drag or shuffle the foot and scrape the toes. With each step, the pelvis tilts upward on the involved side to aid in lifting the toe off the floor **(hip hike)** and the entire extremity swings around in a semicircle from the hip (circumduction). See **gait disorders**.

Circumlocution: Rambling, verbose, roundabout speech often used by patients with **anomia,** who resort to a description of objects when the name escapes recall.

Clasp-knife response: The sudden loss of resistance near the end of the range of motion when a spastic muscle is stretched. See **spasticity**.

Clavicle reflex: Contraction of various muscle groups in the upper limb elicited by percussion over the lateral aspect of the clavicle (see Video A.3). This is not a specific reflex, but an indication of spread of the reflex response. The response is minimal, usually absent, except in the face of upper-extremity hyperreflexia. Normally, the response should be the same on each side. It is useful in comparing the reflex activity of the two upper limbs.

Claude's sign of reflex hyperkinesia: Reflex movements, either extension or retraction, following a painful stimulus to an extremity, even though the part seems totally paralyzed, a type of **associated movement**.

Claw foot: A deformity due to denervation and weakness of the intrinsic foot muscles, causing hyperextension at the metatarsophalangeal joints and flexion at the interphalangeal joins with abnormal toe flexion producing a claw deformity. It may occur with any chronic denervating process, most often polyneuropathy such as CMT disease. See **hammer toes, pes cavus**.

Claw hand: A hand posture most often seen in ulnar neuropathy (ulnar griffe). The interossei and lumbricals flex the metacarpophalangeal (MCP) joints and extend the interphalangeal (IP) joints. Weakness of these muscles causes loss of MCP joint flexion and loss of PIP joint extension. The hand assumes a position of rest in which the MCP joints are held in extension and the PIP and DIP joints are flexed. Since the ulnar nerve innervates all the interossei and both the third and fourth lumbricals, ulnar weakness primarily affects the ring and small fingers because both lumbrical and interosseous functions are lost and these fingers assume a clawed position (Fig. C.13). Clawing is more severe when the ulnar lesion is distal because the unopposed pull of the flexor digitorum profundus exacerbates the deformity; with proximal lesions, the long flexor may itself be somewhat weak and the clawing less severe. When lesions affect both the ulnar and median nerves, all the fingers may be clawed. Other conditions that may superficially resemble ulnar clawing include Dupuytren's contracture and **camptodactyly**. An ulnar griffe is sometimes referred to as a **benediction hand,** but the term is not used consistently and best avoided. See **finger drop.**

Cleckley's sign: See **minor extensor toe signs.**

Clock drawing test (CDT): A test of visuospatial capability and mental status. Originally developed as a test of constructional and visuospatial function, the CDT has evolved into a simple and quick test of general cognitive abilities. Given a circle,

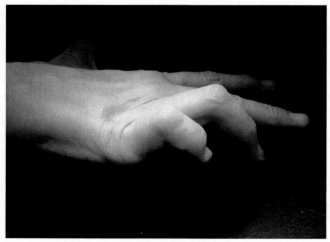

Figure C.13. Clawing of the ulnar digits in low ulnar nerve palsy. (From Rayan G, Akelman E; American Society for Surgery of the Hand. *The Hand: Anatomy, Examination, and Diagnosis.* 4th ed. Philadelphia, PA: Wolters Kluwer Health/Lippincott Williams & Wilkins; 2011, with permission.)

the patient is asked to insert the numbers and draw the hands indicating a specific time. An abnormal CDT increases the probability of dementia. Errors on the CDT develop early in AD and worsen progressively. Studies have shown a sensitivity of 36% to 75%, a specificity of 72% to 98%, and a positive LR of 5.3.[8]

Clonus: A series of rhythmic involuntary muscular contractions induced by the sudden passive stretching of a muscle or tendon. It often accompanies the spasticity and hyperactive DTRs seen in CST disease. Clonus occurs most frequently at the ankle, knee, elbow, and wrist, and occasionally elsewhere. Ankle clonus consists of a series of rhythmic alternating flexions and extensions of the ankle **(Video C.7)**. Unsustained clonus fades away after a few beats, whereas sustained clonus persists as long as the examiner continues to hold slight dorsiflexion pressure on the foot. Unsustained symmetric ankle clonus may occur in normal individuals with physiologically fast DTRs. Sustained clonus is never normal. Patellar clonus consists of a series of rhythmic up-and-down movements of the patella. It may be elicited if the examiner grasps the patella between the index finger and the thumb and executes a sudden, sharp, downward thrust, holding downward pressure at the end of the movement. Clonus of the wrist or of the fingers may be produced by a sudden passive extension of the wrist or fingers. A quick supination movement of the forearm can induce pronator clonus. Ankle clonus usually has a frequency of 5 to 8 Hz. Because of the shorter reflex pathways involved, upper extremity clonus is a bit faster.

Cloverleaf skull: See **craniosynostosis.**

Clubbing: A characteristic change in the shape of the nails seen in a number of cardiopulmonary diseases, particularly cyanotic congenital heart disease **(Fig. C.14)**. The essential finding is loss of the angle between the nail and the proximal soft

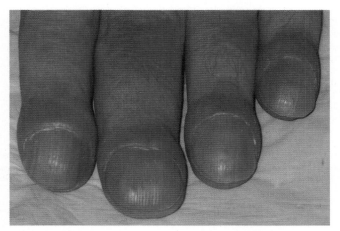

Figure C.14. Clubbing of the fingers. The normal angle between the base of the nail and the distal finger is about 160 degrees. With clubbing, the distal phalanx of each finger becomes rounded and bulbous ("lollipop configuration") and the nail angle exceeds 180 degrees. The proximal nail fold feels spongy. (From Berg D, Worzala K. *Atlas of Adult Physical Diagnosis.* Philadelphia, PA: Wolters Kluwer Health/Lippincott Williams & Wilkins; 2006, with permission.)

tissues. Clubbing may occasionally occur in conditions of potential neurologic interest, including sarcoidosis, Hodgkin's disease, celiac disease, primary biliary cirrhosis, acromegaly, HIV infection, hereditary hemorrhagic telangiectasia, hyperparathyroidism, and both hyper- and hypothyroidism.

Clubfoot (club foot, talipes equinovarus): See **pes cavus.**

Cochleopupillary reflex: Dilation of the pupil in response to a loud noise.

Cogan's lid twitch sign: A brief overshoot twitch of lid retraction following sudden return of the eyes to primary position after a period of downgaze **(Video C.8).** The lid will briefly twitch upward and then settle back to its previous position. This sign should increase suspicion of MG but is not diagnostic; it may be seen in other conditions as well. A similar upward twitch may occur on glancing quickly to the side from primary position (eyelid hopping).

Cogan's rule: See **optokinetic nystagmus.**

Cogan's syndrome: See **oculomotor apraxia.**

Cognitive screening instruments: Any of a number of short screening mental status evaluation instruments developed for use at the bedside and in the clinic. The most widely used of these is the Folstein mini-mental state exam (MMSE); but there are others as well **(Table C.2).** The MMSE takes about 10 minutes to administer and has a series of scored questions that provides a localization-based overview of cognitive function, but it does not assess any function in detail. The maximum score is 30. Minimum normal performance depends on age and educational level, but it has been variously stated as between 24 and 27 **(Table C.3).**[31] One set of

Table C.2. Other Frequently Used Cognitive Screening Instruments

Orientation-memory-concentration test
Short orientation-memory-concentration test
CAMCOG
Cambridge mental disorders of the elderly examination
General practitioner assessment of cognition
Memory impairment screen
Mini-cognitive assessment instrument (Mini-Cog)
Information-memory-concentration test
Short test of mental status
Cognistat
Montreal cognitive assessment

Table C.3. Mean (Standard Deviation) Mini-Mental State Examination Scores

	55–59	60–64	65–69	70–74	75–79	80–84	>85
9–12 y or high school diploma	28 (2.2)	28 (2.2)	28 (2.2)	27 (1.6)	27 (1.5)	25 (2.3)	26 (2.0)
College experience or higher degree	29 (1.5)	29 (1.3)	29 (1.0)	28 (1.6)	28 (1.6)	27 (0.9)	27 (1.3)

Data from Crum RM, Anthony JC, Sassett SS, et al. Population-based norms for the Mini-Mental State Examination by age and education level. *JAMA.* 1993;269:2386–2391, with permission.

criteria for the lower limit of normal is 23 for high school dropouts, 27 for high school graduates, and 29 for college graduates.

The MMSE has limitations in both sensitivity and specificity and should not be used as more than a screening instrument. It is affected by age, education, gender, and cultural background. A cutoff score of 23 has a sensitivity of 86%, a specificity of 91%, and a positive LR of 8.9 for detecting dementia in a community sample.[8] But this score is insensitive and will not detect mild cognitive impairment, especially in well-educated or high-functioning patients (ceiling effect). A normal MMSE score does not reliably exclude dementia. There is also a relatively high false-positive rate. The design of the MMSE makes it insensitive for right hemisphere or frontal lobe pathology. A 15-item extension, the modified MMSE, addresses some of the limitations of the traditional MMSE.

One study found that two brief, simple tests offered similar sensitivity and specificity to the MMSE.[32] These are the recall of a five-item name and address, "John Brown 42 Market Street Chicago" (a component of the Short Orientation-Memory-Concentration test) and the 1-minute verbal fluency for animals (see **category fluency**). These performed similarly to the MMSE in screening for dementia and memory problems in clinical practice.

The Mini-Cog combines the **clock drawing test** with tests of recall using three unrelated words. A Mini-Cog score of ≤2 has a positive LR of 9.5 for the diagnosis of dementia.[8]

Cogwheel pursuit: See **saccadic pursuit**.

Cogwheel rigidity: See **rigidity**.

Coin-in-the-hand test: An apparently, but not really, difficult test to detect malingering or embellishment of memory loss.[33] The examiner shows a coin in one hand to the patient, who then counts backwards from 10 with eyes closed, then opens the eyes and attempts to remember in which now-closed hand the coin was. Patients with real memory deficits perform very well, while those feigning memory loss perform around the random chance level. Subsequent studies have shown the coin-in-the-hand test has potential as a quick and easy screening tool to detect neurocognitive symptom exaggeration and can effectively supplement commonly used **cognitive screening instruments**.[34]

Cold calorics: See **caloric tests**.

Cold hands sign: Cold, dusky, purplish discoloration of the digits due to impaired peripheral vasomotor control, evidence of MSA (Fig. C.15).

Cold pack test: See **ice pack test**.

Cold reversal: See **temperature reversal**.

Collapsing (give-way, breakaway) weakness: A pattern of weakness in which muscular contractions are poorly sustained and may give way suddenly, rather than gradually, as the patient resists the force exerted by the examiner. Collapsing weakness is one of the **functional signs** suggestive of a nonorganic origin of a patient's deficit. Patients with bona fide organic muscle weakness will yield smoothly as the examiner defeats the weak muscle. Some patients with collapsing weakness will give up entirely and allow the muscle or limb to flop at the slightest touch; others will provide variable resistance throughout the range of motion with alternating moments of effort and no effort. At the peaks of contraction, strength is normal; in the valleys there is little or no resistance. This pattern of variable strength is referred to as "ratchety" or "catch and give." Collapsing weakness may improve with encouragement; real weakness does not.

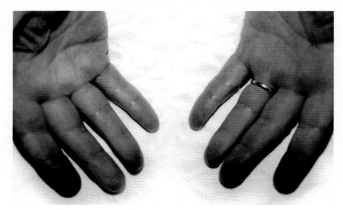

Figure C.15. Dusky, violaceous fingers typical of multiple system atrophy. (From Reich SG. The cold hands sign in MSA. *Neurology.* 2003;60:719, with permission.)

As with all so-called nonorganic signs, the reliability of collapsing weakness has been questioned, may be misinterpreted, and should be kept in clinical context. In one study, one third of 30 consecutive patients admitted with acute structural CNS lesions (25 were stroke) either had or were thought to have collapsing weakness.[35] Some patients have real weakness with an additional element of functional weakness.

Collier's sign (posterior fossa stare): Lid retraction in primary gaze, seen with lesions involving the posterior commissure (Fig. C.16). See **eyelid retraction**.

Color agnosia: The inability to name colors in the absence of any defect in color vision. The patient is not color blind, but cannot name colors or match colors when given a verbal or written list. See **agnosia.**

Color anomia: A similar but less severe condition in which the patient has retained ability to recognize colors and can pick a color from a list, but cannot spontaneously name the color, in the absence of aphasia or other naming difficulty.

Color blindness: An inherited impairment of the ability to perceive color without any other visual impairment. The most common form is X-linked, affects red–green perception (deuteranopia), and may affect as many as 8% of the male population. Acquired impairment of color perception is also common and occurs primarily with disorders involving the anterior visual pathways, but these deficits are not customarily referred to as color blindness. See **achromatopsia.**

Color desaturation: A decrease in the intensity or brightness of a color or hue, seen most often with red, and typically referred to as red desaturation. It is characteristic of optic nerve or optic chiasm disease. Red desaturation, along with other impairments of color vision, may be one of the earliest manifestations of optic neuropathy. Red desaturation in the temporal hemifields may be one of the earliest manifestations of bitemporal hemianopia with optic chiasm disease. See **achromatopsia.**

Combined vertical gaze palsy: The simultaneous presence of both **downgaze palsy** and **upgaze palsy**, with preservation of horizontal gaze. The lesion involves the rostral interstitial nucleus of the MLF in the upper brainstem; the most common cause is infarction of the rostral midbrain. Other etiologies include PSP, CBD,

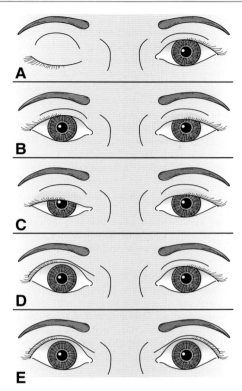

Figure C.16. Characteristics of different causes of abnormal lid position. **A:** Right third cranial nerve palsy with complete ptosis. **B:** Left Horner's syndrome with drooping of upper lid and slight elevation of lower lid. **C:** Bilateral, asymmetric ptosis in myasthenia gravis. **D:** Right lid retraction in thyroid eye disease. **E:** Bilateral lid retraction with a lesion in the region of the posterior commissure (Collier's sign). (From Campbell WW. *DeJong's the Neurologic Examination*. 7th ed. Philadelphia, PA: Wolters Kluwer Health/ Lippincott Williams & Wilkins; 2013, with permission.)

Wernicke's encephalopathy, MS, Whipple's disease, Wilson's disease, and mass lesions causing midbrain dysfunction. In supranuclear disorders, such as PSP, reflex eye movements on testing the oculocephalic response may remain intact (see **Bell's phenomenon**). **Skew deviation** is sometimes present.

Compass gait: See **star walking**.

Complete ophthalmoplegia: Total loss of all external eye movements. This occurs in only a few conditions, such as severe MG, botulism, Miller Fisher syndrome, thyroid eye disease, late progressive external ophthalmoplegia, Kearnes-Sayre syndrome, PSP, **oculomotor apraxia**, Wernicke's encephalopathy, Wilson's disease, anticonvulsant toxicity, pituitary apoplexy, bilateral brainstem ischemia, and, of course, brain death.

Conceptual apraxia: A type of **apraxia** in which a patient seems unable to grasp the concept of how to go about completing a task. The patient may select a wrench to drive a screw, a screwdriver to hammer a nail, or a toothbrush to brush her hair.

Conduction aphasia: A type of **aphasia** characterized primarily by impaired repetition. The typical deficit is poor repetition with relative preservation of other language functions. Speech is relatively fluent, but contaminated by paraphasic errors; comprehension is unaffected, and naming is variable. Repetition is worst for multisyllabic words and sentences, and it is during repetition that paraphasic errors are most apt to appear. Patients are aware of and try to correct the pronunciation errors. The remainder of the neurological examination is often normal, or shows mild hemiparesis, hemisensory loss, or hemianopia. The lesion most often lies in the deep white matter in the region of the supramarginal gyrus and involves the arcuate fasciculus and other fiber tracts that run from the posterior to the anterior language areas. The etiology is usually an embolic occlusion of a terminal branch of the MCA.

Conduction apraxia: **Apraxia** worse when imitating the examiner's gestures than when pantomiming to verbal command; so named because of the perceived similarity between imitation of a gesture and the repetition deficit in conduction aphasia.

Conductive hearing loss: Impaired hearing due to decreased conduction of sound to the cochlea. Conductive hearing loss (CHL) may result from occlusion of the external auditory canal, middle ear disease (e.g., otitis), or abnormality of the ossicular chain (e.g., otosclerosis). **Sensorineural hearing loss** (SNHL) is that due to disease of the cochlea or eighth cranial nerve. As a generality, CHL affects low frequencies or is relatively flat, whereas SNHL affects high frequencies. Speech discrimination is relatively unaffected in CHL. Patients with elements of both CHL and SNHL are said to have mixed hearing loss.

To bedside examination, with CHL there is primarily loss of air conduction; bone conduction is preserved or even exaggerated beyond the normal because the middle ear cavity becomes a resonating chamber. The **Rinne test** is negative, and the **Weber test** lateralizes to the involved side **(Table C.4)**.

Confabulation: A situation in which a patient with memory loss, most classically Wernicke-Korsakoff syndrome, "fills in the gaps" in memory by saying whatever comes to mind, having no idea whether it is actually true or not. There is memory impairment out of proportion to other cognitive functions. Unable to recall

Table C.4. Rinne and Weber Tests

	Auditory Acuity	Rinne Test	Weber Test
Conductive hearing loss	Decreased	BC > AC (Rinne negative or abnormal)	Lateralizes to abnormal side
Sensorineural hearing loss	Decreased	AC > BC (Rinne positive or normal)	Lateralizes to normal side

Normally, the auditory acuity is equal in both ears, air conduction is greater than bone conduction (Rinne test normal or positive) bilaterally, and the Weber test is nonlateralizing (midline). The table depicts the pattern on the involved side with *unilateral* conductive or sensorineural hearing loss.
From Campbell WW. *DeJong's the Neurologic Examination.* 7th ed. Philadelphia, PA: Wolters Kluwer/Lippincott Williams & Wilkins; 2013, with permission.

things, the patient makes up wild tales without an intent to deceive and without any awareness whether the information is or is not true. The confabulation may range from minor deviations from actual events to blatant falsehoods. Two forms are recognized: spontaneous and provoked. The provoked type typically emerges during memory testing.

Congenital (infantile) nystagmus: See **nystagmus.**

Congenital oculomotor apraxia: See **oculomotor apraxia.**

Congruence: The degree to which visual field defects in the two eyes match in a homonymous hemianopia. As a general rule, the more congruent the defect, the more posterior the lesion. When the hemianopia is complete, no judgment about congruence can be made.

Conjunctival reflex: Similar to the **corneal reflex** except elicited by stimulation of the conjunctiva; a much less active and much less useful reflex, unfortunately occasionally confused with and inadvertently done instead of the corneal reflex.

Consensual pupillary light reflex: Pupillary constriction in the eye contralateral to the one receiving a light stimulus.

Consensual reflex: The occurrence of a contralateral or bilateral response to a unilateral stimulus, as in the consensual pupillary response.

Constructional apraxia: An inability to copy geometric forms of any complexity because of impaired visuospatial skills. The patient may be capable of drawing a square but not a three-dimensional cube, or be able to draw individual shapes but not able to synthesize them into a more complex geometric figure. The patient may also lose the ability to draw actual things, such as a three-dimensional house with a roof and chimney, a clock, or a daisy. Constructional apraxia usually occurs with parietal lobe lesions, occasionally with frontal lesions that interfere with the patient's ability to comprehend spatial relationships. See **apraxia, buccofacial apraxia, ideomotor apraxia, ideational apraxia, dressing apraxia, clock drawing test.**

Contraction fasciculation: A type of fasciculation that does not occur spontaneously, but instead is provoked by minimal contraction of a muscle. Contraction fasciculations do not carry the same significance as spontaneous fasciculations, but do suggest underlying enlargement of motor unit territory, especially as occurs in chronic denervating disorders such as SMA. Contraction fasciculations of the chin and perioral muscles are especially characteristic of Kennedy's disease. See **fasciculation.**

Contracture: Fixed limitation of movement that may occur at a joint affected by long-standing weakness, dystonia, or similar conditions. With contracture, a muscle cannot be stretched to its normal limits without considerable resistance and the production of pain. Patients with spasticity are at particular risk for contractures, particularly in the calf muscles, which draw the foot downward, producing a loss of range of motion on attempted passive dorsiflexion ("tight heel cords"). Contractures may ultimately result in periarthritic changes, joint ankylosis, and fixed deformities. They are a major clinical problem in some clinical conditions, especially SCI, TBI, and certain neuromuscular disorders, affecting up to 70% of outpatients with DMD. Contractures not only limit the functional use of the involved limb, but also impair mobility, self-care, and hygiene and may lead to pain and pressure sores.

Convergence insufficiency: An inability to bring the eyes together in a normal convergence movement. The convergence movement of the near reflex is mediated by the vergence subcomponent of the supranuclear ocular motor control system, which consists of a slow dysconjugate eye movement to foveate the near object by contracting both medial rectus muscles. Convergence insufficiency results in inadequate convergence and an inability to focus normally at near.

Convergence retraction nystagmus: One of the core features, along with impaired upgaze, of Parinaud's (dorsal midbrain) syndrome. When the patient attempts to look up, the eyes spasmodically converge and retract backward into the orbits **(Video Link C.5)**. The convergence–retraction movements readily appear during forced upward saccades in response to a down-moving OKN tape. The retraction movement is best seen from the side. See **optokinetic nystagmus**.

Convergence spasm: See **spasm of the near reflex**.

Corectopia iridis: See **eccentric pupil**.

Corkscrew vessels: The dilated, arteriolized, conjunctival, and episcleral blood vessels with a tortuous, corkscrew shape that are characteristic of a carotid cavernous fistula **(Fig. C.17)**. Such fistulas may be traumatic or develop spontaneously because of rupture of an intracavernous carotid aneurysm. Other findings may include cranial nerve palsies, pulsatile **proptosis**, **chemosis**, an ocular **bruit**, and evidence of increased venous pressure in the eye.

Corneal light reflex test (Hirschberg's test): An examination used in the evaluation of **diplopia** and ocular malalignment. The test depends on observing the reflection of an examining light on the cornea and estimating the amount of ocular deviation depending on the amount of displacement of the reflection from the center of the pupil. Each millimeter of light displacement from the center indicates 18° of eye deviation.

Corneal reflex: A reflex elicited by lightly touching the cornea with a wisp of cotton or tissue, used to assess V$_1$ function. The stimulus causes blinking of the ipsilateral (direct reflex) and contralateral (consensual reflex) eyes. The afferent limb of the reflex is mediated by CN V$_1$, the efferent limb by CN VII. With a unilateral trigeminal lesion, both the direct and consensual responses may be absent; neither eye blinks **(Table C.5)**. Stimulation of the opposite eye produces normal direct and consensual responses. With a unilateral CN VII lesion, the direct response may be impaired, but the consensual reflex should be normal. Stimulation of the opposite side produces a normal direct response but an impaired consensual response.

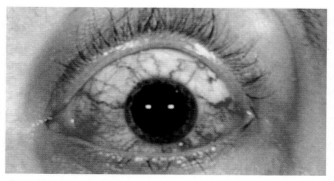

Figure C.17. Corkscrew conjunctival and episcleral vessels in a patient with a carotid-cavernous fistula.

Table C.5. Patterns of Direct and Consensual Corneal Light Reflex Abnormality with Trigeminal and Facial Nerve Lesions

	Direct Corneal Reflex	Consensual Corneal Reflex
Complete trigeminal nerve lesion		
Stimulate involved eye	Absent	Absent
Stimulate opposite eye	Normal	Normal
Complete facial nerve lesions		
Stimulate involved eye	Absent	Normal
Stimulate opposite eye	Normal	Absent

From Campbell WW. *DeJong's the Neurologic Examination*. 7th ed. Philadelphia, PA: Wolters Kluwer Health//Lippincott Williams & Wilkins; 2013, with permission.

Lesions involving the brainstem polysynaptic trigeminofacial connections may produce impairment of both direct and consensual responses. The corneal reflex may be depressed with lesions of the contralateral hemisphere, especially if there is thalamic involvement. Corneal sensation may be impaired in contact lens wearers, even when the lenses are out. See **conjunctival reflex.**

Cornell's sign: See **minor extensor toe signs.**

Corneomandibular (Wartenberg's) reflex: Stimulation of cornea causes contralateral movement of the mandible (Wartenberg's winking jaw phenomenon); indicates supranuclear interruption of the ipsilateral corticotrigeminal tract (**Video Link C.6**). Said to be the only eye sign in ALS.

Cortical blindness: Loss of vision due to bilateral occipital lobe lesions associated with a denial of the disability. Lesions involving the occipital lobes bilaterally that extend to the adjacent parietal and temporal association areas may produce a bilateral hemianopia (biposterior syndrome). These patients may lack awareness of their deficit, or they may have awareness but deny that the deficit exists (Anton's syndrome or denial visual hallucination syndrome, **anosognosia** for blindness). The patient may behave as if he can see—try to walk, bump into objects, and fall over things. There is the belief that the patient **confabulates** or "hallucinates his environment." Cortical blindness may occur after stroke, cardiorespiratory arrest, head trauma, bacterial meningitis, progressive multifocal encephalopathy, and even as a postictal phenomenon.

Cortical deafness: Patients with hearing impairment due to bilateral temporal lobe destruction who are unaware of their deficit in the way in which patients with cortical blindness are unaware of their visual impairment extremely rare.

Cortical dysarthria: See **apraxia of speech.**

Cortical sensory loss: The pattern of sensory loss seen with lesions involving the sensory cortex in the parietal lobe. The deficit primarily involves discriminatory sensation with little if any impairment in the primary sensory modalities, especially with lesions posterior to the primary sensory cortex. There often is severe impairment of position sense resulting in **sensory ataxia** and **pseudoathetosis**, but vibratory sensation is only rarely affected. Other possible findings include **astereognosis**, **agraphesthesia**, impairment of **two-point discrimination**, **autotopagnosia**, **anosognosia**, topagnosia, or Gerstmann's syndrome. Sensory **inattention**, or **extinction**, is often an early and important diagnostic finding in parietal lobe lesions.

Corticospinal tract signs: See **long tract signs.**

Costoclavicular maneuver: See **thoracic outlet syndrome provocative tests.**

Counterpressure sign: See **geste antagoniste.**

Cover tests: Maneuvers used in the evaluation of strabismus, diplopia, and ocular malalignment. The cover tests are predicated on forcing one eye or the other to fixate by occluding its fellow and determining the drift of the nonfixing eye while it is under cover. Varieties of cover testing include the cover–uncover test and the alternate cover test. The cover–uncover test is used primarily by ophthalmologists to evaluate patients with congenital strabismus where there is an obvious squint. When neurological patients have an obvious malalignment, its nature is usually apparent. The alternate cover test is used to evaluate more subtle deviations.

A phoria is a latent deviation held in check by fusion. Breaking fusion by covering one eye causes the covered eye to deviate nasally (esophoria) or temporally (exophoria). If the cover is switched to the other eye (alternate cover), the just uncovered eye is forced to move into position to take up fixation. If an adduction movement occurs, it means the eye had been deviated outward under cover (exophoria). An abduction movement means the eye had been deviated inward (esophoria). Cover test simulators are available on the Internet. For a discussion of strabismus and the cover tests, see **Video Link C.7.** See **strabismus.**

Cozen's sign: See **lateral epicondylitis provocation tests.**

Craniosynostosis: Premature closure of cranial sutures. The primary clinical manifestation of craniosynostosis is an abnormally shaped skull; the configuration depends on which suture(s) have fused prematurely. The skull is unable to expand in a direction perpendicular to the fused suture line. With synostosis of a major suture, the skull compensates by expanding in a direction perpendicular to the uninvolved sutures. Premature closure of the sagittal suture, the most common form of craniosynostosis, produces a skull that is abnormally elongated (scaphocephaly, dolichocephaly). Synostosis of both coronal sutures causes a skull that is abnormally wide (brachycephaly). When the coronal and lambdoid sutures are involved, the skull is tall and narrow (turricephaly, tower skull). Synostosis of the sagittal and both coronal sutures causes oxycephaly (acrocephaly), a pointed, conical skull. Plagiocephaly refers to a flattened spot on one side of the head; it is due to premature unilateral fusion of one coronal or lambdoid suture. Pachycepaly is flattening of the occiput because of closure of the lambdoid sutures. Synostosis involving the metopic suture causes trigonocephaly, a narrow, triangular forehead with lateral constriction of the temples. Synostosis of the posterior sagittal and both lamboidal sutures produces the "Mercedes Benz pattern." Closure of the parieto-temporal sutures causes the cloverleaf skull. Severe craniosynostosis involving multiple sutures may cause increased ICP.

Craniosynostosis usually occurs as an isolated condition, but there are numerous syndromes in which craniosynostosis occurs in conjunction with other anomalies, particularly malformations of the face and the digits, e.g., the Crouzon, Apert, and Carpenter syndromes. Several genetic mutations may cause craniosynostosis. There are many potential causes of nonsyndromic craniosynostosis, including environmental, hormonal, and biomechanical factors.

Cloverleaf skull: See **craniosynostosis.**

Cremasteric reflex: A **superficial reflex** elicited by stroking or lightly scratching or pinching the skin on the upper, inner aspect of the thigh. The response consists of a contraction of the cremasteric muscle with a quick elevation of the homolateral testicle. The innervation is through the ilioinguinal and genitofemoral nerves (L1–L2). The cremasteric reflex must not be confused with the **scrotal reflex**, or dartos reflex, which produces a slow, writhing, vermicular contraction of the scrotal skin on stroking the perineum or thigh or applying a cold object to the scrotum. The cremasteric reflex may be absent in elderly males, in individuals who have a hydrocele or varicocele, in torsion of the testicle, and in those who have had orchitis or epididymitis. The superficial reflexes, especially the abdominal and cremasteric reflexes, have a special significance when their absence is associated with increased DTRs, as this combination suggests the presence of CST dysfunction.

Crocodile tears: A gustatory-lacrimal reflex characterized by tearing when eating, especially highly flavored foods, due to a facial nerve **aberrant regeneration** syndrome in which axons originally innervating the salivary gland are misdirected to the lacrimal gland. **Gustatory sweating** is similar, but with sweating and flushing over the cheek rather than lacrimation.

Crossed adductor reflex: Adduction of the opposite leg when obtaining the **adductor reflex**. A slight crossed adductor response is not necessarily abnormal, but strong crossed adduction, or adduction of the opposite leg when obtaining the knee jerk, suggests CST disease. See **crossed reflexes, inverted reflexes** and **spread of reflexes**.

Crossed aphasia: The presence of aphasia with a right hemisphere lesion in a right-handed patient or a left hemisphere lesion in a left-handed patient, violating the usual rules for hemispheric dominance for language. Such patients apparently have crossed or mixed hemispheric dominance for language.

Crossed body adduction (scarf) test: See **shoulder examination tests.**

Crossed diplopia: A type of **diplopia** based on the location of the true and false images. Diplopia may be divided into crossed (**heteronymous diplopia**) and uncrossed (**homonymous diplopia**). If the false image as determined by red lens or Maddox rod testing is on the same side as the eye that sees it, there is homonymous diplopia; if the image is on the opposite side, there is heteronymous diplopia. If the false image comes from the ipsilateral eye (e.g., red image to the right on right gaze), the diplopia is uncrossed (a line could be drawn directly from the false image to the paretic eye). If the false image comes from the contralateral eye (e.g., white image to the right on right gaze), a line from the false image to the paretic eye would cross a line drawn from the true image to the nonparetic eye and the diplopia is said to be crossed.

Crossed extensor (Phillipson's) reflex: A complex polysynaptic spinal reflex in which a withdrawal reflex of the limb ipsilateral to the stimulus is accompanied by extension of the contralateral limb. The crossed flexor reflex is when the contralateral leg flexes rather than extends. See **pathologic reflexes.**

Crossed reflexes: Reflexes that appear in the homologous limb due to segmental spread at the spinal cord level. This may occur to some degree normally, such as the **crossed adductor reflex**, but when the crossed response is very active, or the reflex is not the same, e.g., eliciting the knee jerk on one side causes adduction on the opposite side, it is usually a sign of CST disease. See **inverted reflexes, spread of reflexes**.

Crossed straight leg raising sign (Fajersztajn's sign): When raising the good leg during the **straight leg raising** test produces pain in the symptomatic leg; if this

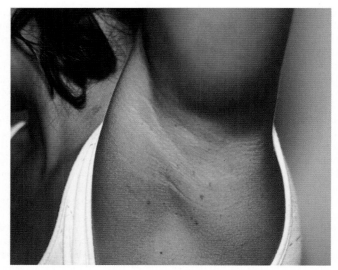

Figure C.18. Neurofibromatosis 1. Crowe's sign (axillary "freckles") is considered pathognomonic for the disease. (From Goodheart HP. *Goodheart's Photoguide of Common Skin Disorders*. 2nd ed. Philadelphia, PA: Wolters Kluwer Health/Lippincott Williams & Wilkins; 2003, with permission.)

sign is present, the likelihood of a root lesion is very high. The test is not sensitive (22% to 43%) but is specific (88% to 98%, LR 3.4).[8]

Crowded optic disc: When the size of the scleral opening in the posterior globe is small, the disc consists entirely of neuroretinal tissue and the optic cup is inconspicuous or nonexistent. Such a small cupless disc is more vulnerable to AION and is termed a crowded disc or "disc at risk."

Crowe's sign: Axillary freckling in NF1 **(Fig. C.18**, Table N-1). Axillary and inguinal freckling is usually noted between 3 and 5 years of age. Freckling can also occur above the eyelids, around the neck, and under the breasts.[1]

Cruciate weakness (paralysis, hemiplegia): A term used in two ways: (1) spastic weakness of one arm and the contralateral leg due to a lesion involving the pyramidal decussation in the lower medulla. At the decussation of the pyramids, the arm fibers lie medial to the leg fibers. Arm fibers decussate first and come to lie in the medial portion of the lateral CST in the upper cervical spinal cord. Leg fibers decussate more caudally and come to lie in the lateral portion of the lateral CST. A strategically placed lesion can involve arm fibers that have already decussated but leg fibers that have not, which causes a crossed pattern of weakness. (2) weakness of both arms, **brachial diplegia**, with relative sparing of the legs, due to a lesion involving the rostral portion of the pyramidal decussation. The findings are similar to those of a central cord syndrome of the cervical spine or the man-in-the-barrel syndrome due to watershed cerebral infarction. Most cases are due to trauma.

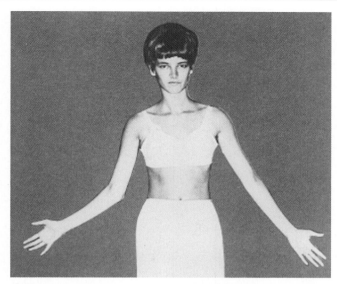

Figure C.19. Residual right cubitus valgus secondary to malunion of a fractured lateral condyle 15 years previously, with the recent development of symptoms and signs of an incomplete tardy ulnar nerve palsy. (From Salter RB. *Textbook of Disorders and Injuries of the Musculoskeletal System.* 3rd ed. Baltimore, MD: Lippincott Williams & Wilkins; 1999, with permission.)

Cubitus valgus: Deviation of the elbow toward the midline and the forearm laterally. The deformity often occurs after an elbow fracture or dislocation and predisposes to ulnar neuropathy at the elbow **(Fig. C.19)**. Rather than following the normal fairly straight or mildly valgus path, the "carrying angle" of the elbow is increased.

Cubitus varus: Deviation of the elbow away from the midline and the forearm medially.

Curtain sign: (1) In MG with bilateral ptosis, usually asymmetric, manually raising the more ptotic lid causes increased ptosis on the opposite side; aka **enhanced ptosis, seesaw ptosis (Fig. C.20)**.[36] This is explained by Hering's law of reciprocal innervation. Both lids receive the same level of innervation. Maximal firing attempting to hold the more ptotic lid open keeps the fellow lid open more, but with manual elevation the level of firing decreases and the previously less ptotic lid suddenly collapses **(Video Link C.8)**. (2) with unilateral pharyngeal weakness, movement of the healthy side across the posterior pharynx toward the weak side on stimulation by the examiner.

Cushing response (triad, reflex): Hypertension, bradycardia, and slow irregular respirations because of increased ICP, a late and ominous development.

Cutaneous reflexes: See **superficial reflexes.**

Cyriax release test: See **thoracic outlet syndrome provocative tests.**

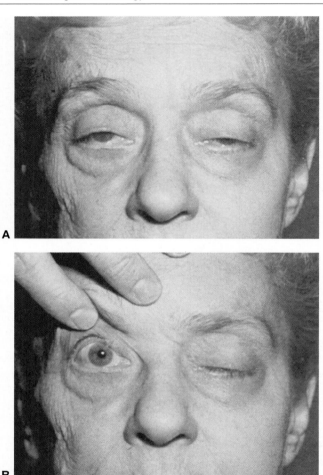

Figure C.20. Enhanced ptosis in a 78-year-old patient with myasthenia gravis. **A:** The patient has bilateral ptosis. **B:** When the right eyelid is elevated, the patient develops increased (enhanced) ptosis on the opposite side. (From Miller NR, Newman NJ, Biousse V, et al, eds. *Walsh and Hoyt's Clinical Neuro-ophthalmology: The Essentials.* 2nd ed. Philadelphia, PA: Wolters Kluwer Health/Lippincott Williams & Wilkins; 2007, with permission.)

Video Links

C.1. CSF rhinorrhea. (From Diekman T, Mees B. Images in clinical medicine. Cerebrospinal fluid leak. *N Engl J Med.* 2009;361(14):e26.) Available at: http://www.nejm.org/doi/full/10.1056/NEJMicm0708178

C.2. Cervical dystonia. (From Francesca Morgante, MD, PhD, Continuum Video Gallery, American Academy of Neurology.) Available at: http://journals.lww.com/continuum/pages/videogallery.aspx?videoId=98&autoPlay=true

C.3. Cheyne-Stokes respirations in a patient with congestive heart failure. Available at: https://www.youtube.com/watch?v=VkuxP7iChYY

C.4. Choreic gait. Note the involuntary, irregular, jerky movements of this woman's body and extremities, especially on the right side. There are also choreiform movements of the face. A lot of her movements have a writhing, snake-like quality, which could be called choreoathetosis. (From Alejandro Stern, Stern Foundation and the University of Utah School of Medicine.) Available at: http://library.med.utah.edu/neurologicexam/html/gait_abnormal.html#13

C.5. Convergence retraction nystagmus and tectal pupils due to a mass in the pretectal region. (From Dr. Jason Barton, Canadian Neuro-Ophthalmology Group.) Available at: http://www.neuroophthalmology.ca/case-of-the-month/eye-movements/diplopia-and-vertical-gaze-problems-in-neurofibromatosis-type-1

C.6. The corneomandibular reflex. (From Heliopoulos I, Vadikolias K, Tsivgoulis G, et al. Corneomandibular reflex (Wartenberg reflex) in coma: a rarely elicited sign. *JAMA Neurol.* 2013;70:794–795.) Available at: https://www.youtube.com/watch?v=iNsx-iLrGG4

C.7. Strabismus and the cover tests. (From Root T, OphthoBook.) Available at: http://www.ophthobook.com/videos/tropias-and-phorias-video

C.8. Video showing enhanced ptosis in a patient with ocular myasthenia gravis. (From Marc Dinkin, MD, Continuum Video Gallery, American Academy of Neurology.) Available at: http://journals.lww.com/continuum/pages/videogallery.aspx?videoId=113&autoPlay=true

References

1. Williams VC, Lucas J, Babcock MA, et al. Neurofibromatosis type 1 revisited. *Pediatrics.* 2009;123:124–133.
2. Reimers CD, Schlotter B, Eicke BM, et al. Calf enlargement in neuromuscular diseases: a quantitative ultrasound study in 350 patients and review of the literature. *J Neurol Sci.* 1996;143:46–56.
3. Coles A, Dick D. Unilateral calf hypertrophy. *J Neurol Neurosurg Psychiatry.* 2004;75:1606.
4. Bland JD. Carpal tunnel syndrome. *BMJ.* 2007;335:343–346.
5. Kaul MP, Pagel KJ, Wheatley MJ, et al. Carpal compression test and pressure provocative test in veterans with median-distribution paresthesias. *Muscle Nerve.* 2001;24:107–111.
6. El MY, Ashour S, Youssef S, et al. Clinical diagnosis of carpal tunnel syndrome: old tests-new concepts. *Joint Bone Spine.* 2008;75:451–457.
7. D'Arcy CA, McGee S. The rational clinical examination. Does this patient have carpal tunnel syndrome? *JAMA.* 2000;283:3110–3117.
8. McGee S. *Evidence Based Physical Diagnosis.* 3rd ed. Philadelphia, PA: Elsevier/Saunders; 2012.
9. Dennis M, Bowen WT, Cho L. *Mechanisms of Clinical Signs.* Sydney, New South Wales, Australia: Churchill Livingstone; 2012.
10. Nord KM, Kapoor P, Fisher J, et al. False positive rate of thoracic outlet syndrome diagnostic maneuvers. *Electromyogr Clin Neurophysiol.* 2008;48:67–74.
11. Amirfeyz R, Gozzard C, Leslie IJ. Hand elevation test for assessment of carpal tunnel syndrome. *J Hand Surg Br.* 2005;30:361–364.
12. Hansen PA, Micklesen P, Robinson LR. Clinical utility of the flick maneuver in diagnosing carpal tunnel syndrome. *Am J Phys Med Rehabil.* 2004;83:363–367.
13. Saddawi-Konefka D, Berg SM, Nejad SH, et al. Catatonia in the ICU: an important and underdiagnosed cause of altered mental status. A case series and review of the literature. *Crit Care Med.* 2014;42:e234–e241.
14. Huh YE, Kim JS. Bedside evaluation of dizzy patients. *J Clin Neurol.* 2013;9:203–213.
15. Nagaratnam N, Singh-Grewal D, Chen E, et al. Cerebral ptosis revisited. *Int J Clin Pract.* 1998;52:79–80.
16. Ziu M, Savage JG, Jimenez DF. Diagnosis and treatment of cerebrospinal fluid rhinorrhea following accidental traumatic anterior skull base fractures. *Neurosurg Focus.* 2012;32:E3.
17. Diekman T, Mees B. Images in clinical medicine. Cerebrospinal fluid leak. *N Engl J Med.* 2009;361:e26.
18. Spurling RG, Segerberg LH. Lateral intervertebral disk lesions in the lower cervical region. *J Am Med Assoc.* 1953;151:354–359.
19. Tong HC, Haig AJ, Yamakawa K. The Spurling test and cervical radiculopathy. *Spine.* 2002;27:156–159.
20. Viikari-Juntura E, Porras M, Laasonen EM. Validity of clinical tests in the diagnosis of root compression in cervical disc disease. *Spine.* 1989;14:253–257.
21. Anekstein Y, Blecher R, Smorgick Y, et al. What is the best way to apply the Spurling test for cervical radiculopathy? *Clin Orthop Relat Res.* 2012;470:2566–2572.

22. De Luigi AJ, Fitzpatrick KF. Physical examination in radiculopathy. *Phys Med Rehabil Clin N Am.* 2011;22:7–40.

23. Johnson I. Bakody sign. *Surg Neurol.* 1977;7:370.

24. Fast A, Parikh S, Marin EL. The shoulder abduction relief sign in cervical radiculopathy. *Arch Phys Med Rehabil.* 1989;70:402–403.

25. Malanga GA, Landes P, Nadler SF. Provocative tests in cervical spine examination: historical basis and scientific analyses. *Pain Physician.* 2003;6:199–205.

26. Tashiro K. Kisaku Yoshimura and the Chaddock reflex. *Arch Neurol.* 1986;43:1179–1180.

27. Chisholm KA, Gilchrist JM. The Charcot joint: a modern neurologic perspective. *J Clin Neuromuscul Dis.* 2011;13:1–13.

28. Sackellares JC, Swift TR. Shoulder enlargement as the presenting sign in syringomyelia. Report of two cases and review of the literature. *JAMA.* 1976;236:2878–2879.

29. Narayan SK, Sivaprasad P, Sahoo RN, et al. Teaching video neuroimage: Chvostek sign with Fahr syndrome in a patient with hypoparathyroidism. *Neurology.* 2008;71:e79.

30. Meneret A, Guey S, Degos B. Chvostek sign, frequently found in healthy subjects, is not a useful clinical sign. *Neurology.* 2013;80:1067.

31. Crum RM, Anthony JC, Bassett SS, et al. Population-based norms for the Mini-Mental State Examination by age and educational level. *JAMA.* 1993;269:2386–2391.

32. Kilada S, Gamaldo A, Grant EA, et al. Brief screening tests for the diagnosis of dementia: comparison with the mini-mental state exam. *Alzheimer Dis Assoc Disord.* 2005;19:8–16.

33. Kapur N. The coin-in-the-hand test: a new "bed-side" test for the detection of malingering in patients with suspected memory disorder. *J Neurol Neurosurg Psychiatry.* 1994;57:385–386.

34. Schroeder RW, Peck CP, Buddin WH Jr., et al. The Coin-in-the-Hand Test and dementia: more evidence for a screening test for neurocognitive symptom exaggeration. *Cogn Behav Neurol.* 2012;25:139–143.

35. Gould R, Miller BL, Goldberg MA, et al. The validity of hysterical signs and symptoms. *J Nerv Ment Dis.* 1986;174:593–597.

36. Gorelick PB, Rosenberg M, Pagano RJ. Enhanced ptosis in myasthenia gravis. *Arch Neurol.* 1981; 38:531.

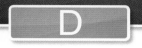
Dalrymple sign: Lid retraction in primary gaze, seen in thyrotoxicosis; may be confused with **Collier's sign**. Due to overactivity of Müeller's muscle related to increased sympathetic tone. See **eyelid retraction**.

Dancing eyes, dancing feet: See **opsoclonus-myoclonus syndrome**.

Dartos reflex: See **scrotal reflex**.

Dazzle reflex: See **menace reflex**.

Decerebrate rigidity and decorticate rigidity: Postures seen in patients with severe CNS damage. In brief, decorticate posturing includes upper extremity adduction and flexion and lower extremity extension (Fig. D.1). In decerebrate posturing, there is extension of both upper and lower extremities (Fig. D.2). Decerebration is traditionally thought to indicate a lesion below the red nucleus, involving the rubrospinal tracts, but above the lateral vestibulospinal tracts. These neuroanatomic correlates do not seem to apply as well in humans as experimental animals. Decerebrate posturing may occur in patients with bilateral cerebral lesions, well above the red nucleus. The distinction is useful prognostically; patients with decorticate posturing in response to pain tend to have a better prognosis than those with decerebrate posturing. With decerebrate rigidity, the arms are internally rotated

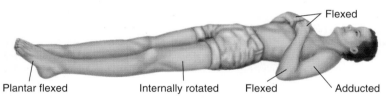

Plantar flexed   Internally rotated   Flexed   Adducted

Figure D.1. In decorticate rigidity, the elbows, wrists, and fingers are flexed with the legs extended and internally rotated. (From Bickley LS, Szilagyi P. *Bates' Guide to Physical Examination and History Taking.* 8th ed. Philadelphia, PA: Wolters Kluwer Health/Lippincott Williams & Wilkins; 2003, with permission.)

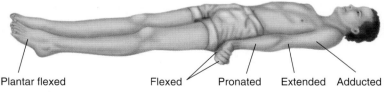

Plantar flexed   Flexed   Pronated   Extended   Adducted

Figure D.2. In decerebrate rigidity, the arms are adducted and extended at the elbows, with the forearms pronated and the wrists and fingers flexed. The legs are extended at the knees and internally rotated with the feet plantar flexed. The posture may occur spontaneously or in response to external stimuli such as light, noise, or pain. (From Bickley LS, Szilagyi P. *Bates' Guide to Physical Examination and History Taking.* 8th ed. Philadelphia, PA: Wolters Kluwer Health/Lippincott Williams & Wilkins 2003, with permission.)

at the shoulders, extended at the elbows, and hyperpronated, with the fingers extended at the metacarpophalangeal joints and flexed at the interphalangeal joints. The legs are extended at the hips, knees, and ankles, and the toes are plantar flexed. Patients with extreme decerebrate rigidity may have opisthotonos, with all four limbs stiffly extended, the head back, and the jaws clenched. When the process extends to involve the medulla, the decerebration disappears. The most common cause of decerebrate rigidity in humans is trauma, and the presence of extensor posturing is a poor prognostic indicator. Decorticate rigidity is characterized by flexion of the elbows and wrists with extension of the legs and feet. The causative lesion is higher than that causing decerebrate rigidity, preserving the function of the rubrospinal tract, which enhances flexor tone in the upper extremities.

Decomposition of movement: The breaking down of a motor act into its component parts so that it is carried out in a jerky, awkward fashion; seen characteristically in cerebellar disease. See **dyssynergia, cerebellar signs.**

Decorticate rigidity: See **decerebrate rigidity** and **decorticate rigidity.**

Deep abdominal reflexes: See **abdominal reflexes.**

Deep tendon reflex (DTR): The reflex caused by sudden stretch of a muscle, usually brought about by percussion of its tendon, occasionally by percussing another structure to which the muscle is attached, such as bone, fascia, or aponeurotic structure, as in the jaw jerk (see Video A.3). Also referred to as the muscle stretch or myotatic reflex. It is fashionable to criticize the term for various reasons, but it is deeply entrenched; Erb introduced it in 1875, and in 1885 Gowers recommended it be discarded.

The DTRs elicited routinely are the biceps, brachioradialis, triceps, knee, and ankle. However, a DTR can be elicited from any muscle with a tendon that can be percussed, directly or indirectly, and other DTRs are occasionally useful (**Table D.1**, see Video A.3).

Defective response inhibition: Impairment of the ability to inhibit a response, described by Luria as a sign of frontal lobe dysfunction. The prefrontal cortex, especially the ventrolateral prefrontal cortex, is important in the control of response inhibition. See **automatic responses, Stroop test, antisaccade task, alternating sequences test, applause sign, echopraxia, imitation** and **utilization behavior, environmental dependency** and **the Go/No-Go test.**

Table D.1. Occasionally Useful DTRs that Are Not Routinely Obtained

Orbicularis oculi
Jaw
Clavicle
Pectoralis
Deltoid
Pronator
Finger flexor
Deep abdominal
Suprapatellar
Hamstring
Adductor
Extensor digitorum brevis
Peroneal (tibialis anterior)
Tibialis posterior
Plantar stretch

Dejerine's sign: Radiating pain on coughing, sneezing, or straining at stool; a significant but seldom elicited sign of radiculopathy. The patient may relate such pain during the history, or radicular pain can sometimes be elicited during the Valsalva test. See **cervical radiculopathy signs, Spurling's sign, straight leg raising test.**

Deltoid reflex: Contraction of the deltoid muscle on tapping over the insertion of the deltoid muscle at the junction of the upper and middle third of the lateral aspect of the humerus, resulting in slight abduction of the upper arm (axillary nerve, C5–C6). Usually difficult to elicit; asymmetry sometimes detectable in patients with C5 radiculopathy (see Video A.3).

Delusion: A strongly held false belief. Delusions are characteristic of psychotic states and other psychiatric disorders, but can occur in neurological illnesses, particularly in dementia.

Denial of disability: See **anosognosia.**

Dermatochalasis: Age-related lax, baggy skin around the eyelids, which can simulate **ptosis**, but levator function is normal. The term *blepharochalasis* is often used synonymously. See **pseudo-Horner's syndrome.**

Dermatomyositis skin changes: The various cutaneous manifestations of DM. The mechanism of these skin changes is unclear, but microvascular injury related to both complement deposition and antibody complex damage is likely involved.[1] Gottron's papules are violaceous, slightly elevated papules and plaques over the

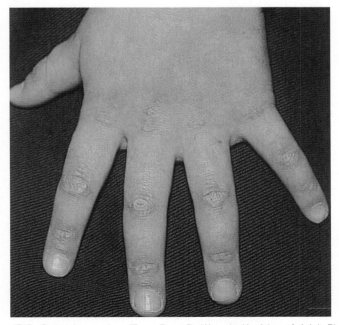

Figure D.3. Gottron's papules. (From Berg D, Worzala K. *Atlas of Adult Physical Diagnosis.* Philadelphia, PA: Wolters Kluwer Health/Lippincott Williams & Wilkins; 2006, with permission.)

extensor surfaces of the DIP, PIP, and MCP joints of the hands (Fig. D.3). Sometimes the lesions are slightly scaly. Similar lesions are often located over the elbows and knees (Gottron's sign). Gottron's papules are said to be pathognomonic for DM, allowing for the diagnosis even in the absence of muscle weakness (dermatomyositis sine myositis, amyopathic dermatomyositis). Patients referred for neuromuscular consultation with the diagnosis of dermatomyositis sine myositis have invariably proven to have muscle weakness on careful examination.

A heliotrope rash is a violaceous to dusky, erythematous, symmetrical, periorbital discoloration with or without edema, also reportedly pathognomic of DM (Fig. D.4). The sign may be subtle, with only slight discoloration along the eyelid margin. A malar rash is a reddish, butterfly-shaped macular rash that spreads over the nose and both cheeks, but spares the nasolabial folds. It is characteristic of DM and SLE. When the typical DM rash is present over the upper back, posterior neck, and shoulders, it is referred to as the "shawl sign," and when in a V-shaped pattern involving the chest and anterior neck in the distribution of the neck of a shirt as the "V sign." Periungual telangiectasias are due to abnormal nail bed capillary loops

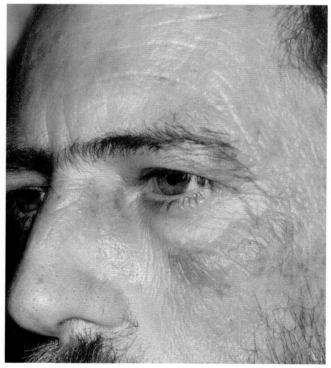

Figure D.4. Heliotrope rash in a patient with dermatomyositis. (From Berg D, Worzala K. *Atlas of Adult Physical Diagnosis.* Philadelphia, PA: Wolters Kluwer Health/Lippincott Williams & Wilkins; 2006, with permission.)

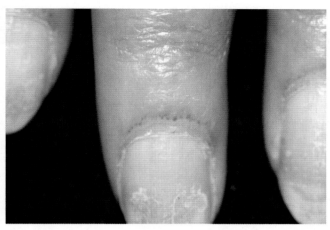

Figure D.5. Periungual telangiectasias due to dilated capillary loops. (From Good-heart HP. *Goodheart's Photoguide of Common Skin Disorders.* 2nd ed. Philadelphia, PA: Lippincott Williams & Wilkins; 2003, with permission.)

(Fig. D.5). These dilated capillaries appear as a fine red line or a punctum with a radiating red line.

Calcinosis (calcinosis cutis) is ectopic calcification in the skin and subcutaneous tissues as a response to inflammation and tissue damage **(Fig. D.6)**. Calcium deposition may occur in a number of conditions and is an occasional complication of DM. As many as 20% of adult DM patients develop calcinosis.[2] Calcinosis is a

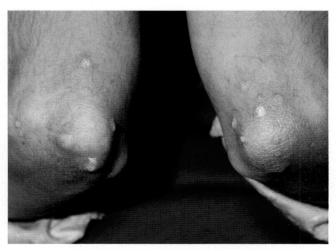

Figure D.6. Calcinosis cutis is seen in both juvenile and adult dermatomyositis. (From Craft N, Fox LP. *VisualDx. Essential Adult Dermatology.* Philadelphia, PA: Wolters Kluwer Health/Lippincott Williams & Wilkins; 2010, with permission.)

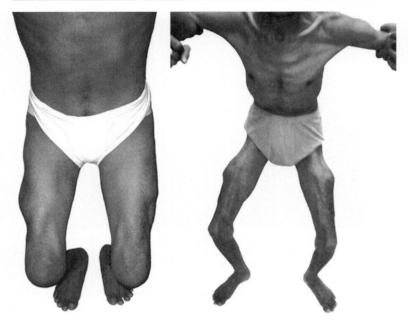

Figure D.7. Diamond on quadriceps sign. (From Pradhan S. Diamond on quadriceps: a frequent sign in dysferlinopathy. *Neurology.* 2008;70:322, with permission.)

major cause of morbidity in juvenile DM. Diagnosis at a young age, disease severity, and the presence of anti-NXP2 autoantibodies substantially increase the risk.[3]

Diamond on quadriceps sign: Asymmetric diamond-shaped bulges seen in the anterolateral thighs of patients with dysferlinopathy (LGMD 2B and Miyoshi myopathy) when standing with the knees slightly bent **(Fig. D.7)**. Proximal and distal atrophy causes the curious island of sparing to stand out. Other unusual muscle shapes have been described as a manifestation of dysferlinopathy, such as selective biceps atrophy causing a "bowl-shaped biceps" **(Fig. D.8)**.

Digit span testing: One of the components of the mental status examination. Forward digit span is a good test of attention, concentration, and immediate memory. Backward digit span is a more complex mental process that involves working memory; it requires the ability to retain and manipulate the string of numbers. Expected performance is 7 ± 2 forward and 5 ± 1 backward. Reverse digit span should not be more than two digits less than the forward span. Forward digit span is also a test of repetition and sometimes impaired in aphasic patients. Supraspan numbers have more than seven digits. Supraspan number recall, like reverse digit span, requires active memory processing.

Digiti quinti sign (fifth-finger sign): With the hands outstretched in drift position, the small finger on the side of a hemiparesis is abducted more than on the normal side **(Fig. D.9)**. One of the **subtle signs of hemiparesis.**

Dilation lag: The tendency of a pupil lacking normal sympathetic innervation to dilate more slowly than normal. The pupil in Horner's syndrome not only dilates less

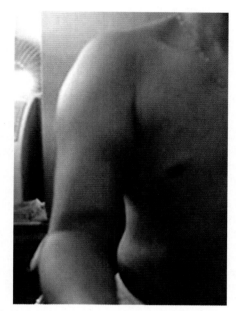

Figure D.8. Bowl-shaped biceps in a patient with a mutation in the dysferlin gene.

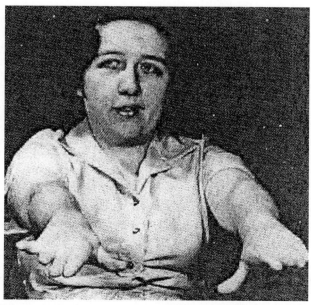

Figure D.9. The digiti quinti sign—slight abduction of the small finger on the side of a mild right hemiparesis. Note the flattened right nasolabial fold and drooping of the corner of the mouth. (From Alter M. The digiti quinti sign of mild hemiparesis. *Neurology.* 1973;23:503–505, with permission.)

fully, but also dilates less rapidly. In the first few seconds after dimming the lights, the slowness of dilation of the affected pupil may accentuate the anisocoria, causing more pupillary asymmetry at 4 to 5 seconds after lights out than at 10 to 12 seconds.[4] Dilation lag is best appreciated photographically or with pupillography, but can be seen with careful bedside observation. Assessing for dilation lag can help in distinguishing Horner's syndrome from physiologic anisocoria.

Dimple sign: A small indentation or concavity that marks the site of pressure that has led to a compression neuropathy. The dimple arises because of habitual leg crossing in peroneal neuropathy or elbowing in ulnar neuropathy.[5,6] Focal discoloration or callus formation carries the same significance.

Diplegia: A term referring to weakness of like parts on the two sides of the body. **Facial diplegia** is weakness of both sides of the face, and **brachial diplegia** is weakness of both arms. **Spastic diplegia** refers to the weakness of both legs that occurs in cerebral palsy (Little's disease).

Diplopia: The perception of two visual images from a single stimulus because of discordant retinal images—one real, one not. Diplopia may be binocular or monocular. Monocular diplopia is often considered a nonorganic symptom, but there are many organic causes, primarily ophthalmologic conditions such as **cataract**, corneal astigmatism, **lens dislocation**, retinal detachment, and macular disease. Binocular horizontal diplopia usually results from dysfunction of the medial or lateral rectus muscles. Vertical diplopia tends to result from disorders of the oblique muscles, less often of the vertically acting recti, or from **skew deviation**. Diplopia is worse with gaze in the direction of the involved muscle.

There are many etiologies. The diplopia of MG varies greatly with time of day and fatigue. Progressive diplopia raises the possibility of a compressive lesion involving a cranial nerve. Patients with a history of congenital strabismus may develop diplopia later in life because of decompensation of the squint, causing failure of fusion. Ocular neuromyotonia causes brief, spasmodic contraction of any extraocular muscle due to abnormal, spontaneous discharges arising in an ocular motor nerve.

There are subjective and objective tests for diplopia and ocular malalignment. The subjective tests depend on the patient's observation of images, the objective tests on the examiner's observation of the corneal light reflections, eye movements during certain maneuvers such as the **cover tests** (see **strabismus**) and the **Bielschowsky head tilt test**.

Diplopia may be divided into **crossed diplopia** and uncrossed diplopia types, depending on the relationship of the false image to the eye that perceives it. If the false image is on the same side as the eye that sees it, there is homonymous (uncrossed) diplopia; if the image is on the opposite side, there is heteronymous (crossed) diplopia. For the patient with maximal separation of images on right horizontal gaze, uncrossed diplopia would imply right lateral weakness and crossed diplopia left medial rectus weakness. Any process that prevents relaxation of the antagonist, such as fibrosis, contracture, infiltrations, entrapment, or co-contraction can simulate weakness of any particular extraocular muscle.

Diplopia rules: Maxims used to identify the false image and deduce the weak muscle in the patient with diplopia. There are three rules to identify the false object: (1) the separation of images is greatest in the direction of action of the weak muscle, (2) the false image is the more peripheral, and (3) the false image comes from the

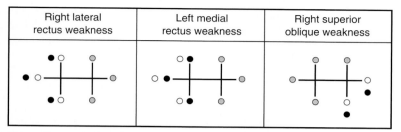

Right lateral rectus weakness	Left medial rectus weakness	Right superior oblique weakness

Figure D.10. Red lens diplopia fields, drawn as seen by the examiner. The red lens is placed over the right eye, and the eyes moved through the six cardinal positions of gaze with the patient looking at an examining light. White circles depict images coming from the left eye (white light), dark circles images from the right eye (red light), and intermediate circles images from both eyes (pink light). (From Campbell WW. *DeJong's the Neurologic Examination.* 7th ed. Philadelphia, PA: Wolters Kluwer Health/Lippincott Williams & Wilkins; 2013, with permission.)

paretic eye. The false image may be identified in different ways. The simplest is to move the patient's eyes into the position with the greatest separation of images, then cover one eye. If the more peripheral image disappears, the covered eye is the paretic eye. The red lens test and Maddox rod test are attempts to be more precise that are especially useful when the diplopia is mild and the weak muscle or muscles not apparent from examination of ocular versions (**Fig. D.10**).

Direction of scratch test: A test of posterior column function (see **posterior column signs**). The patient's ability to detect the direction of a 2-cm vertical scratch over the lower limbs has been described as a sensitive sign of posterior column function, possibly abnormal when more traditional tests, such as position and vibration sensation, are not impaired.[7] The posterior columns carry fibers mediating fine discriminatory and localized tactile sensibility.

Disc edema: See **papilledema.**

Disinhibition: Essentially a lack of impulse control. Disinhibition, ranging from mildly inappropriate social behavior to full-blown mania, may occur with dysfunction of the orbitofrontal cortex, particularly of the right hemisphere. Disinhibition is one of the cardinal manifestations of the behavioral variant of FTD. Common manifestations of a lack of normal impulse control include a lack of judgment and social tact, improper sexual remarks and gestures, and other antisocial acts. Patients often display inappropriate jocularity (see **witzelsucht, moria**) or have angry outbursts. The most common cause of disinhibition by far is of course alcohol ingestion.

Dissociated nystagmus: Nystagmus that is different in the two eyes, e.g., greater in the abducting eye in internuclear ophthalmoplegia (**Video D.1**).

Dissociated sensory loss: A pattern of sensory loss that involves different modalities to different degrees, either in the same or in different body regions. When the sensory pathways run in divergent locations, such as in the spinal cord and brainstem, a disease process may affect one type of sensation and not another. A common example is lateral medullary stroke, which causes a very characteristic pattern of sensory loss that only involves pain and temperature and completely spares light touch. The pain and temperature loss involves the ipsilateral face because of involvement of the spinal tract of cranial nerve V, and the contralateral body because of damage to the lateral spinothalamic tract, sparing the light touch pathways that are running in the midline in the medial lemniscus. A classic but not common cause of dissociated sensory loss is syringomyelia. The pain and temperature sensory fibers crossing in the anterior commissure are affected; light touch sensory fibers running in the posterior columns are well removed from the site of the pathology and remain intact. As a result, syringomyelia characteristically causes isolated, segmental sensory loss to pain and temperature at the involved level with preservation of other sensory functions. In anterior spinal artery infarction, the lesion involves the anterior two-thirds of the cord, sparing the posterior columns, causing dense sensory loss to pain and temperature but normal touch, pressure, position, and vibration. Patients with Brown-Séquard syndrome have extreme dissociation of modalities, with loss of pain and temperature on one side of the body and loss of touch, pressure, position, and vibration on the other side of the body. Dissociated sensory loss may also occur with thalamic lesions (see **thalamic sensory loss**).

Dissociation of reflexes: A difference in the activity level of the **deep tendon reflexes** and the **superficial reflexes**. In addition to causing hyperreflexia, spasticity and the emergence of **pathologic reflexes** CST lesions also often cause a decrease or absence of the superficial reflexes. The increase in DTRs and decrease in superficial reflexes is referred to as reflex dissociation.

Dissociation of the abdominal reflexes: Absent **superficial abdominal reflexes** and exaggerated **deep abdominal reflexes**, suggestive of a CST lesion (see Video A.1).

Disuse atrophy: The type of muscle atrophy that follows prolonged immobilization of a part of the body. Disuse atrophy may occur in an extremity that has been in a splint or cast, one that cannot be moved normally because of joint disease, such as arthritis, one that is paretic following a cerebral lesion, or after prolonged bed rest. It may occur rapidly and can sometimes simulate neurogenic atrophy. The quadriceps femoris is particularly susceptible to disuse atrophy due to bed rest or because of pain in the knee or hip. The degree of muscle wasting is greater than the degree of weakness, which is typically minimal or absent, and the atrophy recovers quickly with resumption of use.

Dix-Hallpike (Nylen-Bárány) maneuver: A maneuver to elicit positional (or positioning) nystagmus in the evaluation of vertigo (Video Link D.1). To perform the Dix-Hallpike maneuver, the patient is moved from a seated position to a supine position with the head extended 45° and turned 45° to one side so that one ear is dependent. The patient is returned to sitting and the maneuver repeated in the opposite direction. The patient should become symptomatic when the affected ear is dependent.

If vertigo or nystagmus occurs, the patient is held in the provoking position until the symptoms subside, and then the movement is repeated to assess its recurrence. In BPPV, nystagmus begins after a latency of about 3 to 10 seconds, occasionally as long as 40 seconds; persists for 20 to 30 seconds, rarely as long as a minute; and then gradually abates (fatigues or habituates) after about 30 seconds, even though the head remains in the provoking position. The nystagmus is commonly torsional with the fast component toward the dependent ear (geotropic).

With BPPV involving canals other than the posterior, the Dix-Hallpike maneuver may be negative. The roll test, rolling the head of the supine patient to one side, may provoke a response with horizontal canal BPPV. In cupulolithiasis, latency and fatigability are absent because the adherent otoconia are in constant contact with the cupula.

The response is transient, and repeating the Dix-Hallpike maneuver several times consecutively provokes less of a response each time until eventually the nystagmus and vertigo are nil, due to **adaptability**. The terms *adaptability, fatigability*, and *habituation* are used inconsistently in regard to failure of the nystagmus to persist when induced and the decrease in the response on repetition. After a period of 10 to 15 minutes, the maneuver again elicits the response.

This type of positional nystagmus is most often due to peripheral vestibular disease. Although rare, positional vertigo can occur with a central lesion, especially one near the fourth ventricle, but the characteristics of the nystagmus are different. With a central lesion, there is typically no latency, and the nystagmus begins as soon as the head is placed in the provoking position. Central positional nystagmus is typically vertical (either up- or downbeating), without the rotatory component seen with peripheral lesions. When torsional nystagmus is present, it may beat away from the ground (**ageotropic nystagmus**). In addition, the nystagmus and associated symptoms may persist for a prolonged period, longer than 30 to 40 seconds, sometimes continuing as long as the head position is maintained. Another characteristic of central lesions is a mismatch in the severity of the nystagmus, vertigo, and nausea, in contrast to peripheral lesions where nystagmus, vertigo, and nausea are generally of comparable intensity.

The characteristics of peripheral versus central positional nystagmus and related findings are summarized in **Table D.2.**

Dolichocephaly: See **craniosynostosis.**

Doll's eye phenomenon (maneuver, test): See **oculocephalic response.**

Dorsal foot response (Mendel-Bechterew reflex): Tapping or stroking over the outer aspect of the dorsum of the foot in the region of the cuboid bone, or over the fourth and fifth metatarsals causes quick plantar flexion of toes, especially the smaller ones (the same response as in **Rossolimo's sign**) in patients with CST disease; in normals there is no movement or slight dorsiflexion of toes. See **pathologic reflexes.**

Double athetosis: See **athetosis.**

Double elevator palsy (monocular elevation deficiency, monocular elevation palsy): A condition in which both muscles that raise one eye, the superior rectus and inferior oblique, are weak, causing a reduced ability to elevate the eye. There is hypotropia in primary gaze, as well as reduced elevation of the involved eye in all positions of gaze. It may result from supranuclear, nuclear, or infranuclear lesions or from mechanical or restrictive conditions in the orbit, particularly involving the inferior rectus, e.g., blowout fracture, thyroid orbitopathy.

Double straight leg raising test: See **O'Connell's test.**

Double ring sign: A common optic disc anomaly, evidence of optic nerve hypoplasia. The disc appears abnormally small with a peripapillary halo, bordered by a ring of increased or decreased pigmentation, creating a "double ring," that facilitates recognition of the anomaly. It is often associated with tortuosity of the retinal veins.

Downbeat nystagmus: A form of **nystagmus** in which the fast component beats down, likely due to dysfunction of the vertical neural integrator or imbalance in

Table D.2. The Characteristics of Central versus Peripheral Positional Nystagmus on Dix-Hallpike Maneuver

Finding	Peripheral	Central
Latency	Yes, typically 3–10 s, rarely as long as 40 s	No
Fatigability* (habituation)	Yes, individual episode typically lasts 10–30 s, rarely as long as 1 min	No
Adaptability* (fatigability)	Yes, maneuver done several times consecutively provokes less of a response each time	No
Nystagmus direction	Direction fixed, typically mixed rotational upbeating with small horizontal component; quick phase of intorsion movement toward the dependent ear, upbeat toward forehead	Direction changing, variable, often purely vertical (either upbeating or downbeating) or purely horizontal
Suppression of nystagmus by visual fixation	Yes	No
Severity	Severe, marked vertigo, intense nystagmus, nausea	Mild vertigo, less obvious nystagmus, inconspicuous nausea
Consistency (reproducibility)	Less consistent	More consistent
Past pointing	In direction of nystagmus slow phase	May be in direction of fast phase

*Adaptability and fatigability are not used consistently in literature.
From Campbell WW. *DeJong's the Neurologic Examination*. 7th ed. Philadelphia, PA: Wolters Kluwer Health/Lippincott Williams & Wilkins; 2013, with permission.

the tone of the central connections of the vertical semicircular canals and otoliths **(Video Link D.2)**. The most common causes are cerebellar infarction, cerebellar and spinocerebellar degeneration syndromes, MS, and developmental anomalies affecting the pons and cerebellum.[8] Downbeat nystagmus in primary gaze is a common manifestation of the Chiari malformation or other structural lesions at the craniocervical junction and in the region of the foramen magnum, when the nystagmus is often greatest in eccentric downgaze.

Downgaze palsy: Difficulty looking down with preservation of other eye movements. Isolated downgaze palsy is rare, but it can occur with critically located lesions in the rostral midbrain tegmentum involving the rostral interstitial nucleus of the MLF bilaterally, or its projections. Difficulty with downgaze is a common early manifestation of PSP. See **combined vertical gaze palsy**.

Dressing apraxia: An inability to don clothing correctly. Dressing requires bimanual cooperation to solve a complex spatial problem. Patients with dressing **apraxia** lose the ability to manipulate their clothing in space and to understand its three-dimensional relationships **(Video Link D.3)**.[9] A useful test is to turn one sleeve of a garment inside out, then ask the patient to put it on; patients with dressing apraxia are often baffled. Dressing apraxia usually occurs with parietal lobe lesions, occasionally frontal lesions, that interfere with the patient's ability to comprehend spatial relationships, frequently in conjunction with **constructional apraxia**. See **buccofacial apraxia, ideomotor apraxia, ideational apraxia.**

Drift: The tendency of a limb to migrate when held horizontally in front with eyes closed. The most commonly seen form is **pronator drift**, but there is also **parietal drift, cerebellar drift,** and **leg drift**.

Dromedary gait: See **gait disorders.**

Drop (dropped) arm sign: See **shoulder examination tests.**

Drop finger: See **finger drop.**

Drop wrist: See **wrist drop.**

Dropped head (head drop, head ptosis, floppy head): A chin-on-chest clinical predicament usually due to severe weakness of the neck extensors leading to an inability to hold the head up (Fig. D.11). The most common causes are inflammatory myopathy, ALS, and MG. In these conditions, posterior paraspinal muscle weakness can occur early and selectively, and head drop may be the presenting manifestation of the disease. It is common in the later stages of FSH dystrophy and some forms of SMA. Some cases are due to a relatively benign isolated neck extensor myopathy, an idiopathic restricted noninflammatory myopathy. The "**bent spine syndrome**," related to thoracic paraspinal weakness, may cause a similar head posture. Patients will sometimes hold the head in their hands (**Rust's sign**) or prop the chin on one fist.

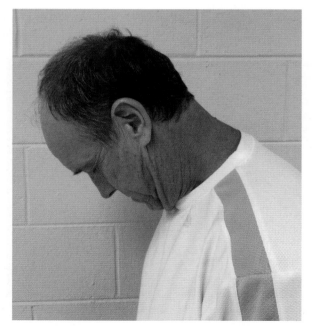

Figure D.11. Dropped head syndrome due to neck extensor weakness.

Rare causes include adult onset acid maltase deficiency, CIDP, desmin myopathy, nemaline myopathy, mitochondrial myopathy, hypothyroid myopathy, hyperparathyroidism, LEMS, and myotonic dystrophy. Dropped head syndrome from neck extensor weakness may be confused with **anterocollis** due to **cervical dystonia** and a neck-flexed posture is also common in PD, but neck extension strength in these conditions is unimpaired. Dropped head syndrome has also been reported in syringomyelia.

Drusen: Acellular, calcified hyaline deposits, also referred to as hyaloid bodies, within the optic nerve that occur in about 2% of the population, bilaterally in 70% of cases, almost exclusively in Caucasians. On the disc surface, drusen have a highly refractile, rock-candy appearance, but when buried beneath the surface, they may produce only disc elevation and blurred margins, causing confusion with papilledema, a condition referred to as **pseudopapilledema** (Fig. D.12). Rarely, drusen may cause scotomas, contraction of the VFs, or sector defects.

Duane's syndrome: A congenital ocular motility disorder caused by aplasia or hypoplasia of the sixth nerve nucleus accompanied by anomalous innervation of the lateral rectus by CN III.

There are three recognized subtypes of Duane's syndrome; type I accounts for about 80% of cases. The core feature of type I Duane's syndrome is a limitation of abduction with otherwise normal eye movements. The patient is unable to abduct the eye, and adduction induces co-contraction of the lateral rectus, causing retraction of the globe into the orbit. Dynamic enophthalmos caused by co-contraction makes the palpebral fissure narrow on adduction (**pseudoptosis**) and widen on abduction (Video Link D.4).

Ductions: Movements of one eye with the other eye covered. Eye movements are divided into ductions (movements of one eye), versions (binocular

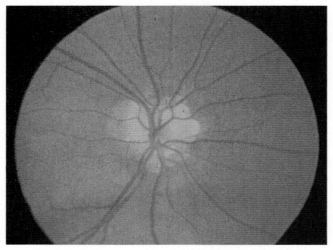

Figure D.12. Drusen of the optic nerve head simulating papilledema. (From Campbell WW. *DeJong's the Neurologic Examination.* 7th ed. Philadelphia, PA: Wolters Kluwer Health/Lippincott Williams & Wilkins; 2013, with permission.)

conjugate movements), and vergences (binocular dysconjugate movements). Vertical movements are sometimes divided into supra-ductions/versions and infra-ductions/versions. The eye may be abducted away from or adducted toward the nose. The terms in-/ex-cycloduction have been largely replaced by intorsion and extorsion to refer to rotational movements.

Forced ductions involve pushing or pulling on an anesthetized globe in order to passively move it through an impaired range. An eye affected by ocular muscle weakness, MG, or an ocular motor nerve palsy moves freely and easily through a full range. An eye affected by restrictive myopathy or an entrapped muscle cannot be moved passively any better than actively.

Dynamic visual acuity: A test of the integrity of the vestibulocular reflex (VOR). When the VOR is functioning normally, the patient can maintain ocular fixation during head rotation and read even while shaking the head. The dynamic visual acuity test is performed by obtaining a baseline acuity and then determining the acuity while shaking the head back and forth. Degradation by more than three lines on the Snellen chart suggests an impaired VOR. A symptomatic corollary of a defective VOR is oscillopsia, a visual illusion of environmental motion causing jiggling while walking or in a car and difficulty reading signs while in motion.

Dysarthria: Defective articulation of sounds or words of neurologic origin.[10] In neurologic patients, the speech abnormalities most often encountered are dysarthria and aphasia. The essential difference is that aphasia is a disorder of language and dysarthria is a disorder of the motor production or articulation of speech. In dysarthria, language functions are normal and the patient speaks with proper syntax, but pronunciation is faulty because of a breakdown in performing the coordinated muscular movements necessary for speech production. A good general rule is that no matter how garbled the speech, if the patient is speaking in correct sentences—using grammar and vocabulary commensurate with his dialect and education—he has dysarthria and not aphasia. Any number of central or peripheral disturbances of the innervation of the articulatory muscles may cause dysarthria. Lesions may involve the peripheral nerves, brainstem nuclei, or the central corticobulbar, extrapyramidal, or cerebellar pathways. A commonly used classification separates dysarthria into flaccid, spastic, ataxic, hypokinetic, hyperkinetic, and mixed types. The two most common types are flaccid and spastic. The different types cause variation in the rate, rhythm, and volume of the patient's speech.

Flaccid dysarthria results from weakness of the soft palate, larynx, and tongue due to such conditions as ALS or MG. Early, the most pronounced difficulty is with pronunciation of linguals and velars; later, the labials are affected. The speech pattern is breathy and nasal **(Video Link D.5)**. The speech is "thick," as though the mouth were filled with soft food. In advanced cases, speech is reduced to unintelligible laryngeal noises. Dysphagia is typically present as well. In MG, the dysarthria becomes more severe with prolonged talking, such as counting, and may reach the point of anarthria. Thomas Willis, who provided one of the first descriptions of MG in 1672, wrote of a woman who, when she tried to talk for a prolonged period, "temporarily lost her power of speech and became mute as a fish." An occasional myasthenic patient must hold his jaw closed with his hand in order to enunciate.

Spastic dysarthria often results from bilateral supranuclear lesions, rendering the muscles that govern articulation both weak and spastic. Phonation is typically strained-strangled, and articulation is slow (see Video Link D.5). The tongue is protruded and moved from side to side with difficulty. There may also be spasticity of the muscles of mastication; mouth opening is restricted and speech seems to come from the back of the mouth. The jaw jerk, gag reflex, and facial reflexes often become exaggerated. ALS may cause dysarthria with both spastic and flaccid features.

Ataxic dysarthria causes a lack of smooth coordination of the tongue, lips, pharynx, and diaphragm (see Video C.3). Ataxic speech is slow, slurred, irregular, labored, and jerky. Words are pronounced with irregular force and speed, with involuntary variations in loudness and pitch lending an explosive quality. There are unintentional pauses, which cause words and syllables to be erratically broken. Excessive separation of syllables and skipped sounds in words produce a disconnected, disjointed, faltering, staccato articulation (**scanning speech**). The speech pattern is reminiscent of a person who is sobbing or breathing hard from exertion. The unusual spacing of sounds with perceptible pauses between words and irregular accenting of syllables may cause a jerky, singsong cadence that resembles the reading of poetry. Ataxic speech is particularly characteristic of multiple sclerosis. It may be accompanied by grimaces and irregular respirations. Ataxia of the voice and scanning speech may be more apparent when the patient repeats a fairly long sentence. In a series of 444 patients with unilateral cerebellar lesions, mostly tumors, dysarthria was present in 10% to 25% and appeared with left hemisphere lesions more often than right.[11]

Dyscalculia: See **acalculia.**

Dyschromatopsia: See **achromatopsia.**

Dysdiadochokinesia: Inability to make rapid repetitive or rapid alternating movements (RAMs). The patient with impaired RAMs has difficulty with such tests as patting the palm of one hand alternately with the palm and dorsum of the other hand, tapping the index finger on the thumb crease, patting alternately with the palm and dorsum of the hand on the thigh, rapid tapping of the fingers, tapping out a complex rhythm, tapping the foot in steady beat, or rapid pronation–supination movements such as imitating screwing in a light bulb or turning a doorknob. Because of the inability to rapidly reverse an action, it is often accompanied by impairment of the **checking reflex** and loss of the **rebound phenomenon.** Dysdiadochokinsia, also called dysrhythmokinseis, is characteristic of cerebellar disease, when it is usually accompanied by **ataxia, dysmetria, dyssynergy,** and **hypotonia,** but loss of such skilled, fractionated distal extremity movements may also occur with CST disease. In an analysis of 444 patients with unilateral cerebellar lesions, mostly tumors, dysdiadochokinesia was present in 47% to 69%.[11]

Dysesthesia: An abnormal, unpleasant, or painful sensation that may occur spontaneously or after a stimulus. Dysesthesias often occur along with paresthesias, which are abnormal but not painful sensations. Dysesthesias occur most often in peripheral nerve disease but may develop in other conditions as well.

Dysgeusia: An aberration, perversion, or distortion of taste. Dysgeusia has many possible etiologies, including drugs, especially chemotherapy, zinc deficiency, xerostomia, as well as facial and glossopharyngeal nerve injuries.

Dysgraphia: See **agraphia.**

Dyskinesia: A type of **abnormal involuntary movement**. The term is often used to encompass complex involuntary movements that do not neatly fit into another category, such as chorea, tremor, or dystonia.[12] Dyskinesia is used most often to refer to abnormal involuntary movements related to drugs and are a common dose-related complication of the treatment of PD with levodopa and dopamine agonists **(Video D.2)**. In some disorders, the dyskinesias occur paroxysmally. Paroxysmal dyskinesias strike suddenly and unexpectedly when the patient is engaged in otherwise normal motor behavior. The dyskinesias may be precipitated by movement (paroxysmal kinesigenic dyskinesia) or by other factors, such as stress, heat, or fatigue (paroxysmal nonkinesigenic dyskinesia). Paroxysmal hypnogenic dyskinesias occur during sleep. See **orofacial dyskinesias** and **tardive dyskinesias**.

Dyskinetic gait: A gait accompanied by a great deal of adventitial, dyskinetic movement and not otherwise fitting into another category of gait disturbance. See **choreic gait**.

Dyslexia: Difficulty reading; see **alexia**. Reading difficulty due to acquired alexia is unrelated to the developmental dyslexia seen most often in school-age boys that may cause severe reading disability.

Dysmetria: One of the components of **cerebellar ataxia** and a characteristic finding in disease of the cerebellum, along with **dyssynergia**, lack of agonist–antagonist coordination, **decomposition of movement, dysdiadochokinesia,** and **tremor** (see **cerebellar signs**). Dysmetria refers to errors in judging distance and gauging the distance, speed, power, and direction of movement. The movement may be carried out too slowly or too rapidly with too much or too little force and the patient may misjudge too long or too short. Hypermetria is more common. Kinesiologic studies show an initial burst of motor activity, which the patient then cannot control and regulate in the normal fashion, explaining the tendency to hypermetria.[13] Disturbances of the timing and intensity of the antagonist activity necessary to brake the movement have also been documented.[14] Studies of multijoint movements show abnormalities in relative timing of motor activity at the different joints, causing incoordination between the shoulder and elbow, or between the knee and ankle. On the **finger-to-nose test**, the patient may stop before reaching the nose, pause, and then complete the act slowly and unsteadily, or overshoot the mark and bring the finger to the nose with too much speed and force. In an analysis of 444 patients with unilateral cerebellar lesions, mostly tumors, dysmetria was present in 71% to 86%.[11] Dysmetria may also involve eye movements, see **ocular dysmetria**.

Dysphasia: A term used in several ways. Some clinicians, particularly in Europe, use it more or less synonymously with aphasia, others use it to refer to mild aphasia. More often in the United States, the term development dysphasia is used in the context of delayed acquisition of language skills in children.

Dysphonia: A change in the volume, quality, or pitch of the voice. Aphonia is complete voice loss. Dysphonia is usually due to a disorder of the larynx; laryngitis is a common example. Vocal cord dysfunction from a polyp or an interference with normal innervation may also cause dysphonia. **Spasmodic dysphonia** is a focal dystonia that produces a striking abnormality of voice production. Recurrent laryngeal nerve weakness causes a flaccid dysphonia with breathiness and mild inspiratory stridor. Dysphonia with a normal cough suggests laryngeal disease or a nonorganic speech disturbance. The most common nonorganic voice disorders are dysphonia and aphonia.[15] Two common functional dysphonias seen in children and adolescents are the whispering syndrome, seen primarily in girls, and mutational falsetto (high-pitched voice), seen primarily in boys.

Dyspnea: See **respiratory failure, signs of.**

Dysprosody: See **aprosodia.**

Dyssynergia: One of the components of **cerebellar ataxia** and a characteristic finding in disease of the cerebellum, along with **dysmetria,** lack of agonist–antagonist coordination, **decomposition of movement, dysdiadochokinesia,** and **tremor.** Cerebellar disease disturbs the normal harmonious, coordinated action between the various muscles involved in a movement so that they contract with the proper force, timing, and sequence of activation to insure smooth, properly coordinated movement. Lack of integration of the components of the act results in **decomposition of movement**—the act is broken down into its component parts and carried out in a jerky, erratic, awkward, disorganized manner. Detrusor-sphincter dyssynergia refers to a specific example of the loss of the harmonious, coordinated action between two muscles that interferes with bladder function.

Dystonia: A term used to describe transient or sustained hypertonia that does not fit into one of the other categories of increased muscle tone, such as **rigidity, spasticity,** or **Gegenhalten.**[16] Dystonia causes spontaneous, involuntary, sustained or intermittent, frequently repetitive muscle contractions that force the affected parts of the body into abnormal movements or postures or both. Dystonia may affect the extremities, neck, trunk, eyelids, face, or vocal cords and may be either constant or intermittent, and generalized, segmental, focal, multifocal, or in a hemidistribution. Dystonic movements are patterned and twisting, tending to recur in the same location, in contrast to the random and fleeting nature of chorea. The speed of dystonia varies widely, from slow, sustained, and cramp-like (athetotic dystonia) to quick and flicking (myoclonic dystonia). When the duration is very brief (less than 1 second), the movement may be referred to as a dystonic spasm; when more sustained (several seconds), as a dystonic movement; and when prolonged (minutes to hours), as a dystonic posture. Occasionally, dystonia is associated with rapid, rhythmic, tremulous movements between the dystonic movements (dystonic tremor). Action dystonia occurs when carrying out a voluntary movement. As in athetosis, **overflow** may occur, with the dystonia brought out by use of another part of the body (see Video Link C.2).

Dystonia has been classified in various ways. Current thinking emphasizes the clinical characteristics, such as age at onset and distribution, and etiology, including nervous system pathology and inheritance.[16]

Generalized dystonia involves large portions of the body, often producing distorted postures of the limbs and trunk. The movements are slow, bizarre, and sometimes grotesque, with an undulating, writhing, twisting, turning character, and a tendency for sustained contraction at the peak of the movement (torsion dystonia, torsion spasm). There is peculiar, axial twisting of the spine, causing marked torsion of the entire vertebral column with lordosis, scoliosis, and tilting of the shoulders and pelvis. Dystonia musculorum deformans is a rare progressive disease causing generalized dystonia that usually begins in childhood; numerous other genetic forms of dystonia exist. Dystonia also occurs in Wilson's disease, in HD as it progresses, in PD, occasionally with structural lesions affecting the basal ganglia, in NMS, and as a drug side effect.

Hemidystonia is along the spectrum of hemichorea and hemiballismus, but due to a lesion of the contralateral striatum. The focal dystonias are disorders causing involuntary contractions in a limited distribution. Common forms include cervical dystonia, oromandibular dystonia, writer's cramp, blepharospasm, and spasmodic dysphonia (see Video Link C.2). A segmental dystonia is more extensive than a focal dystonia and involves contiguous body regions, such as cervical dystonia accompanied by oromandibular dystonia.

Dystonia may also be classified into primary (idiopathic) and secondary forms. The secondary dystonias may result from structural CNS disease, especially involving the striatum, or from drugs or toxins. Dystonia sometimes occurs as a feature of some other neurologic disorder, such as HD, PKAN, X-linked dystonia-parkinsonism (Lubag), or Wilson's disease.

Dystonia is commonly confused with a functional disorder. It is made worse by stress and anxiety. The sensory tricks (geste antagoniste) employed may seem bizarre. Dystonia may only occur with certain acts, such as writing, but not with other acts involving the same muscles. Dystonia of the lower extremities may occur only on walking forward and not on walking backward or running, signs usually associated with a functional gait disorder. The formal neurologic examination with many forms of dystonia is normal. Dystonia may occur as a complication of peripheral nerve injury and in association with a complex regional pain syndrome. All these features can make distinguishing dystonia from nonorganic disease challenging.

Dystonic foot: A foot posture characterized by tonic extension of the great toe with flexion of the other toes, arching of the foot, and inversion of the ankle that may be present at rest or brought on or made worse with ambulation; it is seen primarily

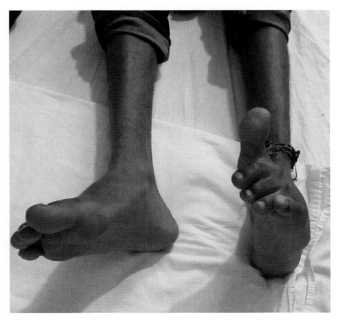

Figure D.13. Dystonic foot, or striatal toe, due to an infarction of the putamen. (From Kumar S, Reddy CR, Prabhakar S. Striatal toe. *Ann Indian Acad Neurol.* 2013;16:304–305, with permission.)

in PD (**Fig. D.13**, see Video Link C.2).[17] In some cases, the great toe is involved primarily and the condition referred to as a **dystonic toe** or **striatal toe**.

Dystonic posture: See **dystonia**.

Dystonic spasm: See **dystonia**.

Dystonic toe: See **dystonic foot**.

Dystonic tremor: See **dystonia**.

Video Links

D.1. A demonstration and discussion of the Dix-Hallpike maneuver. (From the David E. Newman-Toker Collection of the Neuro-Ophthalmology Virtual Education Library (NOVEL), University of Utah.) Available at: http://content.lib.utah.edu/cdm/singleitem/collection/ehsl-dent/id/3

D.2. Downbeat nystagmus caused by lithium toxicity. Note the nystagmus is more prominent with downward and lateral gaze. (From Matthew J. Thurtell, MBBS, FRACP, Continuum Video Gallery, American Academy of Neurology, http://journals.lww.com/continuum/Pages/videogallery.aspx.) Available at: http://journals.lww.com/continuum/pages/videogallery.aspx?videoId=123&autoPlay=true

D.3. Dressing apraxia due to a left parietal lesion. (From Venkatesh Bolegave, 2014.) Available at: https://www.youtube.com/watch?v=mLczBWwx0rs

D.4. Type I Duane's syndrome. (From Kathleen B. Digre, John A. Moran Eye Center, Neuro-ophthalmology Virtual Education Library [NOVEL], University of Utah.) Available at: http://stream.utah.edu/m/dp/frame.php?f=a99b354aceb1a054881

D.5. Examples of flaccid and spastic dysarthria. (From Paul D. Larsen, MD, University of Nebraska Medical Center and Suzanne S. Stensaas, PhD, University of Utah School of Medicine, http://library.med.utah.edu/neurologicexam/html/home_exam.html) Available at: http://library.med.utah.edu/neurologicexam/html/mentalstatus_resources.html#01

References

1. Dennis M, Bowen WT, Cho L. *Mechanisms of Clinical Signs.* Sydney, New South Wales, Australia: Churchill Livingstone; 2012.
2. Valenzuela A, Chung L, Casciola-Rosen L, et al. Identification of clinical features and autoantibodies associated with calcinosis in dermatomyositis. *JAMA Dermatol.* 2014;150:724–729.
3. Tansley SL, Betteridge ZE, Shaddick G, et al. Calcinosis in juvenile dermatomyositis is influenced by both anti-NXP2 autoantibody status and age at disease onset. *Rheumatology (Oxford).* 2014;53(12):2204–2208.
4. Crippa SV, Borruat FX, Kawasaki A. Pupillary dilation lag is intermittently present in patients with a stable oculosympathetic defect (Horner syndrome). *Am J Ophthalmol.* 2007;143:712–715.
5. Carney LR. The dimple sign in peroneal palsy. *Neurology.* 1967;17:922.
6. Massey EW. Dimple sign in mail carrier's ulnar neuropathy. *Neurology.* 1989;39:1132.
7. Hankey GJ, Edis RH. The utility of testing tactile perception of direction of scratch as a sensitive clinical sign of posterior column dysfunction in spinal cord disorders. *J Neurol Neurosurg Psychiatry.* 1989;52:395–398.
8. Yee RD. Downbeat nystagmus: characteristics and localization of lesions. *Trans Am Ophthalmol Soc.* 1989;87:984–1032.
9. Foundas AL. Apraxia: neural mechanisms and functional recovery. *Handb Clin Neurol.* 2013;110:335–345.
10. Enderby P. Disorders of communication: dysarthria. *Handb Clin Neurol.* 2013;110:273–281.
11. McGee S. *Evidence Based Physical Diagnosis.* 3rd ed. Philadelphia, PA: Elsevier/Saunders; 2012.
12. Ha AD, Jankovic J. An introduction to dyskinesia—the clinical spectrum. *Int Rev Neurobiol.* 2011; 98:1–29.
13. Hallett M, Massaquoi SG. Physiologic studies of dysmetria in patients with cerebellar deficits. *Can J Neurol Sci.* 1993;20(suppl 3):S83–S92.
14. Diener HC, Dichgans J. Pathophysiology of cerebellar ataxia. *Mov Disord.* 1992;7:95–109.
15. Roy N. Functional dysphonia. *Curr Opin Otolaryngol Head Neck Surg.* 2003;11:144–148.
16. Albanese A, Bhatia K, Bressman SB, et al. Phenomenology and classification of dystonia: a consensus update. *Mov Disord.* 2013;28:863–873.
17. Nausieda PA, Weiner WJ, Klawans HL. Dystonic foot response of Parkinsonism. *Arch Neurol.* 1980;37:132–136.

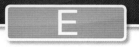

Eccentric pupil (corectopia, Wilson's sign): Displacement of the pupil from the center of the iris; usually seen in severe midbrain disease **(Table E.1)**.[1]

Echographia: The repetition by writing of that overheard, similar to **echolalia**.

Echolalia: The meaningless repetition of heard words (see **perseveration**). The repeating is involuntary and automatic. It often occurs in **transcortical aphasia**, in GTS, in dementia, and as a manifestation of **imitation behavior** in patients with frontal lobe lesions.

Echopraxia: The involuntary, automatic repetition or imitation of the gestures or actions of another person, specifically the patient copying the actions of the examiner, even after specific instructions not to do so. Echopraxia is a prominent feature in many cases of GTS, as a manifestation of **imitation behavior,** and in the startle reflex disorders (see **hyperekplexia**). See **stimulus bound behavior, environmental dependency.**

Elbow flexion test: A test for ulnar neuropathy at the elbow. The elbow flexion test is similar to **Phalen's test** for CTS. The elbow is held fully flexed for 30 to 60 seconds to elicit paresthesias. Variants include elbow flexion plus pressure applied just distal to the ulnar groove, holding the elbow flexed and the wrist flexed in ulnar deviation and combining elbow flexion with internal rotation of the shoulder. In a study of 44 extremities with electrodiagnostically proven ulnar neuropathy at the elbow, with 30 seconds of flexion the sensitivities were as follows: elbow flexion test 0.32, pressure provocation alone 0.55, and pressure plus elbow flexion test 0.91.[2] The elbow flexion test causes paresthesias in 3.6% of normals at 1 minute but in 16.2% at 3 minutes, so continuing flexion beyond 1 minute degrades the usefulness of the test.[3]

Elevated Arm Stress Test (EAST, Roos, "hands up test"): See **carpal tunnel syndrome provocative tests** and **thoracic outlet syndrome provocative tests.**

Elderly gait: See **gait disorders.**

Ely's (heel-to-buttock) sign: A maneuver designed to demonstrate contracture of the rectus femoris, but which will also cause pain in high lumbar radiculopathy or psoas irritation as might occur with pyelonephritis or with psoas abscess or hematoma. The patient is placed prone and the knee flexed to bring the heel to touch the opposite buttock (Fig. E.1). Ely's sign is similar to and often confused with **reverse straight leg raising** or the **femoral nerve stretch test,** but in those the heel is raised straight up.

Table E.1. Unusual Pupil Shapes

Eccentric pupil	Displacement of the pupil from the center of the iris
Oval pupil	Oval shape
Paradoxical pupils	Constrict in darkness
Scalloped pupils	Characteristic of familial amyloidosis
Springing pupil	Intermittent dilation lasting minutes to hours
Tadpole pupil	Intermittent comma shape

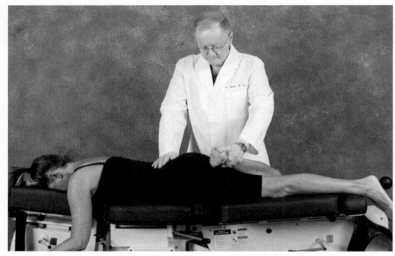

Figure E.1. Ely's sign with the patient prone, the heel is placed on the opposite buttock, pain may be elicited in high lumbar radiculopathy; similar to the femoral nerve stretch test (reverse straight leg raising test). (From Cox JM. *Low Back Pain: Mechanism, Diagnosis, and Treatment.* 7th ed. Philadelphia, PA: Wolters Kluwer Health/Lippincott Williams & Wilkins; 2011, with permission.)

Emotional facial palsy: Facial asymmetry more apparent with spontaneous expression, as when laughing. See **facial palsy.**

Emotional incontinence (emotionalism): Difficulty with emotional control causing spontaneous, unprovoked laughing and crying or emotional display overly extreme for the circumstances. Such emotional lability often occurs in patients with **pseudobulbar palsy.** Patients with **witzelsucht** or **moria** may also seem overly jocular.

Empty can (Jobe) test: See **shoulder examination tests.**

Encephalocele: Herniation of brain contents outside the calvarium. These malformations are usually very obvious and present in infancy. One type, however, may present in adults as recurrent meningitis or CSF rhinorrhea. The nasal encephalocele forms because of a defect between the frontal and ethmoid bones at the site of the foramen cecum. There are three types: nasofrontal, nasoethmoid, and nasoorbital. The first two may betray their presence by causing **hypertelorism** or a slightly elongated nose, causing the patient to appear dysmorphic.

End point nystagmus: The fine **nystagmus** that often occurs in extreme abduction, in about the last 10°. It is a normal physiologic phenomenon; the difficulty lies in distinguishing it from mild instances of abnormal **gaze-evoked nystagmus.** Abnormal nystagmus occurs short of extreme gaze and is more sustained than physiologic end-point nystagmus, which usually dampens after 5 to 6 seconds.[4]

Enhanced physiologic tremor: An exaggeration of the physiologic tremor present but not apparent in everyone. The frequency of physiologic tremor varies from 8 to 12 Hz, averaging about 10 Hz in the young adult, somewhat slower in children and older persons. The tremor may increase because of anxiety, excitement, fright, and other conditions with increased adrenergic activity, such as thyrotoxicosis or pheochromocytoma. Enhanced physiologic tremor (EPT) involves principally the fingers and hands and may be fine and difficult to see yet still very symptomatic when a high degree of manual dexterity is required, such as in a dentist. The tremor is both postural and action but not present at rest. It may be brought out by placing a limb in a position of postural tension, by performing voluntary movements at the slowest possible rate, or holding the index fingertips as close together as possible without touching. The tremor may be better appreciated by placing a sheet of paper on the outstretched fingers; shaking of the paper may be obvious even though tremor is not grossly visible. Similar tremor occurs due to the effects of nicotine, caffeine, and other stimulants. EPT is the most common of the three most common tremors seen in clinical practice; the other two are ET and the tremor of PD. Distinguishing enhanced physiologic tremor from mild forms of ET is difficult and sometimes arbitrary.

Enhanced ptosis: See **curtain sign.**

Enophthalmos: Posterior displacement of the globe in the orbit, which may occur in a variety of circumstances. When bilateral, enophthalmos may simply indicate dehydration. When unilateral, it can be congenital, or due to trauma or maxillary sinus disease. Enophthalmos is frequently mistaken for ipsilateral ptosis or contralateral proptosis. Patients with NF1 may develop pulsatile enophthalmos due to absence of the sphenoid wing and lateral wall of the orbit[5]. In **Horner's syndrome,** there is apparent enophthalmos, but it is an optical illusion and the actual globe position is normal.

Environmental dependency: A tendency to respond to things in the environment in an automatic, uninhibited way, as in **utilization behavior, imitation behavior,** and **echopraxia.** Environmental dependency seems relatively specific for frontal lobe dysfunction and particularly for pathology involving the right orbitofrontal region.[6]

Epicanthic (epicanthic, mongoloid) folds: Vertical, bilateral folds of skin extending from the upper lid to the medial canthi. The folds may create the appearance of esotropia (pseudoesotropia) by covering the inner portion of the eye (Fig. E.2). Epicanthal folds are common in people of Asian ancestry. They also occur in Down's syndrome, fetal alcohol syndrome, and phenylketonuria.

Epidermal nevus: A congenital skin lesion due to hyperplasia of epidermal structures. The lesion is often linear, following the lines of Blaschko, the paths along which skin cells migrate during embryogenesis. An epidermal nevus is usually present at birth or develops in early childhood and with aging becomes thicker and darker. The nevus is classified according to the type of skin cell involved, as keratinocytes (nevus verrucosus) or sebaceous glands (nevus sebaceous).

In an epidermal nevus syndrome, the nevus is associated with neurological manifestations, such as seizures or a focal deficit, for example, a nevus sebaceous (of Jadassohn) of the scalp associated with seizures and mental retardation, known as the Schimmelpenning syndrome (Fig. E.3).[7]

Epiphora: Overflow of tears down the cheek, may occur in Bell's palsy, with **crocodile tears,** or during an attack of cluster headache.

Equine gait: See **steppage gait.**

Equinus (equinovarus) deformity: A plantarflexed foot posture that may result from foot drop due to peroneal nerve palsy, spasm of the calf muscles in foot dystonia, spasticity due to a CST lesion, trauma, arthritis of the ankle joint, or a

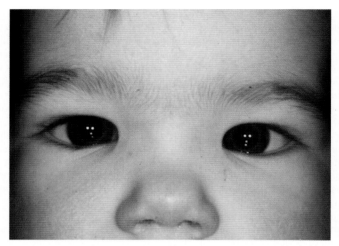

Figure E.2. Infantile-onset essential esotropia, with small-moderate angle deviation of the left eye. Note also the confounding presence of pseudoesotropia caused by conspicuous epicanthal folds. (From Chern KC, Saidel M. *Ophthalmology Review Manual.* 2nd ed. Philadelphia, PA: Wolters Kluwer Health/Lippincott Williams & Wilkins; 2012, with permission.)

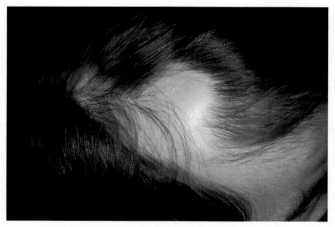

Figure E.3. A linear nevus sebaceous in a child with an ipsilateral ocular lesion, seizures, and developmental delay.

developmental anomaly, such as a congenital clubfoot. Horses walk digitigrade (on the toes), so the equine prefix is used for conditions that throw weight bearing onto the forefoot. See **pes cavus.**

Ergotism: A syndrome due to the effects of ergot alkaloids, characterized by vasoconstriction with a burning skin sensation, gangrene, and CNS symptoms such as hallucinations and convulsions. In the middle ages, epidemics occurred because of fungal contamination of rye and the condition was called St. Anthony's fire because of the burning paresthesias, pruritis, and formication. Vasoconstriction may lead to gangrene, usually of the fingers, hands, toes, feet, ears, and/or nose. Ergotism has most classically been seen as a complication of the treatment of migraine with ergotamine, but can also occur with the use or ergot-derived drugs in the treatment of PD and restless legs syndrome (Fig. E.4).

Erythyma migrans: The skin lesion associated with Lyme disease. The typical skin lesion has an expanding border and a clearing center, often with a punctate central lesion at the site of the tick bite that is intensely erythematous and sometimes vesicular or necrotic, creating a "bull's-eye" appearance (Fig. E.5). Lesions can reach a diameter of 10 to 30 cm, clearing in the center, to create a ring configuration. The lesion disappears in several weeks without treatment. Multiple lesions occur in 15% of patients and suggest systemic spread.

Esophoria: See **strabismus.**

Esotropia: See **strabismus.**

Essential anisocoria: See **anisocoria.**

Essential blepharospasm: See **blepharospasm.**

Essential tremor: The most common of all movement disorders. ET is a postural and action tremor that tends to affect the hands, head, and voice.[8] ET is often familial, the prevalence increases with age, and it tends to slowly worsen. About

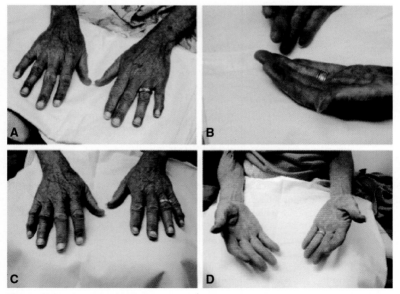

Figure E.4. Ergotism with cyanosis of the fingers bilaterally while on pergolide (**A** and **B**). One week after stopping pergolide and starting ropinirole, the ergotism was remarkably improved (**C** and **D**). (From Morgan JC, Sethi KD. Pergolide-induced ergotism. *Neurology.* 2006;67:104, with permission.)

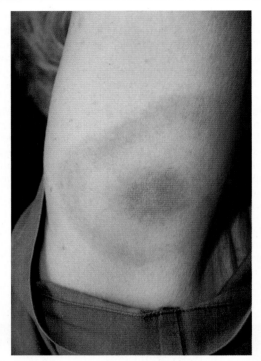

Figure E.5. Erythema migrans, the characteristic rash of Lyme disease. This photograph depicts the "bull's-eye" pattern rash at the site of a tick bite. (From Burkhart CN, Morrell D. *VisualDx. Essential Pediatric Dermatology.* Philadelphia, PA: Wolters Kluwer Health/Lippincott Williams & Wilkins; 2010, with permission.)

two-thirds of ET patients have a family history of the disorder; first-degree relatives of ET patients are 5 to 10 times more likely to develop it. "Senile tremor" is ET occurring during senescence with a negative family history.

ET is typically of medium amplitude and rate but may become coarse when severe **(Video E.1)**. ET tends to oscillate at higher frequency and lower amplitude than does **parkinsonian tremor** (PT). Not all body parts necessarily have identical tremor rates. In ET, the head and voice tremor rate is typically about 4 Hz, the hand tremor a bit faster. Usually, PT is most prominent at rest, while that of ET occurs with a sustained posture, such as with the hands outstretched, or on action. PT may persist with hands outstretched but usually damps, at least transiently, when making a deliberate movement, whereas ET usually worsens. The head and voice are often involved with ET, only rarely with PT, although PT may involve the lips and jaw. The movement of the head may be in an anterior–posterior (affirmative, yes-yes, tremblement affirmatif) or a lateral (negative, no-no, tremblement negatif) direction. Alcohol and β blockers often improve ET but have no effect on PT. Although often thought of as relatively benign, ET can become severe and incapacitating.

While the above textbook description holds in many instances, there are frequently patients where the distinction between ET and PT is far from clear.[9] The two diseases may coexist and having ET seems to increase the risk of developing PD. There can be "overlap" and it is not uncommon for patients with ET to exhibit "PD signs" and for patients with PD to exhibit "ET signs," creating diagnostic uncertainty.

Rest tremor is a cardinal feature of PD, usually resolving with the initiation of movement, and when it is accompanied by bradykinesia and rigidity, PD is the most likely diagnosis. Although rest tremor is highly suggestive of the diagnosis of PD, it may occur in certain ET patients, primarily those with more severe disease and disease of longer duration. It may help to compare the rest tremor walking vs. seated. In most patients with PD, rest tremor increases in intensity while walking, but in ET it decreases.[9] Having the patient perform a mental task, such as counting backward, may bring out the resting tremor in PD while suppressing any resting component of ET. **Action tremor** is the hallmark of ET, while PT classically dampens with activity. However, patients with PD commonly have various forms of action tremor. One form of action tremor is postural tremor, present with the arms outstretched and still. One form of postural tremor characteristic of PD and rarely seen in ET patients is reemergent tremor. When the patient holds the arms out, they remain still for 10 to 20 seconds, after which the tremor reappears. ET in contrast appears as soon as the arms are stretched out. PT tends to involve the more distal structures, especially the fingers; a flexion-extension tremor of the thumb is much more likely to occur in PD than in ET. The postural wrist tremor in ET typically causes flexion-extension movement, while in PD the tremor often includes a component of pronation-supination. The classical teaching is that the tremor of ET is bilateral and symmetric. In fact, the action tremor in ET is often but not necessarily bilateral, and small to moderate side-to-side differences are the rule rather than the exception.

Euphoria: (1) a state of abnormal elation in the face of dire circumstances. Euphoria may be seen in patients who have frontal lobe disease. Some degree of euphoria affects as many as one-third of patients with FTD, and it is relatively common in patients with advanced MS, where it seems to correlate with white matter burden, enlarged ventricles, and impaired cognition. Patients with late-stage MS may seem inappropriately cheerful, optimistic, and unconcerned about the degree of disability. The euphoria is often accompanied by **disinhibition, emotionalism**, and impulsivity. (2) a direct effect of many drugs, and an incidental effect of others, such as steroids, both corticosteroids and anabolic steroids. See **witzelsucht, moria.**

Exaggerated startle response: See **hyperekplexia.**

Executive function: The ability to plan, carry out, and monitor a series of actions intended to accomplish a goal. Executive functions involve planning and organizational skills, the ability to benefit from experience, abstraction, motivation, cognitive flexibility, and problem solving. Executive functions are the "supervisory" cognitive processes that involve high-level organization and execution of complex thoughts and behavior, including such processes as planning, working memory, attention, verbal reasoning, mental flexibility, multitasking, and initiation and monitoring of actions. Patients with impaired executive functions display disorganized actions and strategies for everyday tasks, sometimes without demonstrable deficits on formal tests of cognition, known as the dysexecutive syndrome.[10]

The responsibility for executive function largely resides with the dorsolateral prefrontal cortex and its connections. Disturbed executive function is common with frontal lobe lesions, but may occur with lesions elsewhere because of the extensive connections of the frontal lobes with all other parts of the brain, although other systems, including the cerebellum, are involved.

Frontal lobe dysfunction is often subtle. At the bedside, special techniques designed to evaluate frontal lobe function may be useful. A commonly used executive function measure is the Wisconsin Card Sorting Test. A bedside variation is to ask the patient to detect a pattern when the examiner switches a coin between hands behind her back—e.g., twice in the right hand, once in the left—then to change the pattern and see if the patient detects the new scheme. Patients with frontal lobe dysfunction who do not have **anomia** when tested by other methods may still have difficulty generating word lists. Consistent with its prominent executive demands, **letter fluency** has been found to correlate more with prefrontal lobe functioning than does **category fluency**.

Patients with frontal lesions tend to have **perseveration**, which may be brought out with **alternating sequences tests**, such as Luria's **fist-edge-palm test**. Other useful bedside tests of executive function include **trail-making tests**, working memory tests such as reverse **digit span** and months backward, **abstraction**, tests for **defective response inhibition (Stroop test, antisaccade task, applause sign, and the Go/No-Go test)** and examining for **environmental dependency** by attempting to elicit **imitation** and **utilization behavior**. The Frontal Assessment Battery is a test battery that can be administered in a few minutes that covers five executive tests plus the **grasp reflex**.[11]

In Alzheimer's disease, language function and visuospatial skills tend to be affected relatively early, while deficits in executive function and behavioral symptoms often manifest later in the disease course. In contrast, FTD is characterized by early deterioration in executive functioning compared with patients with AD.

Exophoria: See **strabismus.**

Exophthalmos: The abnormal protrusion of one or both eyes, which may vary from mild to dramatic and develop suddenly or gradually. The most common cause is thyroid eye disease. **Eyelid retraction** may simulate exophthalmos when the globe is in a normal position. **Ptosis** or **enophthalmos** on one side may be mistaken for exophthalmos on the opposite side. With carotid-cavernous fistula, the bulging eye may also pulsate. See **proptosis.**

Exotropia: See **strabismus.**

Expressive aphasia: See **Broca's aphasia.**

Extensor digitorum brevis reflex: A minor DTR difficult to elicit even in normals and under the best of circumstances and of no value in the diagnosis of radiculopathy.[12] One of many reflexes studied in the fruitless search for a reflex that would be helpful in the diagnosis of L5 radiculopathy. See **hamstring reflexes, peroneal reflex.**

Extensor thrust reflex: A complex, polysynaptic spinal reflex designed to help support the body's weight against gravity. Pressure on the plantar surface of the foot causes reflex contraction of the leg extensors. The reflex disappears with maturation but may return in patients with severe but incomplete spinal cord injuries.

Extensor toe signs: See **Babinski signs, Chaddock's sign, Oppenheim's sign, minor extensor toe signs,** and **Table M.3.**

External hamstring reflex: See **hamstring reflexes.**

Extinction: See **attentional deficits.**

Eyelid apraxia: See **apraxia of eyelid opening** and **apraxia of eyelid closure.**

Eyelid hopping: See **Cogan's lid twitch sign.**

Eyelid myotonia: See **myotonia.**

Eyelid position, abnormal: An asymmetry in the width of the palpebral fissures, which should be equal on both sides, although a slight difference occurs in many normal individuals. The normal upper eyelid in primary position crosses the iris between the limbus and the pupil, 1 to 2 mm below the limbus; the lower lid touches or crosses slightly above the limbus. Normally there is no sclera showing above the iris. The palpebral fissures are normally 9 to 12 mm from upper to lower lid margin. With **ptosis,** the lid droops down and may cross at the upper margin of the pupil, or cover the pupil partially or totally. Ptosis may be unilateral or bilateral, partial or complete, and occurs in many neurologic conditions (see Fig. C.17). With **eyelid retraction,** the upper lid pulls back and frequently exposes a thin crescent of sclera between the upper limbus and the lower lid margin. Lid retraction is a classic sign of thyroid disease, but occurs in neurologic disorders as well.

Eyelid retraction: Abnormal lid position due to elevation of the upper lid, with the lid resting at the upper limbus or with a rim of sclera showing above the limbus, indicating either lid retraction **(tucked lid sign)** or **lid lag.** Thyroid disease is a common cause of lid abnormalities, including lid retraction in primary gaze (**Dalrymple's sign**), infrequent blinking (**Stellwag's sign**), and **lid lag** in downgaze (von Graefe's sign). In thyroid eye disease, the increased catecholamine levels cause hypercontraction of the sympathetically innervated accessory levator (Müeller's) muscle, pulling the eyelid open. Lid retraction in primary gaze also occurs with lesions involving the posterior commissure (**Collier's sign, posterior fossa stare**). Lid retraction with posterior commissure lesions is bilateral, but sometimes asymmetric. With Collier's sign, the levators relax appropriately and the lids usually descend normally on downgaze without lagging behind as they do in thyroid eye disease. In addition, the lid retraction may worsen with attempted upgaze. Circumscribed midbrain lesions may cause eyelid retraction with minimal impairment of vertical gaze. In PD, there is infrequent blinking and there may be some lid retraction. Lid retraction may also be mechanical, due to trauma or surgery. Lid retraction may be confused with ipsilateral proptosis or contralateral ptosis.

References

1. Selhorst JB, Hoyt WF, Feinsod M, et al. Midbrain corectopia. *Arch Neurol.* 1976;33:193–195.
2. Novak CB, Lee GW, Mackinnon SE, et al. Provocative testing for cubital tunnel syndrome. *J Hand Surg Am.* 1994;19:817–820.
3. Rosati M, Martignoni R, Spagnolli G, et al. Clinical validity of the elbow flexion test for the diagnosis of ulnar nerve compression at the cubital tunnel. *Acta Orthop Belg.* 1998;64:366–370.
4. Serra A, Leigh RJ. Diagnostic value of nystagmus: spontaneous and induced ocular oscillations. *J Neurol Neurosurg Psychiatry.* 2002;73:615–618.
5. Lehn A, Airey C, Boyle R. Pulsating enophthalmos in neurofibromatosis 1. *JAMA Neurol.* 2013;70:644–645.
6. Besnard J, Allain P, Aubin G, et al. A contribution to the study of environmental dependency phenomena: the social hypothesis. *Neuropsychologia.* 2011;49:3279–3294.

7. Campbell WW, Sorenson G, Buda F. Linear nevus sebaceous syndrome. *Milit Med*. 1978;143:175–180.

8. Elble, RJ. What is essential tremor? *Curr Neurol Neurosci Rep*. 2013;13:353.

9. Thenganatt MA, Louis, ED. Distinguishing essential tremor from Parkinson's disease: bedside tests and laboratory evaluations. *Expert Rev Neurother*. 2012;12:687–696.

10. Godefroy O, Azouvi P, Robert P, et al. Dysexecutive syndrome: diagnostic criteria and validation study. *Ann Neurol*. 2010;68:855–864.

11. Dubois B, Slachevsky A, Litvan I, et al. The FAB: a Frontal Assessment Battery at bedside. *Neurology*. 2000;55:1621–1626.

12. Marin R, Dillingham TR, Chang A, et al. Extensor digitorum brevis reflex in normals and patients with radiculopathies. *Muscle Nerve*. 1995;18:52–59.

FABER (FABERE, Patrick's) test: An acronym for flexed, abducted, and externally rotated, the position in which the hip is placed during the examination (Fig. F.1). Pain from hip disease or SI joint disease is maximal when the hip is flexed, abducted, and externally rotated by putting the patient's foot on the contralateral knee (figure-4 position) and pressing down slightly on the flexed knee. Pain in the groin elicited in this position is suggestive of hip disease; pain posteriorly suggests SI joint disease. Arthritis of the hip usually causes restricted motion, especially in flexion and internal rotation. Studies of the FABER maneuver for SI joint disease have shown a sensitivity of 70% to 75% and a specificity of 100%.[1]

Face–hand test: A test for tactile inattention or extinction thought to be useful in distinguishing organic brain syndrome from schizophrenia. The patient is touched simultaneously on various combinations of the face and the hand. There may be some tendency to ignore the hand stimulus initially, but persistence of face domination over the hand on simultaneous stimulation suggests an organic process. See **attentional deficits**.

Facial diplegia: Weakness, usually due to peripheral facial palsy. Bilateral facial palsy must be differentiated from other causes of bifacial weakness, such as myopathies

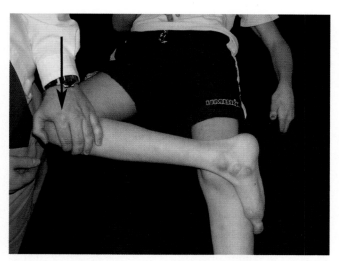

Figure F.1. With the patient supine, the right lower extremity is placed in the figure-4 position with the hip in flexion, abduction, and external rotation (FABER test). While stabilizing the contralateral pelvic brim, the knee is gently pushed toward the examination table. Posterior pain suggests sacroiliac pathology, and anterior pain suggests hip disease. (From Weinstein SL, Flynn JM. *Lovell and Winter's Pediatric Orthopaedics.* 7th ed. Philadelphia, PA: Wolters Kluwer Health/Lippincott Williams & Wilkins; 2014, with permission.)

and MG. In a series of inpatients with facial diplegia, the most common causes were bilateral Bell's palsy, Guillain-Barré syndrome, meningeal tumor, prepontine tumor, and idiopathic cranial polyneuropathy.[2] Differential diagnosis also includes sarcoidosis, Lyme disease, diabetes, head trauma, HIV infection, Miller Fisher syndrome, tuberculous or fungal meningitis, pontine tumor, Melkersson-Rosenthal syndrome, Möebius' syndrome, and a long list of other conditions.

Facial dystonia: An abnormal fixed facial expression; see **procerus sign**.

Facial hemiatrophy (hemifacial atrophy, Parry-Romberg syndrome, Wartenberg's syndrome): A condition causing progressive atrophy of the skin, subcutaneous fat, and musculature of one half of the face, sometimes with trophic changes in the connective tissue, cartilage, and bone **(Fig. F.2)**. Accompanying changes may include trophic changes in the hair, with loss of pigmentation and circumscribed alopecia and vitiligo. The facial atrophy may be accompanied by classic linear scleroderma lesions on the face or elsewhere, and the disorder may be a form of localized scleroderma.

Facial myokymia: A continuous, involuntary muscular quivering that has a rippling, wormlike, appearance[3]. It is usually unilateral. Facial myokymia has been reported with numerous conditions, most intrinsic to the brainstem. It is a classic feature of MS, but may also occur with pontine tumor, CPA tumors, GBS, facial nerve compression, rattlesnake envenomation, SAH, meningeal neoplasia, basilar invagination, syringobulbia, and in association with high titers of voltage-gated K^+ channel (VGKC) antibodies **(Video Links F.1 and F.2)**.

Facial palsy: See **facial weakness**.

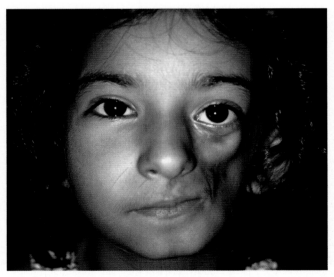

Figure F.2. Facial hemiatrophy (Parry-Romberg syndrome). Atrophy of the skin, subcutaneous fat, and musculature of one half of the face with accompanying changes in the connective tissues and with accompanying atrophy of the ipsilateral tongue. (From Campbell WW. *DeJong's the Neurologic Examination.* 7th ed. Philadelphia, PA: Wolters Kluwer Health/Lippincott Williams & Wilkins; 2013, with permission.)

Facial reflexes: Reflex contractions of facial muscles. There are a number of facial reflexes of relatively minor importance, such as audio- and visuo-palpebral and trigeminofacial. The **orbicularis oculi reflex** and **orbicularis oris (snout) reflex** are more clinically useful. Preservation, even hyperactivity, of reflex facial movements may occur despite loss of voluntary movement in UMN **facial weakness**.

Facial synkinesis (synkinesias): Abnormal muscle contractions of the face, often subtle, synchronous with blinking or mouth movements. They occur most commonly after Bell's palsy with aberrant regeneration but may follow other facial nerve lesions, such as CPA tumors. The most common form is oculo-oral, with subtle perioral movements that occur with blinking. See **inverse jaw winking.**

Facial weakness: Weakness of the muscles of facial expression. The weakness may involve only the lower face or both upper and lower face, unilaterally or bilaterally. Facial weakness can result from UMN or LMN disorders, from myopathy or from neuromuscular junction disorders. See **facial diplegia.**

There are two types of neurogenic facial nerve weakness: peripheral, or LMN; and central, or UMN **(Table F.1)**. Peripheral facial palsy (PFP) may result from a lesion anywhere from the CN VII nucleus in the pons to the terminal branches in the face. Central facial palsy (CFP) is due to a lesion involving the supranuclear pathways before they synapse on the facial nucleus. PFP results from an ipsilateral lesion, whereas CFP, with rare exception, results from a contralateral lesion.

PFP causes flaccid weakness of all the muscles of facial expression on the involved side, both upper and lower face, and the paralysis is usually complete (prosopoplegia). The affected side of the face is smooth, there are no wrinkles on the forehead, the eye is open, the inferior lid sags, the nasolabial fold is flattened, and the angle of the mouth droops (Fig. F.3). The patient cannot raise the eyebrow, wrinkle the forehead, close the eye, bare the teeth, blow out the cheek, or retract the angle of the mouth or the platysma on the involved side. The mouth is drawn to the sound side on attempted movement. The palpebral fissure is open wider than normal, and there may be **lagophthalmos**. During spontaneous blinking, the involved eyelid tends to lag behind, sometimes conspicuously. Very mild PFP may produce only a slower and less complete blink on the involved side. Because of weakness of the lower lid sphincter, tears may run over and down the cheek (**epiphora**).

Table F.1. Upper versus Lower Motor Neuron Facial Weakness

Upper Motor Neuron Facial Weakness	Lower Motor Neuron Facial Weakness
Unilateral weakness of the lower face with relative sparing of the upper face	Equal weakness of both upper and lower face
Possible voluntary/emotional dissociation	No dissociation
Normal lacrimation	Possible decreased lacrimation
Normal taste function on anterior 2/3 of tongue	Possible impaired taste
Normal hearing	Possible hyperacusis/phonophobia
Preserved or exaggerated facial reflexes	Loss of facial reflexes
Usually associated with arm or leg weakness	Possible neighborhood signs depending on location of lesion
Patient frequently unaware of deficit	Patient usually very aware of deficit
No pain	Mild pain common in Bell's palsy
	Vesicles in Ramsay Hunt syndrome
	Bell's phenomenon

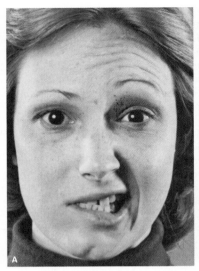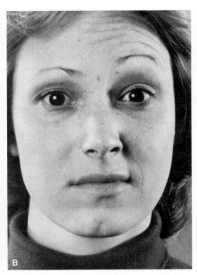

Figure F.3. A patient with a peripheral facial nerve palsy on the right. **A:** Patient is attempting to retract both angles of the mouth. **B:** Patient is attempting to elevate both eyebrows. (From Campbell WW. *DeJong's the Neurologic Examination.* 7th ed. Philadelphia, PA: Wolters Kluwer Health/Lippincott Williams & Wilkins; 2013, with permission.)

The House-Brackmann scale, Burres-Fisch index, and facial nerve function index attempt to quantitate the degree of weakness. See **Bergara-Wartenberg's sign, Babinski's platysma sign.**

The facial weakness in PFP is obvious on both voluntary and spontaneous contraction. There is no dissociation (see below). The **corneal reflex, orbicularis oculi reflex,** and other **facial reflexes** are impaired. In comatose or otherwise uncooperative patients, facial movements can be elicited by painful pressure over the supraorbital nerves, or by other painful stimuli applied to the face to elicit an avoidance response. Facial weakness must be differentiated from a facial contracture on the opposite side, developmental asymmetry, facial hemiatrophy, character lines, and habitual emphasis on the use of one side of the mouth.

Localization of a PFP depends on the associated findings, such as hyperacusis, decreased tearing, impaired taste, and involvement of neural structures beyond CN VII. **Table F.2** summarizes the localization and differential diagnosis of PFP.[4,5] The most common cause of PFP by far is Bell's palsy.

A supranuclear, UMN or CFP, produces weakness of the lower face, with relative sparing of the upper face. The upper face has both contralateral and ipsilateral supranuclear innervation, and cortical innervation of the facial nucleus may be more extensive for the lower face than the upper. The paresis is rarely complete. A lesion involving the corticobulbar fibers anywhere prior to their synapse on the facial nerve nucleus will cause a CFP. Lesions are most often in the cortex or internal capsule. Occasionally, a lesion as far caudal as the medulla can cause a CFP because

Table F.2. Examples of Conditions Causing Peripheral Facial Weakness

Nuclear
  Motor neuron disease
  Möebius' syndrome
  Neoplasm (e.g., pontine glioma)
  Syringobulbia
  Vascular disease
    Ischemic
    Hemorrhagic
  Infection (e.g., poliomyelitis)
Infranuclear
  Intramedullary
    Neoplasm (e.g., pontine glioma)
    Demyelination
    Vascular disease
      Ischemic
      Hemorrhagic
    Trauma
    Infection (e.g., abscess, brainstem encephalitis)
    Syringobulbia
    Central pontine myelinolysis
Extramedullary
  Neoplasm (e.g., acoustic neuroma, meningioma, neoplastic meningitis, parotid tumor)
  Trauma (e.g., petrous fracture)
  Inflammatory/autoimmune/postinfectious (e.g., Bell's palsy, Guillain-Barré syndrome)
  Infection (Herpes zoster, Lyme disease, HIV, tuberculous meningitis)
  Vascular/microvascular (e.g., diabetes)
  Hereditary (e.g., Melkersson-Rosenthal, HNPP)
  Sarcoidosis

HNPP, hereditary neuropathy with liability to pressure palsy.

F

of involvement of the aberrant pyramidal tract. There is considerable individual variation in facial innervation, and the extent of weakness in a CFP may vary from the lower half to two-thirds of the face. The upper face is not necessarily completely spared, but it is always involved to a lesser degree than the lower face. Inability to independently wink the involved eye may be the only demonstrable deficit (**Revilliod's sign**). The **orbicularis oculi reflex** and other **facial reflexes** are frequently preserved, even exaggerated. Separating CFP and PFP is rarely difficult. CFP is typically part of a more extensive deficit due to a lesion of the UMN pathways.

There are two variations of CFP: (1) volitional, or voluntary; and (2) emotional, or mimetic. In most instances of CFP, the facial asymmetry is present both when the patient is asked to smile or show the teeth, and during spontaneous facial movements such as smiling and laughing. However, spontaneous movements and deliberate, willful movements may show different degrees of weakness. When asymmetry is more apparent with one than the other, the facial weakness is said to be dissociated. The dissociation may occur because of bilateral supranuclear innervation for lower facial spontaneous, emotional movements not present for volitional movements, but the anatomical explanation for dissociated facial palsy remains unclear. The most common variant is weakness with voluntary movements becoming less apparent with spontaneous, emotional movements. Facial weakness seen only with emotional movements most commonly results from thalamic or striatocapsular lesions, usually infarction, and rarely with brainstem lesions.

Facilitory paratonia: See **paratonia.**

FAIR test: A maneuver used in the diagnosis of piriformis syndrome, aka the piriformis test. See **piriformis syndrome provocative tests.**

Fajersztajn's sign: See **straight leg raising test.**

False image: The image from the paretic eye in a patient with diplopia. The real image falls on the macula of the normal eye; the false image falls on the retina beside the macula of the paretic eye. The false image is usually fainter than the true image because extramacular vision is not as acute. The clarity, however, depends on the visual acuity in the two eyes. The brain is accustomed to images falling off the macula coming from peripheral vision, so it projects the false image peripherally. The farther away from the macula that the image falls, the farther peripherally the misinterpretation of its origin. As the eye moves in the direction of the paretic muscle, the separation of images increases and the false image appears to be more and more peripheral. See **diplopia rules.**

False localizing signs: Signs not due to a disturbance of function at the site of a lesion, that may cause confusion in clinical localization.[6] False localizing signs occur most often with tumors as they exert mass effect and raise ICP. Sixth nerve palsies are the most common and classic of all false localizing signs; they are nonspecific and bear no necessary anatomical relationship to the central nervous system pathology producing them. Elevated ICP of any cause often produces CN VI dysfunction due to stretching of the nerve over the petrous tip as the increased pressure forces the brainstem attachments inferiorly. Increased ICP with uncal herniation most often compresses the third nerve ipsilaterally. Kernohan's notch syndrome is compression of the contralateral cerebral peduncle against the sharp edge of the opposite side of the tentorium, causing a false localizing hemiparesis ipsilateral to the lesion. Occasionally, the contralateral third nerve is crushed, and the third nerve palsy occurs on the side opposite the herniation. A false localizing hemiparesis is much more common than a false localizing third nerve palsy. Dysfunction of the facial and trigeminal nerves has also been reported due to increased ICP.

False localizing signs also occur with spinal cord lesions. Lesions in the region of the foramen magnum and upper cervical spinal cord, typically compressive extramedullary mass lesions, may cause weakness and wasting of the small hand muscles for reasons that remain unclear; circulatory disturbances affecting the descending distribution of the anterior spinal artery have been invoked. Similarly, weakness and wasting of the predominately C8–T1 innervated small hand muscles may occur with cervical spondylosis at the midcervical level, rather like a very indolent form of central cord syndrome. The reasons remain unclear; arterial, venous, and mechanical factors have been postulated.[6] Although it is common to see a minor discrepancy of two to three segments between the clinical sensory level and the level of the lesion, some patients with cervical cord lesions may have sensory levels many segments lower, as low as the midthoracic level.[7] Similarly, high thoracic lesions may cause signs mimicking lumbosacral-level disease, with a discrepancy of up to 11 segments between the level suggested clinically and the actual level of the lesion.[8]

The notion of false localizing signs has traditionally been limited to the CNS. There is another entire category of peripheral nervous system and neuromuscular disease causing signs that mimic CNS lesions, such as MG causing an ocular motility disorder simulating an **internuclear ophthalmoplegia** (myasthenic pseudo-INO), a small-fiber sensory neuropathy causing selective pain-and-temperature sensory loss (pseudosyringomyelia) or a large-fiber neuropathy causing "pseudotabes." Because of fascicular anatomy, localization of peripheral nerve lesions is frequently not straightforward.[9] For example, sparing of the forearm flexors and lack of sensory loss in the dorsal ulnar cutaneous territory should localize an ulnar neuropathy to the wrist, but these findings occur regularly with ulnar neuropathy at the elbow.[10]

False Rombergism: Sway with eyes closed not due to disease. It is common to see some sway with eyes closed in the absence of any organic neurological impairment, especially in histrionic patients. The swaying is usually from the hips and may be exaggerated. If the patient takes a step, the eyes may remain closed, which never happens with a bona fide **Romberg sign**. The instability can often be eliminated by diverting the patient's attention. Effective distracters are to ask the patient to detect numbers the examiner writes on the forehead with his or her finger, wiggle the tongue, or to perform finger-to-nose testing. Having the shoes off and watching the toe movements may be very informative. The toes of the patient with histrionic sway are often extended; the patient with organic imbalance flexes the toes strongly and tries to grip the floor.

Far point of accommodation: The distance at which a distant image is focused on the retina with no accommodative effort. A person with a perfectly normal eye has a far point of infinity and distant objects are properly focused on the fovea. See **hyperopia and myopia** and **near point of accommodation**.

Fasciculation: Fine, rapid, flickering or vermicular twitching movements due to contraction of a bundle, or fasciculus, of muscle fibers, which vary in size and intensity from so faint and small as to only slightly ripple the surface of the overlying skin to coarse and impossible to overlook (Video F.1). They are random, irregular, fleeting and inconstant. Sometimes fasciculations are abundant, and at other times detection requires a careful search.

Fasciculations are a characteristic feature of motor neuron disease and serve as a very useful marker for the disease; the diagnosis should remain circumspect when they are not demonstrable. Fasciculations can also occur in any chronic denervating process, including radiculopathy and peripheral neuropathy. In chronic denervating disease resulting in an enlarged motor unit territory, slight muscle contraction may activate a larger-than-normal number of muscle fibers, causing a visible twitch referred to as a **contraction fasciculation**. These do not have the same significance as spontaneous fasciculations. Contraction fasciculations may be seen occasionally in normal individuals, especially in the small hand muscles.

Fasciculations unaccompanied by atrophy or weakness do not necessarily indicate the presence of a serious disease process. About 70% of the population have occasional benign fasciculations. Hypercaffeinism is a common cause of fasciculations in normal individuals. Some patients, most often older men, have prominent fasciculations without other abnormality, most often in the calves.

Fast foot maneuver: A quick step trick used by patients with hip and leg weakness when asked to step onto a footstool. Because of feeling unsafe, the patient prefers to get both feet on the stool before attempting to straighten the knees. A normal person steps up with one foot and straightens the knee while simultaneously bringing up the trailing foot. The patient with hip girdle or quadriceps weakness quickly brings up the trailing foot before straightening the knee of the leading leg; this has been referred to as the "fast foot maneuver."

Fatigability: As generally used, a decline in the peak force of contraction of a muscle on repeated testing, or the inability to sustain a contraction, also referred to as fatigable weakness. Fatigability and fatigable weakness are objective signs on examination, as opposed to fatigue, a symptom common in many general medical and neurologic illnesses.[11] A decline in strength on repeated contractions is a cardinal symptom of neuromuscular transmission disorders, especially MG. Fatigable ptosis, another sign common in MG, is brought out or worsened by sustained upgaze. Failure of nystagmus to persist when the head is maintained in the provoking position on **Dix-Hallpike** maneuver is referred to as fatigable nystagmus.

Femoral nerve stretch (traction) test (reverse straight leg raising test): A maneuver to elicit pain in patients with suspected high lumbar radiculopathy. The vast majority, about 85%, of lumbosacral radiculopathies involve either the L5 or S1 roots. Occasional patients present with anterior or lateral leg pain and the possibility arises of L2, L3, or L4 radiculopathy. Just as the **straight leg raising test** is useful for L5 or S1 radiculopathy, this reverse straight leg raising test, more commonly referred to as the femoral nerve stretch test (FNST), may be useful as a way of eliciting root stretch in L2–L4 radiculopathies. With the patient prone and the knee flexed, the examiner pulls upward on the knee or ankle to extend the hip. Reproducing the patient's anterior thigh pain is significant, back pain less so. The femoral nerve stretch test is commonly confused with **Ely's test** but is not the same.

Because the FNST involves hip extension, the patient with SI joint disease, and perhaps facet joint disease, may develop pain in the lower back (Yeoman's test). Theoretically, the patient with SI joint disease should have pain whether the knee is flexed or extended, but in a high lumbar radiculopathy pain should be worse with the knee flexed; it is difficult to find mention of this point in the literature. The FNST is essentially identical to the psoas sign, which is positive in patients with appendicitis and psoas abscess. See **reverse straight leg raising test, Ely's test.**

Festinating gait: The gait characteristic of PD, in which the patient walks with increasing speed but very short steps as if chasing the center of gravity forward; see **gait disorders.**

Fifth finger sign: See **digiti quinti sign.**

Fine motor control: Manual dexterity, the ability to coordinate and control distal extremity movements (Video F.2). Fine motor movements are delicate functions that require smooth interactions between the different components of the motor system as well as normal sensory function. The CST preferentially innervates distal muscles and is in large part responsible for fractionated individual finger movements. Loss of fine motor control is one of the **subtle signs of hemiparesis**. Distal dexterity would also be impossible without normal cerebellar input, as well as normal extrapyramidal function. Examination of fine motor functions is therefore a useful screening motor test, but abnormalities are nonspecific and require further testing to identify the faulty system. Useful fine motor tests include **rapid alternating movements,** such as the **finger tapping test,** asking the patient to simulate flicking water from the fingertips, make piano-playing movements, and alternate touching each fingertip to the thumb as rapidly and repetitively as possible.

Impaired foot tapping may occur as an early manifestation of a CST lesion, and some have suggested that examination of foot tapping is as informative as the Babinski sign in detecting a CST lesion (see **Babinski's plantar sign**).

Finger agnosia: An inability to name or recognize fingers; a type of **autotopagnosia**. It may involve the individual fingers of the patient's own hands or the hands of the examiner. The patient loses the ability to name individual fingers, point to fingers named by the examiner, or move named fingers on request, in the absence of any other naming deficit. Finger agnosia and right–left confusion, along with agraphia and acalculia, make up Gerstmann's syndrome. Finger agnosia alone is not highly localizing, but when all components of the syndrome are present the lesion is likely to lie in the dominant inferior parietal lobule, particularly in the region of the angular gyrus and subjacent white matter.

Some caution is necessary. Many normal individuals cannot name the index, middle, and ring fingers. Some of this is cultural, related to educational level and region of origin. Normal individuals in certain regions of the United States may refer to the index finger as the "dog finger," "poison finger," or "statue of liberty finger."

Finger chase test: See **finger-to-nose test**.

Finger drop: Weakness of finger extension in the absence of weakness of wrist extension. Finger drop without wrist drop is the typical presentation of a posterior interosseous nerve (PIN) lesion. The wrist deviates radially on extension because of weakness of the PIN-innervated extensor carpi ulnaris with preservation of the main trunk–innervated extensor carpi radialis longus, which provides most of the power for wrist extension (Fig. F.4). When all the fingers are equally weak the problem is usually a straightforward PIN palsy, but when only one or two fingers are dropped the problem becomes more complicated and several alternative diagnostic possibilities arise. Tendon rupture in patients with rheumatoid arthritis (Vaughan-Jackson syndrome) tends to drop the small or ring finger first. Even in PIN palsy, some fingers may be affected more than others; most often the ring and small fingers are selectively dropped, producing a posture that superficially resembles an ulnar **claw hand**. This was referred to as a "pseudoulnar claw hand" by turn-of-the-19th-century French neurologists, who pointed out how it could be confused with ulnar neuropathy. A selective thumb drop may also occur in PIN neuropathy (Fig. F.5). Occasionally, cervical radiculomyelopathy will also selectively drop the ring and small fingers, which has been referred to as Ono's hand, myelopathy hand, and the pseudopseudoulnar claw hand.[12] Selective vulnerability of the posterior interosseous fascicles in retrohumeral radial neuropathy may cause confusion with a PIN lesion. Rarely, focal myopathy of the forearm extensors may mimic a PIN lesion. MMN has a predilection for the radial nerve and tends to present as wrist or finger drop without atrophy (Fig. F.6).[13]

Finger escape sign: Drift of the small and ring fingers into abduction with variable flexion within 30 to 60 seconds after holding the hands outstretched. The finger escape sign has been reported as a sign of UMN dysfunction, especially in patients with cervical spondylotic myelopathy. The finger escape sign is widely cited in Orthopedic and Neurosurgery textbooks. It is essentially identical to **myelopathy hand** and similar to the **digiti quinti sign**, which have been long recognized as one of the **subtle signs of hemiparesis** and occur with lesions anywhere along the corticospinal pathway. The same inability to adduct the small finger occurs in ulnar neuropathy (**Wartenberg's sign**).

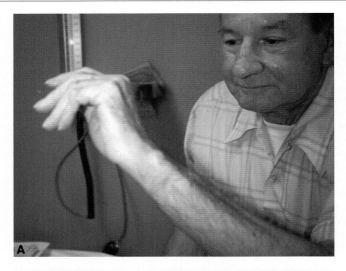

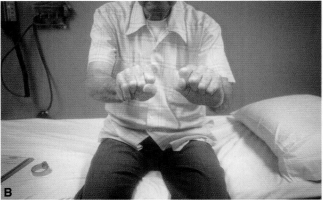

Figure F.4. Posterior interosseous neuropathy causing **(A)** finger drop without wrist drop and **(B)** radial deviation on wrist extension (patient's left hand). (From Campbell WW. *DeJong's the Neurologic Examination.* 7th ed. Philadelphia, PA: Wolters Kluwer Health/Lippincott Williams & Wilkins; 2013, with permission.)

Finger flexor reflex (Wartenberg's sign): A C8–T1 reflex mediated through both the median and ulnar nerves (see Video A.3). It may be elicited in two ways (1) with the patient's hand supinated, e.g., resting on the thigh, with the fingers slightly flexed, the examiner places her fingers against the patient's fingers and taps the backs of her own fingers lightly, or (2) with the patient's hand in the air, palm down, the examiner touches fingers with palm up, with the blow delivered in an upward direction from below. The response is flexion of the patient's fingers and the distal phalanx of the thumb. Wartenberg considered it one of the most important upper

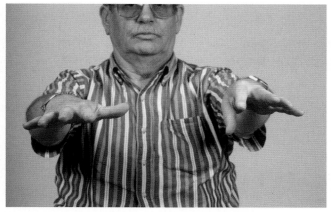

Figure F.5. Weakness primarily affecting thumb and index finger extension in a diabetic with a posterior interosseous nerve palsy.

extremity reflexes. How to elicit the finger flexor reflex is nicely demonstrated at the website for Stanford Medicine 25, An Initiative to Revive the Culture of Bedside Medicine (http://stanfordmedicine25.stanford.edu/the25/tendon.html). The reflex may be exaggerated in CST disease and depressed with C8 or T1 radiculopathy. The **Hoffman's** and **Trömner's** signs are alternative methods of delivering the stretch stimulus. The finger flexor reflex is not elicited routinely but is one of the occasionally useful DTRs (see Table D.1).

Finger rolling test: See **forearm rolling, thumb rolling,** and **subtle signs of hemiparesis.**

Finger tapping test: A test of **fine motor control** and coordination, usually done by having the patient extend the thumb and tap with the index finger on the tip or the crease of the interphalangeal joint as rapidly as possible, comparing the speed and dexterity on the two sides. Loss of dexterity and **fine motor control** are characteristic of CST lesions, **bradykinesia** may be brought out in PD and similar disorders, and cerebellar disease causes clumsiness. In CST lesions, the other fingers may move in concert due to loss of the ability to fractionate individual finger movements (Fisher's sign). Neuropsychologists have more formal versions of the test. Rapid foot tapping accomplishes the same end for the lower extremity. Normals can execute foot taps at 2 to 4 Hz, or 20 to 40 in 10 seconds.

Studies of the finger tapping test have shown a sensitivity of 16% to 79%, a specificity of 88% to 98%, positive LR of 4.7, and negative LR of 0.5 in the detection of contralateral hemispheric disease.[14] Studies of the foot tapping test have shown a sensitivity of 11% to 23%, a specificity of 89% to 94%, and insignificant LRs in the detection of contralateral hemispheric disease.[14]

Finger-to-nose (FTN, finger-nose-finger) test: A test used primarily to screen for **intention tremor,** incoordination, and **past pointing.** With the arm extended, the patient touches the tip of the index finger to the tip of his nose, then to the tip of the examiner's finger, then back to the tip of his nose, slowly at first, then rapidly, with the eyes open and then closed. The examiner's finger may be moved about during

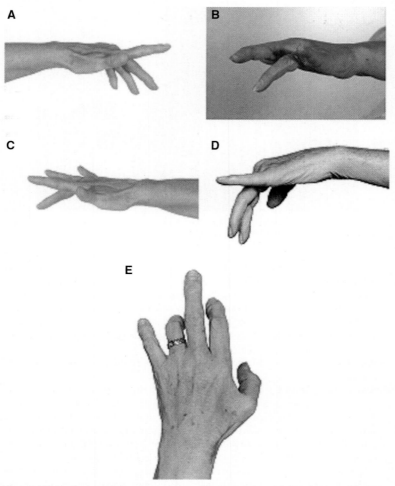

Figure F.6. Typical weakness of extension of individual fingers in multifocal motor neuropathy **(A–E)**. This implies differential conduction block in the terminal motor branches of the posterior interosseous nerve.

the test, and the patient asked to try to touch the moving target as it is placed in different locations at different distances and to move both slowly and quickly. The examiner may pull his finger away and make the patient chase it (**finger chase test**); fully extending the arm in this way can bring out mild **intention tremor** (see Video C.3).

During the FTN test, an **intention tremor** becomes more marked, coarse, and irregular as the finger approaches the target. There may be little tremor during the midrange of the movement, but near the end the tremor erupts. A patient with severe **appendicular ataxia** may not be able to touch hand to head, much less finger to nose. Performing the FTN test against slight resistance may cause mild ataxia to become more obvious, or latent ataxia evident. In a series of 444 patients with unilateral cerebellar lesions, mostly tumors, intention tremor was present in 29%.[14]

Patients with sensory ataxia also have an interesting constellation of findings. Because of neuropathic tremor and sensory ataxia, the FTN test is abnormal, but in a little recognized and reported phenomenon, the tremor actually *improves* with eyes closed.[15] Some of the tremor in sensory ataxia appears to be due to visually guided voluntary corrections of deviations from the intended track with eyes open. Eyes closed, the tremor may abate because the patient cannot see that a deviation is occurring and does not attempt to correct it. He may grope wildly off target but move in a straighter line.

The FTN test done eyes closed may also bring out **past pointing** in the presence of vestibular imbalance or a cerebellar hemispheric lesion. The **heel-to-shin** and toe-to-finger tests are similar maneuvers done to evaluate the lower extremity.

Finkelstein's test: A maneuver to elicit pain in the presence of DeQuervain's disease, a cause of hand pain sometimes confused with CTS. DeQuervain's disease is an inflammatory tenosynovitis that involves the extensor muscles of the thumb, primarily the extensor pollicis brevis. Patients develop pain in the wrist and thumb, primarily involving the radial aspect of the wrist, with tenderness to palpation over the anatomical snuff box. Extension of the thumb against resistance causes pain, but passive extension is painless. In Finkelstein's test, the patient places the thumb in the palm and wraps the fingers around it. The examiner then slowly pushes the wrist in an ulnar direction (Fig. F.7). This stretching of the inflamed thumb extensor tendons reproduces the pain. Mild discomfort with forced ulnar deviation is expected. Patients with active DeQuervain's disease have exquisite pain with Finkelstein's test.

Fist-edge-palm (fist-palm-side, Luria three step, Luria manual sequencing) test: One of the **alternating sequences tests,** which are particularly useful in the evaluation of suspected frontal lobe disease. The patient is asked to repetitively place the hand down in a series of motions: fist, edge of hand, palm, over and over. There is a tendency to **perseveration** and difficulty accurately executing the sequences of hand positions. The examiner demonstrates the task, and then the patient should reproduce it at least 6 times without error.

Fistula test: A test used to reproduce vertigo and nystagmus by increasing and decreasing the pressure in the external ear canal in patients with a perilymphatic fistula or superior canal dehiscence. The test is usually done with a pneumatoscope by an otorhinolaryngologist, but sometimes simple digital pressure against the tragus closing the ear canal can reproduce dramatic nystagmus and vertigo (Hennebert's sign). For a video showing the development of nystagmus in response to the application of pressure on the external auditory canal, see Video Link F.3[16].

Fixation instability: A disorder in which there is an inability to maintain steady fixation because of the intrusion of movements that interrupt fixation and move the eyes away from primary position and then return; see **saccadic intrusions.**

Fixed dystonia (traumatic dystonia, peripherally induced dystonia, complex region pain syndrome dystonia): An uncommon, but severely disabling, condition that usually follows a minor peripheral injury, producing a fixed posture and a pain syndrome. The abnormal postures typically involve flexion of the fingers, wrists, and

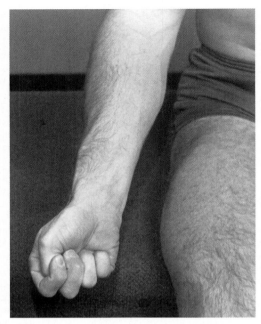

Figure F.7. Finkelstein's test for DeQuervain's thumb extensor tendonitis. With the thumb trapped, forceful ulnar deviation of the wrist stretches the thumb extensor tendons. (From Cipriano JJ. *Photographic Manual of Regional Orthopaedic and Neurological Tests*. 5th ed. Philadelphia, PA: Wolters Kluwer Health/Lippincott Williams & Wilkins, 2010; with permission.)

elbows; plantar flexion of the toes; plantar flexion and inversion of the ankle; and flexion of the knee.[17] There is apparently a psychogenic component in some cases.

Flail arm(s): Complete flaccid paralysis of one or both upper extremities; may be seen in motor neuron disease or brachial plexopathy. Patients who have suffered a severe, panplexus traumatic plexopathy may be left with a completely flaccid and useless upper extremity. In motor neuron disease, the monomelic variant (Hirayama's disease) may lay waste to one upper extremity, especially in young men. Sporadic ALS often begins in one upper extremity and may then spread to the other, leaving the patient with severely weak and wasted arms with little involvement elsewhere (flail arm variant, brachial amyotrophic diplegia, Vulpian-Bernhart syndrome, man in the barrel syndrome).[18] See **flail leg**.

Flail foot: A foot with minimal or no movement in any direction, usually the result of a sciatic nerve injury or severe polyneuropathy.

Flail leg: Similar to the **flail arm** syndrome, ALS may remain strikingly limited to the lower extremities for a prolonged period of time (pseudo-polyneuritic variant).[18]

Flapping tremor: See **asterixis**.

Flexion-adduction sign: A posture of flexion at the elbow and adduction at the shoulder, characteristic of neuralgic amyotrophy.[19] Abduction and lateral rotation of the arm, with the elbow in extension, increases the pain (Fig. F.8).

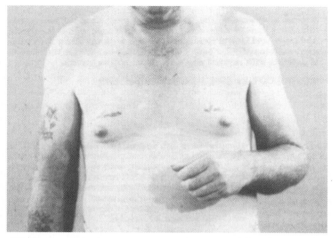

Figure F.8. Flexion adduction posture maintained by patient with neuralgic amyotrophy. (From Waxman SG. The flexion-adduction sign in neuralgic amyotrophy. *Neurology.* 1979;29:1301–1304, with permission.)

Flexion reflex: A primitive, polysynaptic, segmental avoidance or withdrawal reflex. The flexion response includes flexion of the hip and knee, and dorsiflexion of the ankle and toes, all serving to remove the threatened part from danger. The response is suppressed with maturation of the nervous system, but may reappear in various forms in the presence of disease. **Babinski's plantar sign** is a component of this reflex. In patients with SCI, the flexion reflex may reappear in the form of violent **flexor spasms**. See **paraplegia in flexion, triple flexion response.**

Flexor spasms: (1) Violent attacks of lower extremity flexion in SCI patients when the primitive **flexion reflex** is triggered, often along with an episode of autonomic dysreflexia; (2) a type of epileptic spasm, most often seen in infants with West syndrome.[20] The attacks are usually bilateral and symmetrical with a brief phasic event followed by a slower tonic event. Classic salaam attacks or jackknife spasms produce flexion of the neck, waist, arms, and legs with abduction or adduction of the arms. Mixed flexor-extensor spasms are more common than pure flexor spasms.

Flick sign: A sign elicited when taking the history in suspected CTS. See **carpal tunnel syndrome provocative tests.**

Fluent aphasia: See **aphasia.**

Flycatcher tongue: See **trombone tongue.**

Foot drop: Weakness of foot dorsiflexion. The term is used for moderate to severe weakness that is noticeable on watching the patient walk. Mild foot drop may cause no more than a subtle failure of the toes on the affected side to clear with the same margin as the normal side, so asymmetry of toe lift may be the earliest evidence of foot drop. Asymmetry in the wear of the toes of the shoes may help confirm the suspicion. With severe foot drop, the patient walks with a **steppage gait**, raising the affected leg higher off the ground by exaggerated flexion at the hip and knee, to

permit the toes to clear during the stride phase, often with the foot dangling use-
lessly (Video F.3). In normal walking, heel strike occurs first. With a foot
drop, there may be an audible double slap as the toes contact the floor first,
followed by the heel.

Common causes of unilateral foot drop include peroneal nerve palsy and L5 radiculopathy. Weakness of ankle inversion is a key clinical sign indicating that a foot
drop is due to L5 radiculopathy and not peroneal neuropathy at the knee. Causes
of bilateral foot drop include ALS, CMT, and other severe peripheral neuropathies
and certain forms of muscular dystrophy.

Foot dystonia: See **dystonic foot.**

Foot tapping test: See **finger tapping test, fine motor control.**

Foraminal compression test: See **Spurling's sign.**

Forced ductions: Pushing and pulling on the anesthetized globe in order to passively move it through an impaired range. An eye affected by ocular muscle weakness, MG, or an ocular motor nerve palsy moves freely and easily through a full
range. An eye affected by restrictive myopathy, such as thyroid eye disease, or an
entrapped muscle cannot be moved passively any better than actively. Forced ductions are sometimes done in the investigation of ocular motility disorders.

Forced grasping: See **grasp reflex.**

Forearm rolling test: One of the **subtle signs of hemiparesis** and a sensitive indicator of neurological pathology.[21] The patient is instructed to make fists, hold the
forearms horizontally so that the fists and distal forearms overlap with the palms
pointed more or less toward the umbilicus, and then rotate the fists around each
other, first in one direction and then the other (**Fig. F.9, Videos** F.2, **F.4, and F.5**).
Normal patients will have about an equal excursion of both forearms so that the
fists and forearms roll about each other symmetrically. With a unilateral CST lesion, the involved side does not move as much as the normal side, so the patient
will appear to plant, fix, or "post" one forearm and to rotate the opposite forearm
around it. Finger roll is a version of the same test, with the patient rotating just the
index fingers; again the finger on the abnormal side will move less than its fellow.
In the thumb rolling test, the patient rotates only the thumbs. In a series of patients
with mild hemiparesis, thumb rolling was more sensitive (88%) than pronator drift
(47%), forearm rolling (65%), or index finger rolling (65%).[22] Patients with bradykinesia or rigidity from extrapyramidal disease may also show decreased excursion
of the affected limbs.

Studies of forearm rolling have shown a sensitivity of 17% to 87%, a specificity of
97% to 98%, positive LR of 15.6, and negative LR of 0.6 in the detection of contralateral hemispheric disease.[14] Studies of index finger rolling have shown a sensitivity
of 33% to 42%, a specificity of 92% to 98%, positive LR of 6.0, and negative LR of
0.7 in the detection of contralateral hemispheric disease.[14]

Foreign accent syndrome: An unusual speech disorder causing the patient to
sound as though he has developed a foreign accent. The foreign accent syndrome
usually affects patients with some form of aphasia, dysarthria, dysprosodia, or
speech apraxia. It has been reported as the only manifestation of a cortical lesion,
without any clearly definable **dysarthria, aphasia,** or **apraxia** of speech, but with a
sufficiently altered speech rhythm and melody to create the impression the patient
was not speaking the native language.

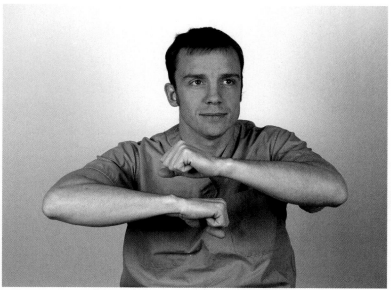

Figure F.9. Testing for a corticospinal tract lesion using forearm rolling. The involved extremity tends to have a lesser excursion as the forearms roll about each other so that the normal extremity tends to rotate around the abnormal extremity, which tends to remain relatively fixed. Patients with mild corticospinal tract lesions may have an abnormal arm roll test in the absence of clinically detectable weakness to formal strength testing. (From Campbell WW. *DeJong's the Neurologic Examination.* 7th ed. Philadelphia, PA: Wolters Kluwer Health/Lippincott Williams & Wilkins; 2013, with permission.)

Freezing: A phenomenon common in PD. In the midst of a motor act, the patient will suddenly freeze in place, unable to move for a short time. Freezing may occur when first starting to walk (start-hesitation), when approaching an obstacle, even when talking or eating.

Freiburg's test: A maneuver used in the diagnosis of piriformis syndrome; see **piriformis syndrome provocative tests.**

Frey's auriculotemporal syndrome: See **gustatory sweating.**

Froment's sign: (1) A substitution movement to compensate for weakness of thumb adduction, seen most often in ulnar neuropathy. When trying to hold a piece of paper tightly between the thumb and the radial aspect of the hand as the examiner tries to extract it, the patient flexes the interphalangeal joint of the thumb with the flexor pollicis longus, trying to secure the paper with the tip of the thumb rather than the side **(Fig. F.10, Video F.6)**; (2) increased tone in the examined limb as it is passively moved while another body part, usually the opposite limb, is contracted, such as by having the patient use the other hand to make a fist, draw circles in the air, or imitate screwing in a lightbulb. The maneuver is used as a way to bring out subtle increased resistance to passive movement. PD often begins

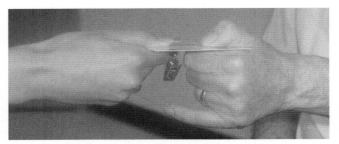

Figure F.10. Froment's sign. The patient attempts to grasp a piece of paper between the thumb and the radial border of the hand. In ulnar neuropathy, the IP joint flexes to compensate for weakness of the adductor pollicis. (From Berg D, Worzala K. *Atlas of Adult Physical Diagnosis*. Philadelphia, PA: Wolters Kluwer Health/Lippincott Williams and Wilkins; 2006, with permission.)

unilaterally, frequently in one limb, and a positive Froment's sign is very helpful in confirming one's suspicions.[23] Such a reinforcement-related tone increase may also be seen in other disorders, including ET and normal aging; (3) a cogwheel phenomenon without rigidity; (4) weakness of the flexor pollicis longus and flexor digitorum profundus to the index finger in anterior interosseous nerve palsy (the same as the **OK sign**).

Frontal bossing: Protuberance of the forehead, usually a sign of congenital hydrocephalus **(Fig. F.11)**. Bossing of the calvarium may also result from a meningioma because of hyperostosis, the site depending on the location of the tumor;

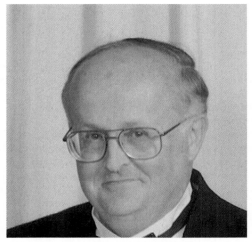

Figure F.11. A patient with frontal bossing due to hydrocephalus since early childhood. (From Orient JM, Sapira JD. *Sapira's Art & Science of Bedside Diagnosis*. 4th ed. Philadelphia, PA: Wolters Kluwer Health/Lippincott Williams & Wilkins; 2010, with permission.)

e.g., parasaggital tumor causing midline bossing. Frontal bossing also occurs in **acromegaly**, fragile X syndrome, extramedullary hematopoiesis as might occur in thalassemia (chipmunk facies), cleidocranial dystosis, Cruzon's syndrome, and Hurler's syndrome.

Frontal lobe gait disorders: Abnormal gait due to disease of the frontal lobe or its connections; see **gait disorders.**

Frontal release signs (FRSs): Responses that are normally present in the developing nervous system, but disappear to a greater or lesser degree with maturation. While normal in infants and children, when present in an older individual they may be evidence of neurological disease. The responses most often included as FRS include the **palmomental, grasp, snout,** and **suck reflexes.** Since these signs are frequently present in normal infants, they are referred to as **primitive reflexes.**

These signs occur most often in patients with severe dementias, diffuse encephalopathy, after head injury, and in other states in which the pathology is diffuse but involves particularly the frontal lobes or the frontal association areas. The significance and usefulness of some of these release signs has been questioned. Studies have found that the **palmomental reflex** and the **Hoffman reflex** and its variants, which are sometimes classified as FRS and sometimes as corticospinal signs, are present in a significant proportion of normal individuals.

An investigation of the PMR, snout, and **corneomandibular reflexes** found at least one of these was present in 50.5% of normal subjects in the third through ninth decades of life.[24] The PMR was the most frequent reflex at all ages, occurring in 20% to 25% of normal individuals in the third and fourth decades. In 20% of the group, more than one of the reflexes was elicited, and in about 2% all three were present. A study of 240 healthy subjects found that FRS were present at a low frequency: PMR (24.5%), suck (3.3%), persistent glabellar (2.5%), grasp (0.83%), snout (0%). In 2% of subjects there were two reflexes, and 0.42% had three reflexes.[25] In patients without neurologic disease, the responses are an isolated finding and are weak and fatigable, disappearing with repetitive stimuli.

Clearly, these reflexes are a normal phenomenon in a significant proportion of the healthy population. They must be interpreted with caution and kept in clinical context. Even when such reflexes are briskly active in an appropriate clinical setting, these responses do not have great localizing value, suggesting instead the presence of diffuse and widespread dysfunction of the hemispheres. See **pathologic reflexes.**

Frozen shoulder (adhesive capsulitis): A common cause of upper extremity pain that may present to the neurologist because of confusion with cervical radiculopathy or entrapment neuropathy.[26] It is characterized by the insidious onset of pain, often worse at night, and loss of motion of the shoulder and occurs more commonly in women. Loss of range of motion of the glenohumeral joint is the key finding, often most significant for external rotation with sharp pain at the end of the range. The etiology is unknown.

Functional (nonorganic, hysterical, psychogenic) gait disorder: See **gait disorders.**

Functional (nonorganic, hysterical, psychogenic) signs: Clinical signs not due to organic neurologic disease. Even the terminology used to describe such symptoms is unsatisfactory. Certainly the term *hysteria/hysterical* is perjorative and outdated, but whether it is best for the consulting neurologist to state the findings are nonorganic, functional, psychogenic, psychosomatic, medically unexplained, nonphysiologic, conversion disorder, supratentorial or stress related is far from clear and many physicians use a personally preferred code or state there is no evidence or neurologic disease.[27]

There are three elements in reaching such a diagnosis: excluding neurologic disease, demonstrating "positive signs" of nonorganicity, and establishing the presence of psychopathology severe enough to explain the symptomatology. The latter cannot be stressed enough. Patients who have a psychiatric condition severe enough to produce a symptomatic neurologic deficit require a psychiatric evaluation. If the psychiatrist disagrees there is substantial emotional morbidity present, the neurologist would be well advised to rethink the diagnosis. In addition, the patient needs treatment of the psychiatric condition. Obtaining psychiatric evaluation and treatment, however, often becomes a delicate matter. Even when accomplished, it seems psychiatrists exercise an abundance of caution in rendering their opinions.

Organic and functional deficits may coexist: the problem of functional or psychogenic overlay.[28] Some patients embellish by nature, others may exaggerate a real deficit for fear the physician may not take them seriously. The dilemma lies in performing an adequate workup to exclude organic disease versus overtesting or overtreatment of a functional disorder, which may reinforce and entrench the symptoms.

Functional disorders fall into the categories of somatoform disorder (somatic symptom disorder in *DSM-5*), where the physical symptoms are produced unconsciously, and factitious disorder or malingering, where there is an intent to deceive. Reliably distinguishing deficits produced unconsciously from those knowingly feigned is practically impossible. *DSM-5* has renamed "conversion disorder" as "conversion disorder (functional neurologic symptom disorder)."

Practicing with an attitude of "guilty until proven innocent," presumes any condition is functional until proven otherwise. This attitude is especially common if the patient is young, female, or has a history or depression or anxiety. When confronted with an enigmatic patient, physicians are often quick to conclude the problem is nonorganic. But many diseases, particularly neurologic ones, may present with puzzling manifestations. With MS presenting as nonspecific sensory symptoms, the majority of misdiagnoses in women are psychiatric, and those in men orthopedic, suggesting a gender-dependent bias in the way physicians interpret sensory complaints.[29] An "innocent until proven guilty" practice style often permits finding disease where none was previously thought to exist.

Misdiagnosis creates medicolegal risk. Malpractice litigation, sometimes with psychiatrists as codefendants, has involved patients diagnosed as psychogenic who proved to have very real neurological conditions. Less common is a suit due to subjecting a patient with a functional deficit to risky diagnostic procedures or treatments, such as TPA.

Estimates are that as many as two-thirds of neurologic patients have some symptomatic psychiatric comorbidity, most commonly depression, anxiety, and personality disorder.[30] Depression occurs both as a coincidental, endogenous disorder and in reaction to a disturbing medical illness. Studies have shown that between 10% and 30% of patients seen by neurologists have symptoms for which there is no current pathophysiological explanation; the higher figure is most often quoted, with statements such as that up to one-third of neurologic outpatients have a functional disorder. For experienced neurologists practicing "innocent until proven guilty," the lower figure is likely more realistic.

All investigators seem to agree that the most common functional neurologic disorder is psychogenic nonepileptic seizures, and this common disorder only accounts for 10% to 20% of patients referred to epileptologists.[31] Even assuming the one-third figure is accurate, a clinician is twice as likely to encounter a patient with organic disease and a coincidental emotional disturbance than one with purely psychogenic complaints. These odds increase for any concern other than seizures or a pain syndrome.

The error rate has declined with modern neuroimaging, but misdiagnoses continue to occur with regularity. Studies from the 1960s suggest that on follow-up more than half the patients with a diagnosis of a functional deficit ultimately developed clearly explanatory neurological or psychiatric conditions.[31] Influential papers by Slater in 1965 cautioned about the misdiagnosis of "hysteria."[32,33] More recent studies, "Slater revisited," suggest that an organic neurological diagnosis does not often subsequently emerge for medically unexplained symptoms. In a study with 6-year follow-up, 3 of 64 patients (4.7%) developed a neurological disorder that explained the original symptoms.[34] In a 12-year longitudinal study, only 1 of 42 patients (2.4%) developed a neurological disorder that explained the original presentation.[35] But in a similar study with 10-year follow-up, a clear neurological diagnosis was subsequently made for the original symptom in 11 of 73 patients (15%) thought to have conversion disorder causing pseudoneurological symptoms.[36] A study of 4,470 neurologic inpatient admissions concluded that only 9% had a purely functional disorder, and these patients were accumulated prior to or at the dawn of the MRI era.[37]

Before drawing conclusions, we must recognize the clinical acumen of clinicians of Slater's era and the limitations of neuroimaging. MRI is of no utility in dealing with many of the conditions neurologists frequently encounter, including most neuromuscular disease, many neuro-ophthalmologic disorders, movement disorders, and the early stages of degenerative conditions, not to mention migraine and other paroxysmal disorders. It has been said the modern neurologist practices "MRI-negative neurology." Patients with abnormal scans are usually straightforward; the real work begins when the initial scan is read as normal. Mistakes are made with some regularity because the wrong part of the neuraxis is scanned, contrast is not given, the scan is misread, or the distinction not made between central and peripheral nervous system disease. Spinal cord disease is a particularly difficult and diagnostically treacherous area with subtle clinical and radiologic findings that require a high level of expertise.

Major neurologic illnesses often initially diagnosed as conversion disorder, malingering, depression, anxiety, neurasthenia, or some other "functional" disorder include MG, MS, porphyria, GBS, **dystonia,** and botulism. The average patient with MG sees five to seven physicians before the correct diagnosis is made. Similar difficulties with diagnosis occur with MS. In a study of 50 consecutive MS patients, 58% had initially been given 41 wrong diagnoses, the patients had been referred to 2.2 ± 1.3 specialists before seeing a neurologist, and learned about their disease 3.5 years after the onset of symptoms.[29] It is axiomatic that the patient with acute intermittent porphyria sees, in sequence, the surgeon, the psychiatrist, and then the neurologist. Patients with GBS have died while the physicians caring for them continued to presume the shortness of breath and paresthesias represented hyperventilation, and many patients with GBS are sent out from the emergency department one or more times before the diagnosis is made. In one cooperative study on plasmapheresis in GBS, young women with the illness were diagnosed as "hysterical" 4 times more frequently than men or older women.

The issue of positive signs of nonorganicity is problematic. Many authors emphasize that the diagnosis of a functional deficit requires the presence of positive evidence of nonorganicity rather than simply the absence of evidence of organic disease. Techniques to "prove" a deficit is nonorganic have held a cherished place in neurology since the days of Charcot. But nearly all the examination techniques touted as proof of nonorganicity are fallible, particularly for sensory findings (see below). Many of the history and examination findings purported as helpful in separating functional and organic deficits are unreliable[31, 38]. The attitude of *la belle indifference* may be misleading. Some patients, especially with nondominant hemisphere lesions, have neglect syndromes, whereas others are stoic. It is not of value in discriminating real from nonorganic disease.[38] Either things such as apparent secondary gain, nonanatomic deficits, and variability of findings on examination have not been studied or investigations have shown they are neither sensitive nor specific for functional disorders.[31] A study of 30 consecutive neurology service admissions with acute structural nervous system damage were evaluated for the presence of seven of the most accepted features of nonorganicity: history of hypochondriasis, secondary gain, la belle indifference, nonanatomical sensory loss, **midline splitting** of pain or vibration, changing boundaries of hypalgesia, and giveaway weakness.[39] All subjects showed at least one of these findings, and most had three or four. The authors concluded that the presence of these "positive" findings of nonorganicity in patients with acute structural brain disease invalidates their use as pathognomonic evidence of a functional deficit. Movement disorders and paralysis were most often mislabeled as nonorganic. Women, homosexual men, those with psychiatric comorbidities, and patients with a seemingly plausible psychogenic explanation for the deficit were most at risk for misdiagnosis. Even the seemingly ironclad finding of spontaneous movement of an extremity in sleep that does not move as well during wakefulness could occur because of motor neglect (see **attentional deficits**). As summarized by McGee,[14] in studies of patients with known organic disorders, 8% have midline sensory splitting, 85% feel vibration in numb areas, 48% have sensory findings that change between examinations or do not make anatomical sense, and 33% have **collapsing weakness.** The long-held but erroneous belief that functional motor and sensory symptoms, such as weakness, tremor, and numbness, are more common on the left side of the body than the right has been convincingly disproven in a systematic review of 1,139 patients.[40]

See **coin-in-the-hand test, mirror test for functional visual loss, sunglasses sign, tubular visual fields,** and **Waddell signs.**

Functional (nonorganic, hysterical, psychogenic) sensory signs: Sensory disturbance not due to organic neurologic disease. The various methods and tricks for detecting nonorganic sensory loss are not entirely reliable, and this diagnosis should be made with caution. In one study of 30 consecutive patients admitted with acute structural CNS lesions, 29 had at least one nonphysiologic sensory finding on examination, including 23% with nonanatomical sensory loss and 70% with **midline splitting.**[39] See **functional signs.** Others have reported midline splitting in patients with organic disease; this is especially prone to occur with thalamic lesions.[41]

One of the obvious clues that sensory loss is nonorganic is failure to follow any sort of anatomical distribution. The demarcation between normal and abnormal often occurs at some strategic anatomical point that has no neurologic significance, such as a joint or skin crease, causing a finding such as numbness circumferentially below the elbow, wrist, shoulder, ankle, or knee. Nonorganic facial sensory loss often stops at the hairline and the angle of the jaw, a nonanatomic distribution. A real spinal sensory level on the trunk slants downward from back to front, but a functional level may be perfectly horizontal; nonorganic sensory loss may be much different on the front and back.

The term *stocking-glove* is used to describe both nonorganic sensory loss and peripheral neuropathy. The key to understanding this confusing usage is the type of stocking. When sensory loss due to length-dependent peripheral neuropathy extends to about the level of the knees, it appears in the hands, causing loss in a glove–knee sock distribution; with nonorganic sensory loss, the impairment may be distal to the wrists and ankles: a glove–ankle sock distribution.

With nonorganic sensory loss, the border between normal and abnormal is usually abrupt and well demarcated, more discrete than in organic sensory loss, and may vary from examination to examination, or even from minute to minute. Responses are typically inconsistent. In spite of complete loss of cutaneous sensibility, the patient may have intact stereognosis and graphesthesia, or in spite of complete loss of position sense the patient may be able to perform skilled movements and fine acts without difficulty, and have no Romberg sign. On finger-to-nose testing, the examiner may touch one finger of the "anesthetic" hand and ask the patient to touch her nose with it. A patient with organic exteroceptive sensory loss will not know which finger was touched; a patient with functional sensory loss uses the correct finger but has trouble finding the nose. The hand wandering widely before eventually finding the nose suggests histrionic tendencies. In the search test, the patient holds the involved hand in the air and searches for it with the unaffected hand. In nonorganic loss the patient may have no difficulty with this task, but with bona fide proprioceptive loss, performance is poor with either hand.

Sensory changes along the midline may provide useful clues. On the trunk, organic sensory loss typically stops short of midline because of the overlap from the opposite side, and splitting of the midline suggests nonorganicity. With nonorganic loss, the change may take place abruptly at the midline or even beyond it. This finding is not reliable on the face because there is less midline overlap on the face, so organic facial sensory loss may extend to the midline. With functional hemi-anesthesia, the midline change may include the penis, vagina, and rectum, and this finding is rare with organic lesions. There may even be midline splitting of vibration, so that the patient claims to perceive a difference in the intensity of vibration when the fork is placed just to right or left of the midline over the skull, sternum, or symphysis pubis, each a single bony structure, or comparing the medial ends of the clavicles or the medial incisor teeth. In all these locations, the vibration is transmitted to both sides, and patients with organic hemi-anesthesia do not perceive any difference in vibration along the midline. The reliability of this sign has not been validated; it can be misleading. Other signs suggestive of nonorganicity include a dissociation between pinprick and temperature, variability from trial to trial, history of hypochondriasis, secondary gain, nonanatomical sensory loss, and changing boundaries of hypalgesia. Gould et al have appropriately cautioned about the validity of hysterical signs and symptoms.[39]

Clinical subterfuge is often used to establish that sensory loss is nonorganic, such as asking the patient to respond "yes if you feel it, no if you don't" (yes–no or touch–no touch test). It is often possible to confuse the patient and confirm the absence of organic changes by checking sensation while the hands are in some bewildering position where it is difficult to tell which side is which, such as crossed behind the back or rotated with fingers interlocked (Bowles-Currier test).

The author has seen all of these "tricks" fail (i.e., indicate the sensory loss is not real when it is), at one time or another, save one: the SHOT syndrome. In the SHOT syndrome, the patient claims to have no Sight in the eye, no Hearing in the ear, no Olfaction in the nose, and no Touch sensation on the body, all on the same side. This pattern is of course utterly impossible on an anatomic basis, and its presence reliably indicates that hemi-body numbness is nonorganic.

Functional (nonorganic, hysterical, psychogenic) weakness: A pattern of weakness seen in patients whose motor deficit is "functional" and is not the result of neurologic disease. Some things are often useful in distinguishing organic from nonorganic weakness. The patient with functional weakness often displays **collapsing weakness** (give way or ratchety) on testing. The patient with bona fide weakness gives uniform resistance throughout the movement; if the examiner decreases his resistance, the patient will begin to win the battle. In functional weakness, if the examiner drops the resistance level, the patient with nonorganic weakness will not continue to push or pull. Instead, the patient will also stop resisting so that no matter how little force the examiner applies, there is an absence of follow-through and the patient never overcomes the examiner.

With functional weakness, there may be an increase or a decrease in strength with repeated testing. Contraction of the apparently weak muscle may be felt when the patient is asked to carry out movements with synergistic muscles, or the antagonists may be felt to contract when the patient is asked to contract the agonist (e.g., the triceps muscle twitches when the patient is told to flex the elbow). Functional testing may fail to confirm weakness suspected during strength testing. For example, there may be apparent foot dorsiflexion weakness, yet the patient is able to stand on the heel without difficulty. Coaching is often helpful in functional weakness. Strength improves if the examiner exhorts the patient not to give up, to keep pushing or pulling no matter what. Patients with nonorganic hemiparesis are more likely to have weakness of the sternomastoid, usually ipsilateral, but this muscle is rarely involved in bona fide hemiparesis because of its bilateral innervation. Evidence does not support the notion that functional weakness is more common on the left.[40]

In patients with weakness of one or both legs, **Hoover's sign,** the **abductor sign,** and the **Spinal Injuries Center test** may help to distinguish functional from bona fide weakness. It is very unusual for functional weakness to present in a peripheral nerve, plexus, or root distribution or to display a proximal/distal gradient.

With the **arm dropping test,** transient voluntary contraction in functional weakness may cause a brief hang-up before the arm collapses. The patient with functional weakness cannot control **associated movements,** which forms the basis of the Hoover and abductor signs. On the **Babinski trunk-thigh test,** a leg with nonorganic weakness fails to flex as expected. The latissimus dorsi that contracts with cough but not voluntarily is suspect. The patient with functional weakness may have a dramatic display of effort, grimacing and grunting when trying to contract the weak muscle. A movement such as a squat may be executed in a slow and laborious manner that actually requires greater than normal strength. Dynamometers have been used in various ways in an attempt to prove weakness is nonorganic.

Normal tone, normal DTRs, normal facial movements in the face of hemiparesis, an absence of trophic changes, normal sphincter function despite paraparesis or quadriparesis, **aphonia**, and a monoplegic dragging gait (see **gait disorders**) all suggest that weakness is nonorganic.

Fukuda stepping test: See **Unterberger-Fukuda stepping test.**

Video Links

F.1. Dramatic facial myokymia due to a rattlesnake bite. (From Kobayashi, SA. Images in clinical medicine. Perioral myokymia. *N Engl J Med.* 2013;368:e5.) Available at: http://www.nejm.org/doi/full/10.1056/NEJMicm1202778

F.2. Facial myokymia. (From Kathleen B. Digre, John A. Moran Eye Center, Neuro-ophthalmology Virtual Education Library [NOVEL], University of Utah.) Available at: http://stream.utah.edu/m/dp/frame.php?f=f50e328860fca754890

F.3. Development of nystagmus in response to the application of pressure on the external auditory canal. (From Chu H, Chung WH. Images in clinical medicine. Perilymph fistula test. *N Engl J Med.* 2012;366:e8.) Available at: http://www.nejm.org/doi/full/10.1056/NEJMicm1010568

References

1. Dennis M, Bowen WT, Cho L. *Mechanisms of Clinical Signs.* Sydney, New South Wales, Australia: Churchill Livingstone; 2012.
2. Keane JR. Bilateral seventh nerve palsy: analysis of 43 cases and review of the literature. *Neurology.* 1994;44:1198–1202.
3. Kobayashi SA. Images in clinical medicine. Perioral myokymia. *N Engl J Med.* 2013;368:e5.
4. May M, Klein SR. Differential diagnosis of facial nerve palsy. *Otolaryngol Clin North Am.* 1991;24:613–645.
5. James DG. Differential diagnosis of facial nerve palsy. *Sarcoidosis Vasc Diffuse Lung Dis.* 1997;14:115–120.
6. Larner AJ. False localising signs. *J Neurol Neurosurg Psychiatry.* 2003;74:415–418.
7. Hellmann MA, Djaldetti R, Luckman J, et al. Thoracic sensory level as a false localizing sign in cervical spinal cord and brain lesions. *Clin Neurol Neurosurg.* 2013;115:54–56.
8. Jamieson DR, Teasdale E, Willison, HJ. False localising signs in the spinal cord. *BMJ.* 1996;312:243–244.
9. Stewart JD. Peripheral nerve fascicles: anatomy and clinical relevance. *Muscle Nerve.* 2003;28:525–541.
10. Campbell WW, Pridgeon RM, Riaz G, et al. Sparing of the flexor carpi ulnaris in ulnar neuropathy at the elbow. *Muscle Nerve.* 1989;12:965–967.
11. Kluger BM, Krupp LB, Enoka RM. Fatigue and fatigability in neurologic illnesses: proposal for a unified taxonomy. *Neurology.* 2013;80:409–416.
12. Campbell WW, Buschbacher R, Pridgeon RM, et al. Selective finger drop in cervical radiculopathy: the pseudopseudoulnar claw hand. *Muscle Nerve.* 1995;18:108–110.
13. Slee M, Selvan A, Donaghy M. Multifocal motor neuropathy: the diagnostic spectrum and response to treatment. *Neurology.* 2007;69:1680–1687.
14. McGee, S. *Evidence Based Physical Diagnosis.* 3rd ed. Philadelphia, PA: Elsevier/Saunders; 2012.
15. Campbell WW. Some observations on sensory ataxia. *Ann Neurol.* 1984;16:151.
16. Chu H, Chung WH. Images in clinical medicine. Perilymph fistula test. *N Engl J Med.* 2012;366:e8.
17. Munts AG, Mugge W, Meurs TS, et al. Fixed dystonia in complex regional pain syndrome: a descriptive and computational modeling approach. *BMC Neurol.* 2011;11:53.
18. Wijesekera LC, Mathers S, Talman P, et al. Natural history and clinical features of the flail arm and flail leg ALS variants. *Neurology.* 2009;72:1087–1094.
19. Waxman SG. The flexion-adduction sign in neuralgic amyotrophy. *Neurology.* 1979;29:1301–1304.
20. Engel, J. *Seizures and Epilepsy.* 2nd ed. Oxford: Oxford University Press; 2013.
21. Sawyer RN Jr, Hanna JP, Ruff RL, et al. Asymmetry of forearm rolling as a sign of unilateral cerebral dysfunction. *Neurology.* 1993;43:1596–1598.

22. Nowak DA. The thumb rolling test: a novel variant of the forearm rolling test. *Can J Neurol Sci.* 2011;38:129–132.
23. Rodriguez-Oroz MC, Jahanshahi M, Krack P, et al. Initial clinical manifestations of Parkinson's disease: features and pathophysiological mechanisms. *Lancet Neurol.* 2009;8:1128–1139.
24. Jacobs L, Gossman MD. Three primitive reflexes in normal adults. *Neurology.* 1980;30:184–188.
25. Brown DL, Smith TL, Knepper LE. Evaluation of five primitive reflexes in 240 young adults. *Neurology.* 1998;51:322.
26. Robinson CM, Seah KT, Chee YH, et al. Frozen shoulder. *J Bone Joint Surg Br.* 2012;94:1–9.
27. Friedman JH, LaFrance WC Jr. Psychogenic disorders: the need to speak plainly. *Arch Neurol.* 2010;67:753–755.
28. Carter AB. The functional overlay. *Lancet.* 1967;2:1196–1200.
29. Levin N, Mor M, Ben Hur T. Patterns of misdiagnosis of multiple sclerosis. *Isr Med Assoc J.* 2003;5:489–490.
30. Reuber M, Mitchell AJ, Howlett SJ, et al. Functional symptoms in neurology: questions and answers. *J Neurol Neurosurg Psychiatry.* 2005;76:307–314.
31. Lanska DJ. Functional weakness and sensory loss. *Semin Neurol.* 2006;26:297–309.
32. Slater ET, Glithero E. A follow-up of patients diagnosed as suffering from "hysteria". *J Psychosom Res.* 1965;9:9–13.
33. Slater E. Diagnosis of "hysteria". *Br Med J.* 1965;1:1395–1399.
34. Crimlisk HL, Bhatia K, Cope H, et al. Slater revisited: 6 year follow up study of patients with medically unexplained motor symptoms. *BMJ.* 1998;316:582–586.
35. Stone J, Sharpe M, Rothwell PM, et al. The 12 year prognosis of unilateral functional weakness and sensory disturbance. *J Neurol Neurosurg Psychiatry.* 2003;74:591–596.
36. Mace CJ, Trimble MR. Ten-year prognosis of conversion disorder. *Br J Psychiatry.* 1996;169:282–288.
37. Lempert T, Dieterich M, Huppert D, et al. Psychogenic disorders in neurology: frequency and clinical spectrum. *Acta Neurol Scand.* 1990;82:335–340.
38. Gould R, Miller BL, Goldberg MA, et al. The validity of hysterical signs and symptoms. *J Nerv Ment Dis.* 1986;174:593–597.
39. Stone J, Smyth R, Carson A, et al. La belle indifference in conversion symptoms and hysteria: systematic review. *Br J Psychiatry.* 2006;188:204–209.
40. Stone J, Sharpe M, Carson A, et al. Are functional motor and sensory symptoms really more frequent on the left? A systematic review. *J Neurol Neurosurg Psychiatry.* 2002;73:578–581.
41. Stone J, Zeman A, Sharpe M. Functional weakness and sensory disturbance. *J Neurol Neurosurg Psychiatry.* 2002;73:241–245.

G

Gaenslen's test: See **sacroiliac joint signs.**

Gag reflex: Constriction of the pharyngeal musculature with elevation of the soft palate elicited by touching the pharynx or palate, comparing the activity on the two sides. The reflex is obtained by touching the lateral oropharynx in the region of the anterior faucial pillar with a tongue blade, applicator stick, or similar object (pharyngeal reflex), or by touching one side of the soft palate or uvula (palatal reflex). The pharyngeal reflex is the more active of the two. When unilateral pharyngeal weakness is present, the raphe will deviate away from the weak side and toward the normal side (**curtain sign**). This movement is usually dramatic (**Video Link G.1**). Minor movements of the uvula and trivial deviations of the midline raphe are not of clinical significance. In normal adults, both palatal and pharyngeal reflexes are usually present, but there may be inter- and intra-individual variation in the intensity of the stimulus required. The gag reflex may be bilaterally absent in some normal individuals.[1] Unilateral absence usually signifies a lower cranial neuropathy. Like most bulbar muscles, the pharynx receives bilateral supranuclear innervation, and a unilateral cerebral lesion does not cause detectable weakness.

The gag reflex is often used to predict whether or not a patient will be able to swallow, especially after acute stroke. In fact, the gag reflex has little to do with normal swallowing. Higher cortical centers have to inhibit the gag response during normal swallowing. The gag reflex is useful but limited in assessing airway protection. Patients with an apparently intact gag reflex may still aspirate, and a patient with a depressed gag reflex may not.[2] A hyperactive gag reflex may occur with bilateral cerebral lesions, as in pseudobulbar palsy and ALS.

Gait apraxia: See **gait disorders.**

Gait disorders: Abnormalities of gait that may occur for many reasons. Some are primarily neurologic; others are not but are often confused with neurologic disorders. A nosology has been suggested that classifies abnormal gait syndromes into low-, mid-, and high-level disorders.[3] Low-level disorders are due to peripheral motor or sensory abnormalities, such as a myopathic gait or a steppage gait due to foot drop. Midlevel disorders result from disease involving the motor pathways and control centers, such as the basal ganglia and cerebellum. Examples include hemiplegic, paraplegic, cerebellar ataxic, parkinsonian, and choreic gait. Highest level disorders are due to disease of the integrative parts of the nervous systems, such as the frontal lobe. Examples include cautious gait, subcortical and frontal disequilibrium, isolated gait ignition failure, frontal gait disorder, and psychogenic gait disorder. Higher level gait disorders are characterized by various combinations of disequilibrium and impaired locomotion.[4] In contrast to the low- and midlevel gait disorders, there is typically a paucity of findings on formal neurologic examination. Description of the clinical semiology of gait disorders remains the most common approach. The common gait abnormalities are beautifully demonstrated at the website for Stanford Medicine 25, An Initiative to Revive the Culture of Bedside Medicine (**Video Link G.2**).

A patient with **foot drop** has weakness of the dorsiflexors of the foot and toes. When mild, this may be manifest only as a decrease in the toe clearance during the stride phase (see Video F.3). With more severe foot drop, the patient is in danger of tripping and may drag the toe when walking, characteristically wearing out the toe of the shoe. When foot drop is severe, the foot dangles uncontrollably during the swing phase. To compensate, she lifts the foot as high as possible, hiking the hip and flexing the hip and knee (steppage gait). The foot is thrown out and falls to the floor, toe first. The touching of toe followed by heel creates a "double tap" that has a different sound than the heel-first double tap of sensory ataxia. The patient is unable to stand on her heel, and when standing with her foot projecting over the edge of a step, the forefoot drops. Foot drops and steppage gait may be unilateral or bilateral. Common causes of unilateral foot drop and steppage gait include peroneal nerve palsy and L5 radiculopathy. Causes of bilateral foot drop and steppage gait include motor neuron disease, severe polyneuropathy and muscular dystrophy. In severe polyneuropathies, the steppage gait may have components of both sensory ataxia and foot drop.

The term *steppage (equine) gait* refers to a manner of walking in which the patient lifts one or both legs high during their respective stride phases, as if walking up steps though the surface is level. These unusually high steps may occur under two very different circumstances. Sensory ataxia is one of the causes of a steppage gait, sometimes referred to as a slapping or stamping gait because the patient lifts the feet up high and then slaps them down smartly to improve proprioceptive feedback. Patients with foot drop may also lift the knee high in order to help the foot clear the floor and avoid tripping. Since both of these gaits are "high stepping," both have been referred to as steppage gaits, but the causes and mechanisms are quite distinct.

In addition to the steppage gait that accompanies foot drop, weakness limited to other muscle groups may cause gait difficulties. With paralysis of the gastrocnemius and soleus muscles, the patient is unable to stand on the toes and unable to push off to enter the swing phase with the affected leg. This may cause a shuffling gait that is devoid of spring. In weakness of the quadriceps muscle (e.g., femoral neuropathy), there is weakness of knee extension, and the patient can only accept weight on the affected extremity by bracing the knee. When walking the knee is held stiffly, there is a tendency to fall if the knee bends. To avoid depending on the weak quadriceps, the knee may hyperextend (**genu recurvatum**). The patient has less difficulty walking backward than forward. Patients may experience particular difficulty extending the knee to enable weight-bearing while descending stairs. Lumbosacral radiculopathy may cause either foot drop or a unilateral **Trendelenburg gait**, or both. In addition, the patient with acute radiculopathy may walk with a list or pelvic tilt, accompanied by flattening of the normal lumbar lordosis. The patient may walk with small steps; if the pain is severe, she may place only the toes on the floor, since dorsiflexion of the foot aggravates the pain. Patients commonly use a cane to avoid bearing weight on the involved leg.

A myopathic (waddling) gait occurs when there is weakness of the hip girdle muscles, most often due to myopathy, and most characteristically due to muscular dystrophy. If the hip flexors are weak, there may be a pronounced **lordosis**. The hip abductor muscles are vital in stabilizing the pelvis while walking (see **Trendelenburg's sign**). When the weakness is bilateral, there is an exaggerated pelvic swing that results in a waddling gait. The patient walks with a broad base, with an exaggerated rotation of the pelvis, rolling or throwing the hips from side to side with every step to shift the weight of the body. In extreme forms, this gait pattern has a bizarre appearance. The patient walks with a pronounced waddle, shoulders thrown back and pelvis thrust forward. This posture places the center of gravity behind the hips so the patient doesn't fall forward because of weak paraspinal extensor musculature. This form of gait is particularly common in FSH muscular dystrophy (Video Link G.3).

Sensory ataxia occurs when the nervous system is deprived of the sensory information, primarily proprioceptive, necessary to coordinate walking. Deafferentation may result from disease of the posterior columns (e.g., tabes dorsalis or subacute combined degeneration), or disease affecting the peripheral nerves (e.g., sensory peripheral neuropathy) or dorsal root ganglia. The patient is extremely dependent on visual input for coordination (Video G.1). When deprived of visual cues, as with eyes closed or in the dark, the gait deteriorates markedly. The difference in walking ability with and without visual input is the key feature of sensory ataxia. If the condition is mild, locomotion may appear normal when the patient walks eyes open; more commonly it is wide based and poorly coordinated. Sensory ataxia can be differentiated from predominantly cerebellar ataxia by accentuation of the difficulty with eyes closed, as with the **Romberg sign**.

The only sign of mild cerebellar ataxia may be the inability to walk tandem or stand on one leg (Video G.2).[5] Sudden stopping or turning may bring out a stagger. Steps lack the normal rhythm and vary in length and trajectory and the base is widened (see Video C.3). With more severe disease, there is a clumsy, staggering, unsteady, irregular, lurching, wide-based gait, and the patient may sway to either side, back, or forward (Video Link G.4).

With severe ataxia, there may be tremors and oscillatory movements involving the entire body (see **titubation, truncal ataxia**). Ataxia of the lower extremities when tested separately usually accompanies cerebellar gait ataxia, except when disease is limited to the vermis. Cerebellar ataxia is present with eyes both open and closed; it may increase slightly with eyes closed, but not so markedly as in sensory ataxia. With a lesion of the cerebellar vermis, the patient will exhibit a lurching, staggering gait, but without laterality, the ataxia will be as marked toward one side as the other. With a hemispheric lesion, the patient will stagger and deviate toward the involved side. Cerebellar gait ataxia is common in MS, alcoholic cerebellar degeneration, cerebellar tumors, stroke, paraneoplastic syndromes, and cerebellar degenerations. With alcoholic cerebellar degeneration, pathology is restricted to the vermis. Nystagmus, dysarthria, and appendicular ataxia, even of the legs, are typically absent.

A lesion of one cerebellar hemisphere affects gait very little, although the patient may exhibit **star walking** and related signs. The episodic ataxias cause gait disturbances that last only minutes to hours. Between attacks, cerebellar function is normal.

The gait of spastic hemiparesis is caused by a lesion interrupting the corticospinal pathways to one half of the body, most commonly stroke. The patient stands with a hemiparetic posture, arm flexed, adducted, and internally rotated, and leg extended (Video Link G.5).

There is plantar flexion of the foot and toes, either due to foot dorsiflexion weakness or to heel cord shortening, rendering the lower extremity on the involved side functionally slightly longer than on the normal side. When walking, the patient holds the arm tightly to the side, rigid and flexed, extends it with difficulty, and does not swing it in a normal fashion. She holds the leg stiffly in extension and flexes it with difficulty. Consequently, the patient drags or shuffles the foot and scrapes the toes. With each step, she may tilt the pelvis upward on the involved side to aid in lifting the toe off the floor (hip hike), lean toward the uninvolved side, and swing the entire extremity around in a semicircle from the hip (**circumduction gait**). Loss of normal arm swing and slight circumduction of the leg may be the only gait abnormalities in very mild hemiparesis.

When spasticity is present bilaterally, hypertonicity in the legs leads to a stiff-legged, slow, clumsy gait. Both legs may circumduct. It is essentially a bilateral hemiplegic gait affecting the legs. The gait in spasticity has been likened to that of a wooden soldier and the gait of cerebellar ataxia to that of a drunken sailor. Scissoring is a gait pattern seen in patients who have severe spasticity of the legs. It occurs in patients who have congenital spastic diplegia (Little's disease, cerebral palsy) and related conditions and in chronic myelopathies due to conditions such as multiple sclerosis and cervical spondylosis. There is characteristic tightness of the hip adductors causing adduction of the thighs, so that the knees may cross, one in front of the other, with each step **(Video G.3)**.

Some conditions, most often MS, cause both spasticity and cerebellar ataxia. The spastic ataxic gait is both wide based and stiff legged. It may have a characteristic bouncing or springing quality due to spontaneous clonus provoked by weight bearing. Spastic ataxia also occurs in spinocerebellar ataxia type 1 and type 7, Machado-Joseph disease, and some cases of Friedreich's ataxia. The gait in parkinsonism is characterized by rigidity, bradykinesia, and loss of associated movements **(Video G.4)**. The patient is stooped, with head and neck forward and knees flexed; the upper extremities are flexed at the shoulders, elbows, and wrists, but the fingers are usually extended and trembling. The gait is slow, stiff, and shuffling; the patient walks with small, mincing steps. Shuffling is particularly evident on starting to walk, stopping, and turning corners. Slowing of turns and decomposition of turns into multiple steps are often the earliest signs. Other features include involuntary acceleration (see **festinating gait**), decreased arm swing, en bloc turning, start hesitation, and **freezing** when encountering obstacles such as doorways. The festinating gait is common in PD but not in other akinetic rigid syndromes. Impaired postural reflexes and a tendency to fall occur earlier in symptomatic parkinsonism, especially in PSP and MSA, than in PD.

A hyperkinetic gait occurs in conditions such as Sydenham's chorea, HD, other forms of transient or persistent chorea, athetosis, and dystonia (see Video Link C.4). The abnormal movements may become more marked while the patient is walking, and the manifestations of the disease more evident. Walking may accentuate not only the hyperkinesias, but also the abnormalities of power and tone that accompany them. In HD, the **choreic gait** may appear grotesque, with dancing or prancing and abundant extraneous movement. It may look histrionic but is all too real. See **dyskinetic gait**.

In athetosis the distal movements and in dystonia the proximal movements, may be more marked when walkiing; in both there are accompanying grimaces. Dystonic syndromes can produce bizarre gait disturbances. Primary torsion dystonia in children often presents as an action dystonia of one foot or leg that first appears on running. The "dromedary gait" is characterized by exaggerated lumbar lordosis and pronounced hip flexion with each step. The term was originally used by Oppenheim to describe the gait in dystonia musculorum deformans. The dystonia causes bizarre postures and with the hips bulging backward and sideways due to the lumbar hyperlordosis, accompanied by compensatory turning of the shoulders and neck with the head held vertically, the gait was judged to resemble that of the camel, which is a stretch.

A number of gait disorders have been ascribed to dysfunction of the frontal lobes. Lesions of the frontal lobe, or of the frontal lobe connections with the basal ganglia and cerebellum, may lead to a gait disorder characterized by a slightly flexed posture, short, shuffling steps, a widened base, and an inability to integrate and coordinate lower-extremity movements to accomplish normal ambulation. There is particular difficulty with starts and turns. Some of these gait disturbances are poorly understood and the relationship between them unclear. In some, the frontal lobe "dysfunction" has been attributed to normal aging. Many terms have been used, which refer to more or less the same phenomenon, including gait apraxia, frontal disequilibrium or ataxia, Bruns' apraxia/ataxia, magnetic gait, and lower half/body or vascular (arteriosclerotic) parkinsonism. Other conditions often included under this rubric include the gait of NPH, marche à petit pas, and the cautious (senile) gait.

The marche à petit pas (walk of little steps) gait resembles that of parkinsonism, but lacks the rigidity, tremor, and bradykinesia. Locomotion is slow, and the patient walks with very short, mincing, shuffling, and somewhat irregular footsteps. The length of the step may be less than the length of the foot. There is often a loss of **associated movements**. This type of gait may be seen in normal elderly persons, but also occurs in patients who have diffuse cerebral hemispheric dysfunction, particularly involving the frontal lobes. It may also occur as part of the syndrome of NPH and in other types of hydrocephalus.

Apraxia of gait is the loss of the ability to use the legs properly in walking, without demonstrable sensory impairment, weakness, incoordination, or other apparent explanation (**Video G.5**). Gait apraxia is seen in patients with extensive cerebral lesions, especially of the frontal lobes. It is a common feature of NPH and may occur in frontal lobe neoplasms, Binswanger's disease, FTD, and other conditions that cause diffuse frontal lobe dysfunction. In rising, standing, and walking there is difficulty in initiating movement, and the automatic sequence of component movements is lost. The gait is slow and shuffling, with short steps. The patients may have the greatest difficulty initiating walking, making small, feeble, stepping movements with minimal forward progress. Eventually the patient may be essentially unable to lift the feet from the floor as if they were stuck or glued down or may raise them in place without advancing them (magnetic gait, gait ignition failure, start hesitation, Petren's gait). After a few hesitant shuffles, the stride length may increase (slipping clutch gait). When trying to turn, the patient may freeze (turn hesitation). In the syndrome of isolated gait ignition failure, or freezing of gait, patients have difficulty starting to walk, but with continued stepping, the gait improves. They may again freeze when turning or encountering an obstacle.

Gait difficulty is typically a prominent symptom in normal-pressure hydrocephalus (NPH). The primary changes are slow walking, widened base, short steps, and shuffling, all nonspecific features and natural compensations seen in patients with various gait disorders (see Video G.5). The gait disturbance in NPH may range from mild, with only a cautious gait or difficulty with tandem walking, to severe, when unaided gait is impossible. It has been referred to as a gait apraxia. As with other disorders of frontal lobe function, patients may mimic stepping motions while supine or sitting.

A cautious ("senile") gait is seen in older patients who have no neurological disease but are uncertain of their balance and postural reflexes. The gait takes on the characteristics seen when a healthy person walks on an icy surface: velocity slows, steps shorten, and the base widens. The posture is stooped and the arms held apart with reduced swing, as if guarding against an imminent fall.[6] The foot–floor clearance is not decreased, and the patient does not shuffle. There is no difficulty with gait initiation, nor is there freezing. The cautious gait is common but has no localizing value and can occur with central or peripheral disorders, due to fear of falling in the elderly and on a psychogenic basis. There is an ostensible "multimodal" gait disorder in the elderly, attributed to aging of the vestibular system, impaired proprioceptive function caused by distal neuropathy and impaired vision. The "reckless gait" occurs when patients have both dementia and gait difficulties. Impaired cognition leads to a lack of recognition and acceptance of the gait disorder; lack of prudence leads to frequent falls.

Many other gait disorders have been described, and some given colorful names. The "gunslinger" or "penguin" gait occurs because of impaired balance and a tendency to fall and is particularly prominent in PSP. Some have likened the hypererect gait with abducted arms to that of a gunslinger or penguin. Patients with unilateral thalamic lesions may have an inability to stand or sit out of proportion to weakness or sensory loss, with a tendency to fall backward or to the side contralateral to the lesion (see **thalamic astasia**). A toppling gait refers to a tendency to totter and fall seen with brainstem and cerebellar lesions, perhaps due to a failure of righting reflexes and slow motor responses. Primary progressive freezing gait causes early and progressive gait freezing; it is not a distinct disorder but a syndrome with diverse causes.

Nonneurologic Gait Disorders

Abnormalities of gait occur for many other reasons and may be confused with neurologic disorders. An antalgic gait is one in which walking is disordered because of pain **(Video G.6)**. Pain in a lower extremity, for whatever reason, causes a shortening of the stance phase on the involved limb as the patient seeks to avoid bearing weight. An antalgic gait may also occur with a neuropathy that causes painful dysesthesias and allodynia of the feet; the patient walks as if on hot coals.

Arthritis may cause difficulties with gait that are secondary to both pain and deformity. A lordosis that resembles that seen in the muscular dystrophies may occur because of pregnancy, ascites, and abdominal tumors. Hip disease can result in a variety of gait compensations. Dislocation of the hips may cause waddling suggestive of a myopathic gait. A waddling gait is also typical of advanced pregnancy. Marked stooping in ankylosing spondylitis resembles parkinsonism.

Nonorganic Gait Abnormalities

A functional (nonorganic, hysterical, psychogenic) gait disorder is one not due to neurologic or other disease.[7] Affected patients may be unable either to stand or walk, despite the absence of weakness or other objective neurological abnormalities.

Testing for strength, tone, and coordination is normal if carried out supine. The patient is able to make bicycling movements when recumbent. A gait abnormality with a normal resting exam may also occur with disease limited to the cerebellar vermis, such as alcoholic cerebellar degeneration or medulloblastoma, in patients with frontal lobe disease and in NPH. In some patients with a spastic gait, the findings at rest may seem minor compared with the gait disturbance. Because of the unusual gait pattern and normal exam at rest, a dystonic gait is commonly mistaken for a functional, nonorganic gait disturbance. In patients with **orthostatic tremor**, the symptoms and findings only appear with weight bearing.

In functional gait disorders, the gait is typically bizarre and does not conform to a specific organic disease pattern. It may take any number of forms. In nonorganic gait disorders, the gait is usually irregular and variable, with a great deal of superfluous movement and often marked swaying from side to side. The patient may appear in great danger of falling, but rarely does so, oftentimes demonstrating superb balance during the contortions. If falling does occur, it is in a theatrical manner without injury. The bizarre movements often require better than normal coordination. There may be skating, hopping, dancing, or zigzagging; the legs may be thrown out wildly, or there may be a tendency to kneel or crumple every few steps because of sudden knee buckling. The gait pattern may appear monoparetic, hemiparetic, or paraparetic. A common nonorganic gait is for the patient to balance on the stance leg for a prolonged period of time, bringing up the swing leg with a great show of effort. This is the "monoplegic dragging pattern" in which the patient drags the affected leg along like a sack of potatoes without the circumduction typical of organic hemiparesis, usually internally or externally rotated, then often hauls the leg onto the bed with both hands **(Fig. G.1)**.[8]

Other features suggestive of nonorganicity include a dramatic fluctuation in the degree of impairment in a short period of time, excessive slowness of movement or hesitation, a "walking on ice" pattern with cautious, broad-based steps and shortened stride length with the arms wide apart as if on a tightrope and occasionally a rapid recovery.[9] The gait may improve with distraction. A "psychogenic" **Romberg sign** is often present as well (see **false Rombergism**).

A characteristic and telltale finding is the preservation of the ability to walk backward or to one side or to run without difficulty. The patient may be able to walk sideways crossing one foot over the other. The ability to perform these more complicated gait maneuvers when the patient cannot walk forward in the normal manner is difficult to ascribe to any organic disorder, although **dystonia** may have some of these features. In the chair test, the patient with difficulty walking can use the legs normally when asked to move around in a wheeled swivel chair (sensitivity 85%, specificity 95%, positive LR 17.0, negative LR 0.2).[10] In most patients with functional gait disorder, the similarity to neurologic disease is slight. Hyperkinetic gait disorders are most likely to be confused with functional conditions. In Keane's[11] series of 60 patients, 23 mimicked paresis and most of the remainder had various ataxic or histrionic patterns. Several authors have noted that knee buckling is a common type of functional gait disorder.

The term **astasia-abasia** originated in an 1888 monograph by Blocq, and the condition is sometimes referred to as Blocq's syndrome. He described patients who were able to jump, or walk on all fours, but unable to stand upright (astasia) or to

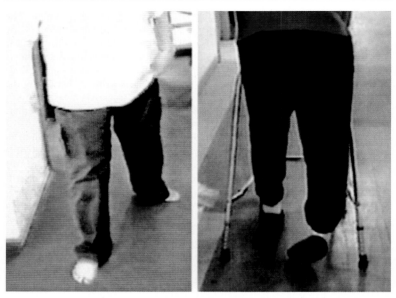

Figure G.1. Monoplegic dragging gait. In both cases, the leg is dragged at the hip. External or internal rotation of the hip or ankle inversion/eversion is common. (From Stone J, Zeman A, Sharpe M. Functional weakness and sensory disturbance. *J Neurol Neurosurg Psychiatry.* 2002;73:241–245, with permission.)

walk (abasia). Astasia-abasia is sometimes used to refer to any inability to either stand or walk normally, but generally refers to a histrionic and dramatic gait disturbance with wild lurching and near falls.

Gait ignition failure: See **gait disorders.**

Galactorrhea: Lactation in a male or nonbreastfeeding female. The condition occurs because of hyperprolactinemia. Normally prolactin secretion is inhibited by dopamine, which is secreted by the hypothalamus and inhibits lactotrophs in the anterior pituitary to stop prolactin production. Hyperprolactinemia and galactorrhea occur because of excess prolactin secretion, a lack of the normal inhibitory dopamine, or impaired prolactin excretion. A common cause of galactorrhea is a prolactin-secreting pituitary adenoma. Galactorrhea occurs in the majority of women with prolactinomas, but is less common in males. Galactorrhea may also occur as a medication side effect from dopamine antagonists, such as psychotropics, H2 antagonists, tricyclic antidepressants, SSRIs, and oral contraceptives. Less common neurologically relevant conditions include acromegaly, MS, hypothyroidism, sarcoidosis, and spinal cord lesions.

Galloping tongue: Unusual episodic, rhythmic tongue movements that may occur after head and neck trauma.

Gaze apraxia (apraxia of gaze, optic apraxia): An acquired inability to voluntarily direct gaze in response to command or a visual stimulus. It is seen most often as a component of **Balint's syndrome.**

Gaze deviation: When the eyes at rest are not aligned straight ahead. The gaze deviation may result because the eyes are forced into the abnormal position because of seizure activity in the frontal lobe, or the abnormal position may be a compensation for a **gaze palsy**.

Gaze-evoked nystagmus (GEN): **Nystagmus** produced by horizontal or vertical gaze; it is the most common form of nystagmus seen in clinical practice and may be either physiologic or pathologic.

Gaze evoked tinnitus: Tinnitus associated with eye movements; it may be due to abnormal communications between the cochlear and vestibular nuclei.

Gaze palsy: A conjugate paralysis of gaze. The frontal eye fields (FEF) move the eyes into contralateral conjugate horizontal gaze, and the eyes at rest normally remain straight ahead because of a balance of input from the FEF in each hemisphere. Seizure activity in one frontal lobe drives the eyes contralaterally. With destructive frontal lobe lesions, the patient is unable to move the eyes contralaterally—a gaze palsy, or, if less severe, a gaze paresis. The intact, normal hemisphere maintains its tonic input, the imbalance causing the eyes to move contralaterally, toward the diseased side—a **gaze deviation**. Patients may have gaze palsy without gaze deviation. The presence of gaze deviation usually means gaze palsy to the opposite side, but it may occasionally signal seizure activity. About 20% of patients with acute hemispheric stroke have transient gaze deviation. In some patients, the gaze deviation due to a structural lesion is to the side opposite that expected. The wrong-way eyes phenomenon is particularly likely to occur in thalamic hemorrhage.[12]

Similar considerations apply to disease of the pons. The pontine paramedian reticular formation (PPRF) governs ipsilateral, conjugate horizontal gaze, drawing the eyes ipsilaterally, in contrast to the frontal eye fields, which push the eyes contralaterally. Destructive lesions of the PPRF impair the ability to gaze ipsilaterally, resulting in a gaze deviation toward the intact side as the normal PPRF pulls the eyes over **(Video Link G.6)**.

When faced with a patient whose eyes rest eccentrically to one side, the possibilities are (1) frontal lobe seizure activity, (2) frontal lobe destructive lesion, and (3) pontine destructive lesion. Patients with destructive frontal lesions gaze away from the side of the hemiparesis (Prévost's or Vulpian's sign); patients with pontine lesions gaze toward the hemiparesis. Frontal lobe gaze deviations are generally large amplitude, pronounced and clinically obvious, whereas pontine gaze deviations are often subtle and easily missed.

Some conditions produce gaze palsies that are bilateral and affect both saccades and pursuit and both horizontal and vertical gaze; see **complete ophthalmoplegia**.

Gaze paretic nystagmus: See **nystagmus**.

Gegenhalten (inhibitory paratonia, paratonic rigidity, Foerster's syndrome): A form of rigidity in which the tone in a limb increases as the examiner attempts to passively move it. The resistance of the patient increases in proportion to the examiner's efforts to move the part; the harder the examiner pushes, the harder the patient seems to push back, despite exhortations to relax. It seems as though the patient is actively fighting, but the response is involuntary. Gegenhalten is usually associated with other abnormal neurologic signs depending on the etiology. The opposite of gegenhalten is **mitgehen**, or facilitory paratonia; see **paratonia**.

Genu recurvatum (back kneeing): The hyperextended position of the knee adopted in the face of quadriceps weakness to compensate for knee instability and avoid knee buckling. It occurs particularly in patients with muscular dystrophy. See **gait disorders.**

Genu varus/valgus: Deviation of the knee away/toward the midline. Patients with varus deformity are bow-legged, with valgus deformity knock-kneed. These deformities are usually developmental or due to degenerative arthropathy, but except for a **Charcot joint** are not generally seen in neurological patients.

Geographic tongue (benign migratory glossitis): An unusual pattern on the tongue surface with areas of depapillation that create reddish islands in a random pattern resembling a map. The inflammatory lesions heal in one area and develop in another, migrating over the tongue surface. Geographic tongue is benign and not related to any neurological conditions. It should not be mistaken for the **glossitis** of nutritional deficiency. See **scrotal tongue.**

Geotropic nystagmus: See **ageotropic nystagmus.**

Geste antagoniste (sensory trick, counterpressure sign, proprioceptive trick): Something done by patients to control dystonic movements and posture.[13] Many if not most patients with cervical dystonia learn they can straighten their head by placing a hand or finger somewhere on the face, chin, or back of the head or performing some other maneuver to provide sensory stimulation or light counterpressure. Many patients have multiple sensory tricks, and sometimes merely the thought of executing the trick may reduce the dystonia **(Video Link G.7).**

Gibbus: Marked kyphosis, due to vertebral collapse with the formation of a wedge vertebra. The deformity can be associated with spinal cord compression. The differential diagnosis includes tuberculosis, trauma, achondroplasia, NF, and mucopolysaccharidoses.

Give-way weakness: See **collapsing weakness.**

Glabellar (glabellar tap) reflex: A reflex contraction of the orbicularis oculi causing an eye blink, elicited by tapping with a finger or percussing with a reflex hammer over the forehead in the midline just above the eyebrows. Normal individuals are able to inhibit the reflex; patients with parkinsonism are unable to inhibit the response and continue to blink with repeated taps (Myerson's sign). A slight decrease in the ipsilateral glabellar reflex is sometimes detectable with early, mild, or resolving unilateral facial weakness. See **orbicularis oculi reflex.**

Glissade: See **ocular dysmetria.**

Global (total, expressive-receptive, complete) aphasia: A type of nonfluent **aphasia** in which comprehension is also impaired. In global aphasia, most commonly a large lesion has destroyed the entire perisylvian language center, or separate lesions have destroyed both the posterior inferior frontal and posterior superior temporal language regions. Grossly nonfluent speech is combined with a severe comprehension deficit and inability to name, repeat, read, or write. Speech is often reduced to expletives or **monophasia.** Typically there is both a hemiplegia and a field cut. Global aphasia is usually due to internal carotid or proximal MCA occlusion. In some patients, comprehension improves, leaving a deficit resembling **Broca's aphasia.** Patients with aphasic syndromes producing deficits in all language modalities, but involvement less severe than global aphasia are said to have mixed aphasia.

Glomus tumor (paraganglioma, chemodectoma): A neoplasm that arises from the glomera of the chemoreceptor system. They commonly arise in the jugular bulb (glomus jugulare), the middle ear (glomus tympanicum), and the nodose ganglion

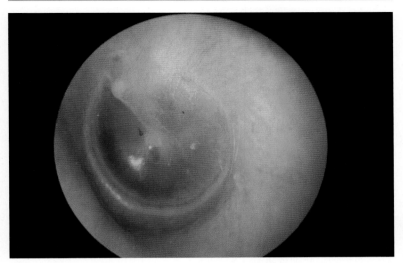

Figure G.2. A vascular, reddish mass in the ear canal. A glomus tympanicum remains contained to the middle ear. With a glomus jugulare, the majority of the tumor may be intracranial and only a nubbin appears behind the eardrum. Dilated blood vessels may course toward the mass along the eardrum or ear canal. (From http://otologytextbook. com/glomus_tumoursP.htm, accessed February 7, 2015.)

G

of the vagus nerve (glomus vagale). On examination, a vascular polyp may be found in the auditory canal or behind the tympanic membrane in a patient with a lower cranial nerve palsy (Fig. G.2). Glomus jugulare tumors are a common cause of jugular foramen syndrome. These tumors grow slowly, may erode bone, and may extend intracranially.

Glossitis: A red, beefy appearance of the tongue, usually the result of vitamin deficiency, most notably B12 deficiency (Fig. G.3). Cells of the tongue papillae have a high proliferation rate. Nutritional deficiencies may impair replication and lead to depapillation.

Glossoplegia: Weakness of the tongue. Conditions causing glossoplegia range from ALS causing severe tongue atrophy, creating a completely paralyzed, fasciculating "bag of worms," to a small cortical infarction causing contralateral tongue weakness as a relatively isolated clinical finding (Fig. G.4).[14]

Gluteal skyline test: A method to detect atrophy of the gluteal musculature, which is most likely to occur with lesions of the S_1 root or inferior gluteal nerve. With the patient lying prone, the examiner observes the contour of the gluteal muscles from the head or foot of the bed. The examiner can sometimes detect subtle atrophy or flattening of the contour of one gluteal muscle by comparing one buttock with the other (Fig. G.5).

Go/No-Go test: A test to detect **defective response inhibition**. The patient is asked to perform an action in response to a stimulus (Go) and do nothing in response to a different stimulus (No Go). If Go stimuli exceed No Go stimuli, the patient with frontal lobe disease has difficulty inhibiting the response on the No Go stimuli.

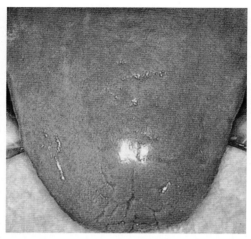

Figure G.3. Atrophic glossitis. A smooth and often sore tongue that has lost its papillae suggests a deficiency in riboflavin, niacin, folic acid, vitamin B12, pyridoxine, or iron. Specific diagnosis is often difficult. Anticancer drugs may also be responsible. (From Cawson RA. *Oral Pathology.* London, UK: Gower Medical Publishing; 1987, with permission.)

Then the rules are changed and the patient is challenged to adapt. Any number of stimulus–responses paradigms are possible. See also **automatic responses, Stroop test,** the **antisaccade task, alternating sequences test,** and **applause sign.**

Gonda's sign: See **minor extensor toe signs.**

Gordon's sign: See **minor extensor toe signs.**

Gordon's flexion sign: An upper extremity **pathological reflex** seen with CST disease; squeezing muscles of forearm causes adduction and flexion of thumb, sometimes with flexion of adjacent digits, more rarely with extension of little finger.

Gordon's extension sign: An upper extremity **pathological reflex** seen with CST disease; pressure on radial side of pisiform bone causes extension and occasionally fanning of the fingers.

Gottron's papules: Skin lesions sometimes seen in DM, see **dermatomyositis skin changes.**

Gower's sign (maneuver): A maneuver used by patients with hip girdle weakness, particularly in the muscular dystrophies where there is marked weakness of the hip extensors, to rise from a stooped position by using the hands to "climb up the legs." Numerous examples of Gower's sign are available on YouTube.

Graphesthesia: See **agraphesthesia.**

Grasp reflex (forced grasping): An involuntary flexor response of the fingers and hand following stimulation of the skin of the palmar surface of the fingers or hand. The grasp reflex is usually classified as a **frontal release sign** and classified with the other **primitive reflexes.**[15] See **pathologic reflexes.**

To examine for a grasp reflex, instruct the patient not to hold onto the examiner's hand as the examiner's fingers are placed in the patient's hand, especially between the thumb and forefinger, or the palmar skin is stimulated gently. If there is slow

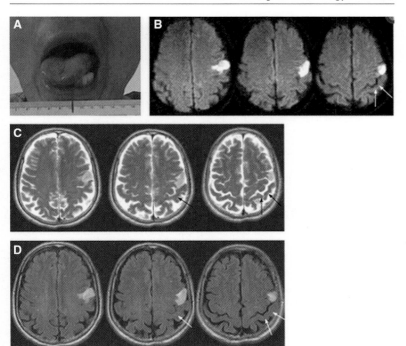

Figure G.4. A: The protruded tongue deviating to the right about 1.5 cm from the midline. **B:** Diffusion weighted. **C:** T2-weighted image. **D:** Fluid-attenuated inversion recovery (FLAIR) magnetic resolution images of the brain showed a small cortical infarction in the precentral gyrus of the left frontal lobe. White and black arrows indicate the precentral knob representing the motor hand area. (From Yoon SS, Park KC. Neurological picture. Glossoplegia in a small cortical infarction. *J Neurol Neurosurg Psychiatry.* 2007;78:1372, with permission.)

flexion of the digits or the patient's fingers close around the examiner's fingers in a gentle grasp that can be relaxed on command, this is the simple grasp reflex, an exaggeration of the normal **palmar reflex**. If the patient's fingers flex against the examiner's fingers in a "hooking" or traction response as they are gently extended by the fingers of the examiner, this is a more developed grasp reflex. With a more marked response, the strength of the grasp increases with attempts to withdraw the examiner's hand or to extend the patient's fingers passively, and there is loss of ability to relax the grasp voluntarily or on command. The grip may be so firm that the patient can be lifted from the bed by the examiner. This is the forced grasping reflex and is a part of the counterholding, or **gegenhalten (paratonia)**, phenomenon. If the sight of the examiner's hand near but not touching the patient's hand, or even a very light touch on the patient's hand between the thumb and forefinger while the patient's eyes are closed, leads to groping movements, this is termed the groping response. Other things may be substituted for the examiner's fingers to elicit the grasp response, such as the handle of the reflex hammer. Stimulation of the dorsum

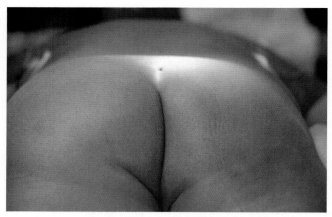

Figure G.5. Atrophy of the right buttock with loss of the normal, rounded contour compared with the left. Note the skin tag at the upper gluteal cleft, which was the clue to the presence of a tethered cord. Photo done preoperatively.

of the hand can inhibit the response, making it more difficult to elicit if the examiner holds the patient's hand in his own palm or rests it on the bed or patient's thigh.

In a study of 491 patients admitted to a neurology service, grasping was found in 8% of patients with CNS lesions.[16] It occurred predominantly in patients with single (14) or multiple (10) hemispheric lesions; the lesion was either in the frontal lobe or the deep nuclei and subcortical white matter. Grasping never occurred when the disease was confined to the retrorolandic regions. In 44 patients with either grasping or CT-documented frontal damage, grasping was found in 70% of patients with involvement of the medial areas and was always associated with damage to the cingulate gyrus. It occurred in only 26% with lesions of the lateral motor and premotor areas. Overall, the grasp reflex had a sensitivity of 13%, specificity of 99% and a positive LR of 20.2 in predicting a lesion of the frontal lobe, deep nuclei, or white matter. Grasping usually affected both hands, even when the lesion was unilateral, and in most patients was not a forced phenomenon but could be modified by will, although it showed up again as soon as the patient's attention was diverted.

Grasp reflex of the foot: See **plantar grasp.**

Grasset-Gaussel phenomenon: A manifestation of CST dysfunction seen in the lower extremities in hemiparetic patients. The normal supine patient can raise either leg separately or raise both together. In CST lesions, the patient may still be able to raise either one separately, but cannot raise them together. If he first raises the paretic leg, raising the normal leg causes the paretic leg to fall. Passively raising the normal leg also causes the paretic leg to fall. If the patient first raises the normal leg, and then the paretic leg is passively raised, the sound one remains elevated.

Grey Turner sign: Ecchymosis of the flank; may be evidence that a lumbosacral plexopathy is due to retroperitoneal hematoma. Retroperitoneal hemorrhage also sometimes causes periumbilical ecchymosis (Cullen's sign). These signs may also appear with ectopic pregnancy and a number of other conditions, none of which are likely to cause lumbosacral plexopathy.

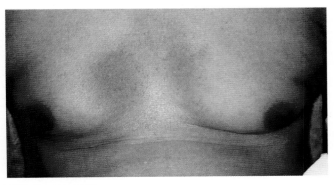

Figure G.6. Gynecomastia.

Gray hair: Loss of hair pigmentation. Premature graying may be a clue to pernicious anemia, ataxia-telangiectasia, Down's syndrome, progeria, myotonic dystrophy, myotonia congenita, hyperthyroidism, Vogt-Kayanaga-Harada syndrome, and Waardenburg's syndrome.

Groping response (reflex): See **grasp reflex.**

Gum hypertrophy: An adverse effect of phenytoin, now fortunately rare. Gingival overgrowth also occurs with calcium-channel blockers and cyclosporine.

Gunn phenomenon: See **jaw winking.**

Gunn pupil: See **afferent pupillary defect.**

Gunslinger gait: See **gait disorders.**

Gustatory sweating (Frey's auriculotemporal syndrome): Sweating in the region of the cheek after the ingestion of food, particularly spicy food, due to aberrant regeneration of autonomic branches in the auriculotemporal branch of the facial nerve damaged by injury or surgery.[17] Parasympathetic axons innervating salivary glands become misdirected into facial sweat glands **(Video Link G.8).**

Gynecomastia: Enlargement of the male breast **(Fig. G.6).** Gynecomastia is one of the features of Kennedy's disease (spinobulbar muscular atrophy), where it is present in 60% to 90% of patients. There are many other causes.[18] It may also occur in cirrhosis, hyperthyroidism, hyperprolactinemia, chronic kidney disease, male hypogonadism of any cause, POEMS, Wilson's disease, Kugelberg-Welander disease, and as a paraneoplastic syndrome due to ectopic HCG production. Gynecomastia occurs as a side effect of certain drugs, particularly spironolactone, calcium-channel blockers, cimetidine, ketoconazole, digitalis, phenytoin, and androgen blockers used for prostate carcinoma. Lipomastia, or pseudogynecomastia, is the accumulation of fat rather than breast tissue and is common in obese men.

Video Links

G.1. Curtain sign. Available at: http://www.youtube.com/watch?v=S9s5ZHCzOXM

G.2. Common gait abnormalities. (From Stanford School of Medicine. Stanford Medicine 25.) Available at: http://stanfordmedicine25.stanford.edu/the25/gait.html

G.3. A patient with a myopathic gait, waddling, toe walking, and hyperlordosis. (From Paul D. Larsen, MD, University of Nebraska Medical Center and Suzanne S. Stensaas, PhD, University of Utah School of Medicine, http://library.med.utah.edu/neurologicexam/html/gait_abnormal.html.) Available at:_____http://library.med.utah.edu/neurologicexam/html/video_window.html?vidurl=../movies/gait_ab_11.mov&vidwidth=320&vidheight=240

G.4. Severe ataxia. (From Paul D. Larsen, MD, University of Nebraska Medical Center and Suzanne S. Stensaas, PhD, University of Utah School of Medicine, http://library.med.utah.edu/neurologicexam/html/gait_abnormal.html.) Available at: http://library.med.utah.edu/neurologicexam/html/video_window.html?vidurl=../movies/gait_ab_14_x2.mov&vidwidth=640&vidheight=480

G.5. Spastic hemiparesis. (From Paul D. Larsen, M.D., University of Nebraska Medical Center and Suzanne S. Stensaas, Ph.D., University of Utah School of Medicine (http://library.med.utah.edu/neurologicexam/html/gait_abnormal.html.) Available at: http://library.med.utah.edu/neurologicexam/html/video_window.html?vidurl=../movies/gait_ab_08.mov&vidwidth=320&vidheight=240

G.6. Bilateral horizontal gaze palsy with intact vertical gaze and convergence in a patient with a pontine lesion. (From the Robert B. Daroff Collection, Neuro-ophthalmology Virtual Education Library (NOVEL), University of Utah.) Available at: http://stream.utah.edu/m/dp/frame.php?f=e500253f509b9b54662

G.7. Geste antagoniste in oromandibular dystonia. Available at: http://www.youtube.com/watch?v=b9roso9B1F0

G.8. Gustatory sweating after resection of a parotid tumor. (From Reich SG, Grill SE. Gustatory sweating: Frey syndrome. *Neurology.* 2005;65:E24.) Available at: http://www.neurology.org/content/suppl/2005/12/05/65.11.E24.DC1/Video.mpg

References

1. Davies AE, Kidd D, Stone SP, et al. Pharyngeal sensation and gag reflex in healthy subjects. *Lancet.* 1995;345:487–488.
2. Leder SB, Espinosa JF. Aspiration risk after acute stroke: comparison of clinical examination and fiberoptic endoscopic evaluation of swallowing. *Dysphagia.* 2002;17:214–218.
3. Nutt JG. Classification of gait and balance disorders. *Adv Neurol.* 2001;87:135–141.
4. Nutt JG. Higher-level gait disorders: an open frontier. *Mov Disord.* 2013;28:1560–1565.
5. Morton SM, Bastian AJ. Mechanisms of cerebellar gait ataxia. *Cerebellum.* 2007;6:79–86.
6. Snijders AH, van de Warrenburg BP, Giladi N, et al. Neurological gait disorders in elderly people: clinical approach and classification. *Lancet Neurol.* 2007;6:63–74.
7. Sudarsky L. Psychogenic gait disorders. *Semin Neurol.* 2006;26:351–356.
8. Stone J, Zeman A, Sharpe M. Functional weakness and sensory disturbance. *J Neurol Neurosurg Psychiatry.* 2002;73:241–245.
9. Lempert T, Brandt T, Dieterich M, et al. How to identify psychogenic disorders of stance and gait. A video study in 37 patients. *J Neurol.* 1991;238:140–146.
10. McGee S. *Evidence Based Physical Diagnosis.* 3rd ed. Philadelphia, PA: Elsevier/Saunders; 2012.
11. Keane JR. Hysterical gait disorders: 60 cases. *Neurology.* 1989;39:586–589.
12. Messe SR, Cucchiara BL. Wrong-way eyes with thalamic hemorrhage. *Neurology.* 2003;60:1524.
13. Poisson A, Krack P, Thobois S, et al. History of the 'geste antagoniste' sign in cervical dystonia. *J Neurol.* 2012;259:1580–1584.
14. Yoon SS, Park KC. Neurological picture. Glossoplegia in a small cortical infarction. *J Neurol Neurosurg Psychiatry.* 2007;78:1372.
15. Schott JM, Rossor MN. The grasp and other primitive reflexes. *J Neurol Neurosurg Psychiatry.* 2003;74:558–560.
16. De RE, Barbieri C. The incidence of the grasp reflex following hemispheric lesion and its relation to frontal damage. *Brain.* 1992;115(pt 1):293–313.
17. Reich SG, Grill SE. Gustatory sweating: Frey syndrome. *Neurology.* 2005;65:E24.
18. Ladizinski B, Lee KC, Nutan FN, et al. Gynecomastia: etiologies, clinical presentations, diagnosis, and management. *South Med J.* 2014;107:44–49.

Hairy patch: One of the possible cutaneous stigmata of occult spinal dysraphism (Fig. H.1). Other cutaneous abnormalities manifestations include **hemangioma,** lipoma, dimple, and skin tag (see Fig. G.5). These dermatologic abnormalities may indicate the presence of significant underlying spinal abnormalities, such as tethered cord, diastometamyelia, dermal sinus, anterior meningocele, or an intraspinal cyst or lipoma.[1] Other common manifestations include pain and foot deformities (see **pes cavus**).

Hamartoma: See **retinal lesions.**

Hammer toes: A deformity of one or more of the lesser four toes that creates flexion of the PIP joint (Fig. H.2). The PIP deformity may be fixed or supple. With some hammer toes, the MTP joint is hyperextended. DIP joint involvement is variable. The terms *claw toe* (see Fig. C.13) and *hammer toe* are sometimes used synonymously. At other times, a distinction is made by such criteria as (1) claw toes tend to affect all the toes but a hammer toe may only affect one or two, (2) MTP extension is always present with claw toes but variable with hammer toes, or (3) claw toes have a flexion deformity at the DIP joint, but this usually does not occur with hammer toes. Schrier et al[2] attempted to bring some consistency to the situation.

Clawing is associated with denervating conditions that cause weakness of the intrinsic foot muscles. An imbalance results between the extrinsic extensor tendons that extend the MTP joints and the intrinsics that flex them, resulting in the claw toe deformity. Atrophy of the foot with guttering of the dorsum and prominence of the tendons is commonly present as well. Hammer toes (strictly defined) develop for a number of reasons, most being nonneurologic.

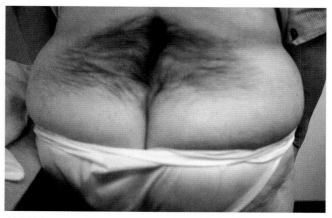

Figure H.1. Hairy patch. (From Campbell WW. *DeJong's the Neurologic Examination.* 7th ed. Philadelphia, PA: Wolters Kluwer Health/Lippincott Williams & Wilkins Health; 2013, with permission.)

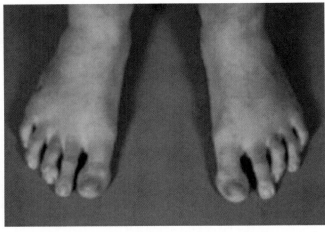

Figure H.2. Hammer toes. (From McCarthy JJ, Drennan JC. *Drennan's the Child's Foot and Ankle.* 2nd ed. Philadelphia, PA: Wolters Kluwer Health/Lippincott Williams & Wilkins Health; 2010, with permission.)

Hamstring reflexes: The medial and lateral hamstring reflexes are reflexes that are difficult to elicit but occasionally useful, especially in the evaluation of patients with suspected radiculopathy (see Table D.1, Video B.4).

The medial hamstring (internal hamstring, semimembranosus, and semitendinosus) reflex is elicited by striking the semitendinosus and semimembranosus tendons just above their insertions on the tibia with the patient seated or recumbent, with the leg abducted and slightly rotated externally and the knee flexed. The examiner's fingers are placed over the tendons on the medial posterior aspect of the knee and the fingers tapped with the reflex hammer. The response is knee flexion. The reflex is mediated by tibial portion of the sciatic nerve, primarily by the L5 nerve root.

While formal studies of "the elusive L5 reflex" have not shown any utility, there are occasional situations where asymmetry of the medial hamstring reflexes in the appropriate clinical setting is definitely useful (**Video Links H.1 and H.2**).[3,4] A decreased medial hamstring reflex has an LR of 6.2, a PPV of 85% to 89% and an NPV of 51% to 61% for the diagnosis of L5 radiculopathy.[5,6]

The lateral hamstring (external hamstring, biceps femoris) reflex is elicited by striking the biceps femoris tendon just above its insertion with the patient sitting, recumbent or lying on the opposite side, and the knee moderately flexed. The examiner's fingers are placed over the tendon on the lateral posterior aspect of the knee and tapped (**Fig. H.3**). The response is knee flexion. The reflex is mediated by tibial portion of the sciatic nerve, primarily by the S1 nerve root. The lateral hamstring reflex is sometimes quite helpful in sorting out whether a depressed or absent ankle jerk is due to peripheral neuropathy or radiculopathy. If the abnormal ankle reflex is due to axonal neuropathy, the lateral hamstring reflex is usually preserved, but in radiculopathy it is depressed or absent in concert with the ankle reflex.

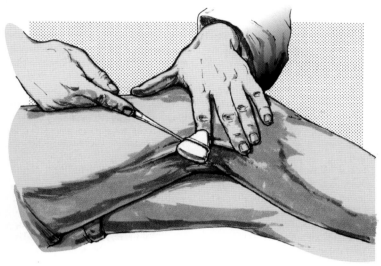

Figure H.3. Method of obtaining the biceps femoris reflex. (From Campbell WW. *DeJong's the Neurologic Examination.* 7th ed. Philadelphia, PA: Wolters Kluwer Health/ Lippincott Williams & Wilkins Health; 2013, with permission.)

Hand elevation test: See **carpal tunnel provocative tests.**
Hand flexor reflex: See **wrist flexion reflex.**
Hand-on-head sign: See **Bakody's sign.**
Hand position test: A term used to describe either Luria's **fist-edge-palm** test, or a test of motor function used in the Full Outline of Responsiveness (FOUR) score evaluation of coma. In the latter, as a motor function test, the patient is asked to make a fist, thumbs up, or peace sign.[7]
Hannington-Kiff sign: An absent thigh **adductor reflex** with a normal **knee reflex;** described as a sign of strangulated obturator hernia.
Harlequin sign: See **hyperhidrosis.**
Head drop: See **dropped head.**
Head impulse test: A bedside examination to help identify an impaired **vestibulo-ocular reflex** (VOR) in patients with acute peripheral vestibulopathy. The examiner briskly rotates the patient's head while having the patient fixate on a target, usually the examiner's nose. Normally, the VOR is able to match the velocity of head rotation, but when impaired the eyes lag behind and a corrective "catch-up" saccade back to the target occurs after head rotation, indicating peripheral vestibular hypofunction on the side toward which the preceding head rotation occurred. The test is useful in evaluating patients with acute spontaneous vertigo since it is positive, revealing a catch-up saccade in acute peripheral vestibulopathy, but usually, although not invariably, negative with central vestibular lesions. For the diagnosis of peripheral vestibular disease, defined by an abnormal caloric response, the presence of a corrective saccade on the head impulse test has a sensitivity of 35%

to 57%, a specificity of 90% to 99%, a positive LR of 6.7, and a negative LR of 0.6.[5] A reliable three-step bedside examination to distinguish brainstem stroke from acute peripheral vestibulopathy is the HINTS: Head impulse, **nystagmus**, test of skew.[8]

The video by Bassani[9] **(Video Link H.3)** demonstrates an abnormal head impulse test with a very obvious catch-up saccade, as well as an abnormal **Unterberger-Fukuda stepping test**, in a patient with vestibular neuritis. The video depicts spontaneous right-beating nystagmus with vertical and counterclockwise components. The nystagmus increases with gaze shift toward the pathological left side and decreases while gazing toward the right side. Performing the head impulse test, the quick rotation of the patient's head toward the pathological left side causes an eye lag, followed by a catch-up saccade to refixate on the target. The last part of the video shows a 45-degree rotation toward the pathological left side during the stepping test.

For a demonstration and discussion of the HINTS from the Neuro-Ophthalmology Virtual Education Library (NOVEL) at the University of Utah, see http://stream.utah.edu/m/dp/frame.php?f=9a1d813e7a4f9c53097.

Head retraction reflex: One of the trigeminal-mediated reflexes. A sharp tap with the reflex hammer just below the nose with the head bent slightly forward produces a quick, involuntary, backward jerk of the head. The head retraction reflex is present in bilateral CST lesions rostral to the cervical spine, e.g., ALS; it is not present in normals.

Head-shaking nystagmus: A type of nystagmus induced by shaking the patient's head, best performed using Frenzel lenses.[10] The examiner tilts the patient's head about 20 degrees downward to bring the axis of rotation close to parallel for the lateral canals, then grasps the head and shakes it horizontally at a frequency of about 2 Hz and a displacement of about 30 degrees to either side, continuing for 20 cycles. In normals or patients with symmetrical vestibular loss, no nystagmus occurs, but with vestibular imbalance contralesional nystagmus may occur that decays over about 30 seconds, sometimes followed by a second phase of nystagmus in the opposite direction. With CNS pathology, there may be strong nystagmus with minimal head shaking, head-shaking nystagmus in the direction opposite to the spontaneous nystagmus or vertical or torsional nystagmus in response to horizontal head shaking.

Head tilt: A tendency to hold the head canted to one side. Causes for a head tilt include CN IV palsy, the **ocular tilt reaction**, **laterocollis**, and the presence of a posterior fossa mass.

Head tilt test: See **Bielschowsky head tilt test.**

Head-turning sign: A clue to the presence of cognitive impairment, when the patient repeatedly turns to the caregiver for help answering questions when giving the history.

Heel-to-shin (HTS) test: A maneuver analogous to the **finger-to-nose test**. In the HTS, the patient is asked to place the heel of one foot on the opposite knee, rest it there momentarily to bring out any postural tremor, tap it up and down on the knee several times, then push the point of the heel (not the instep) along the shin in a straight line to the foot, and then bring it back to the knee. The patient with cerebellar disease is likely to raise the foot too high, flex the knee too much, and place the heel down above or below the knee. The excursions along the shin are jerky and unsteady with the heel sliding back and forth as it slides down (see Video C.3). In the toe-to-finger test, often done along with the HTS, the patient tries to touch the great toe, knee bent, to the examiner's finger. Dysmetria may cause undershooting or overshooting of the mark; intention tremor and oscillations may also be evident.

Heel walking: A test for dorsiflexion weakness of the foot and toes by having the patient stand or walk on the heels, raising the toes as high as possible. The foot and toes on the weak side cannot be lifted as far. See **foot drop.**

Heimann-Bielschowsky phenomenon: See **nystagmus.**

Heliotrope rash: See **dermatomyositis skin changes.**

Hemangioma: A proliferation of blood vessels, usually in the skin. Cutaneous hemangiomas have a red, blue, or purple color depending on the extent and depth of the lesion. The most common type is the capillary hemangioma, or nevus flammeus. Since these lesions do not proliferate, capillary malformation is a better term. Cavernous hemangiomas are more extensive, with large, dilated vascular channels that involve deeper structures and do not regress. A hemangioblastoma is a circumscribed, cystic tumor that arises from blood vessels. Von Hippel-Lindau disease is an autosomal-dominant disorder that causes cavernous hemangiomas and hemangioblastomas in the retina and the CNS, primarily the cerebellum, less commonly the brainstem and spinal cord (see **retinal lesions**). In encephalotrigeminal angiomatosis (Sturge-Weber syndrome), there is a congenital hemangioma over one side of the face (port wine stain) in the trigeminal distribution with associated ipsilateral leptomeningeal angiomas and intracortical calcifications with attendant neurologic complications (Fig. H.4). A hemangioma may be one of the cutaneous stigmata of occult spinal dysraphism (see **hairy patch**).

Capillary malformations are usually located on the head and neck, but may occur on the trunk or extremities. They darken over time and may develop cobblestoning and nodularity. A capillary malformation in any location may be a cutaneous reflection of an underlying spinal cord AVM. Cobb's syndrome is a capillary

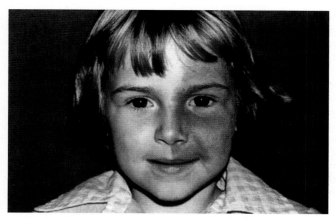

Figure H.4. Child with the Sturge-Weber syndrome, causing the typical port-wine hemangioma of the skin along the distribution of the left trigeminal nerve. (From Allingham RR, Damji KF, Shields MB. *Shields' Textbook of Glaucoma.* 6th ed. Philadelphia, PA: Wolters Kluwer Health/Lippincott Williams & Wilkins; 2011, with permission.)

malformation on the posterior thorax associated with an underlying AVM of the spinal cord. About 20% of high-flow spinal AVMs have an accompanying metameric cutaneous capillary malformation.[11]

Other conditions associated with cutaneous or retinal vascular lesions include Wyburn-Mason syndrome, Gass syndrome, Klippel-Trenaunay-Weber syndrome, and hereditary hemorrhagic telangiectasia (Osler-Weber-Rendu disease).

Hemiachromatopsia (dyschromatopsia): Loss (or impairment) of color vision in one hemifield. Colors appear grayed out to a greater or lesser degree. The responsible lesion usually lies in the contralateral inferotemporal region.[12] Careful testing is required to pick up such deficits and to exclude color anomia or color agnosia.

Hemiakinesia: Bradykinesia or akinesia limited to one side of the body. Greater involvement on one side is the rule in early PD (see hemiparkinsonism). Hemiakinesia may also occur with CBD and with structural lesions of the basal ganglia. Motor neglect may result in bradykinesia of the limbs contralateral to a nondominant brain lesion (see **attentional deficits).**

Hemianopia: See **visual field defects.**

Hemiataxia: Ataxia on one side. Ipsilateral ataxia occurs with lesions of one cerebellar hemisphere. Hemiataxia also occurs in the ataxic hemiparesis syndrome due to lacunar infarction and in the hemiataxia-hypesthesia syndrome due to a thalamic lesion (see **thalamic ataxia).**

Hemiatrophy: Atrophy of one side of the body. Cerebral lesions dating from birth or early childhood may cause a failure of normal growth of the contralateral body. Such hemiatrophy may be subtle; comparing the size of the thumbnails is a traditional technique for detecting mild hemiatrophy. Congenital hemihypertrophy is rarer than hemiatrophy, and there are usually other anomalies. Hemiatrophy may also complicate hemiparkinsonism. Rarely, hemiatrophy is idiopathic. See also **facial hemiatrophy.**

Hemiballismus (hemiballism): A dramatic syndrome of wild, high amplitude, incessant movements on one side of the body **(Video H.1).**[13] The movements resemble those of chorea but are more pronounced; the distinction between severe hemichorea and hemiballismus becomes arbitrary. Like chorea, hemiballistic movements are involuntary and purposeless, but they are much more rapid and forceful and involve the proximal portions of the extremities. When fully developed, there are continuous, violent, swinging, flinging, rolling, throwing, flailing movements of the involved extremities. The movements are ceaseless during the waking state and disappear only with deep sleep. They are usually unilateral and involve one entire half of the body. Rarely, they are bilateral (biballismus or paraballismus) or involve a single extremity (monoballismus). The movements may spare the face and trunk. Hemiballismus is difficult to treat, incredibly disabling, and sometimes fatal because of exhaustion and inanition.

Hemichorea: See **hemiballismus.**

Hemidystonia: See **dystonia.**

Hemifacial atrophy: See **facial hemiatrophy.**

Hemifacial spasm (HFS): Transient, involuntary spasms involving all or part of one-half of the face. Spontaneous muscle twitching usually begins in one orbicularis oculi, less often the oris. Over months to years, HFS usually spreads to involve all the facial muscles on one side, but remains strictly limited to the muscles supplied by the facial nerve. Fully developed HFS causes repetitive, paroxysmal, involuntary, spasmodic, tonic and clonic contractions of the muscles innervated by the facial nerve on the involved side of the face **(Video H.2)**. The mouth twists to the affected side, the nasolabial fold deepens, the eye closes, and there is contraction of the frontalis muscle. The spasms may become very disfiguring and disabling. The spasms persist in sleep and are often exacerbated by chewing or speaking. See **brow lift sign.**

Hemihypertrophy: See **hemiatrophy.**

Hemimasticatory spasm: Brief, sometimes painful, involuntary contractions or spasms of the jaw-closing muscles unilaterally. It may eventually result in masseter hypertrophy. It may be associated with other conditions, including scleroderma and facial hemiatrophy.

Hemiparesis (hemiplegia): Weakness to varying degrees involving one side of the body.

Hemiparkinsonism: Signs of **parkinsonism** greater on one side of the body. Asymmetric involvement with more pronounced abnormalities on one side is typical of early PD.

Hemiplegic gait: See **gait disorders.**

Hemispatial neglect: See **attentional deficits.**

Hemorrhagic rash: See **purpura.**

Hemotympanum: Blood or blood-stained fluid in the middle ear. The tympanic membrane appears bright red, dark red, brown, or bluish depending on the color of the fluid in the middle ear **(Fig. H.5)**. Hemotympanum usually results from a fracture of the temporal bone, usually longitudinal, that cracks the roof of the middle ear (see **Battle's sign**).

Hennebert's sign: See **fistula test.**

Herpes zoster rash: The skin changes produced by *H. zoster* infection. Acutely there are vesicles on an erythematous base. Straightforward zoster infections are readily

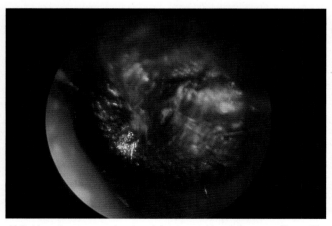

Figure H.5. Hemotympanum due to a left temporal bone fracture. (From Chung EK, Atkinson-McEvoy LR, Lai N, Terry M. *Visual Diagnosis and Treatment in Pediatrics.* 3rd ed. Philadelphia, PA: Wolters Kluwer Health/Lippincott Williams & Wilkins Health; 2015, with permission.)

apparent, and the neurologist is seldom involved. With atypical zoster, the situation is more challenging. Some patients develop a pain syndrome with no rash (zoster sine zoster, zoster sine herpete) or with a subtle rash. The ability to recognize subtle but typical changes becomes important. Postinflammatory depigmentation may provide a clue to past zoster infection in the patient with an unexplained pain syndrome (Fig. H.6). Although involvement of thoracic dermatomes is typical, zoster may strike anywhere (Fig. H.7). When motor neurons are adjacent, zoster may cause weakness, at times severe. Zoster occasionally causes cervical or lumbosacral radiculopathy with a marked motor deficit; the diagnosis becomes apparent with recognition of the zoster skin lesions (Fig. H.8). In Ramsay Hunt syndrome (geniculate herpes), the cause of the facial palsy becomes apparent with finding zoster lesions in the external canal or on the tympanic membrane, which are not always conspicuous (Fig. H.9). See **Hutchinson's sign.**

Heterochromia iridis: A lack of uniformity in the color of the iris. Heterochromia may result from Horner's syndrome, usually congenital or from an insult very early in life. As the child matures, the affected iris fails to darken normally and becomes variegated in color (Fig. H.10). There is often a history of birth trauma, especially brachial plexus injury, or cardiovascular surgery early in life. Although less common, acquired Horner's syndrome in older children and adults may occasionally cause iris heterochromia.[14]

Heteronymous diplopia: See **crossed diplopia.**

Heterophoria: See **strabismus.**

Heterotropia: See **strabismus.**

HINTS: See **head impulse test.**

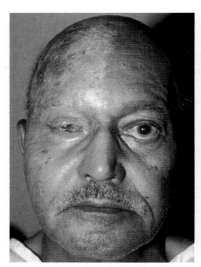 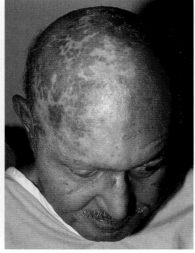

Figure H.6. Scarring due to *H. zoster* involvement of the ophthalmic division of the trigeminal nerve. (From Campbell WW. *DeJong's the Neurologic Examination.* 7th ed. Philadelphia, PA: Wolters Kluwer Health/Lippincott Williams & Wilkins Health; 2013, with permission.)

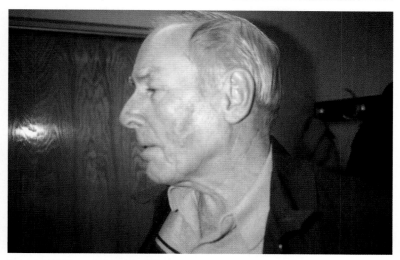

Figure H.7. *H. zoster* involving V2.

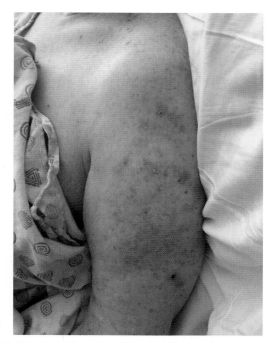

Figure H.8. Healing *H. zoster* rash outlining the C5 dermatome in a patient who presented with a severe C5 radiculopathy that caused near total paralysis of C5 innervated muscles.

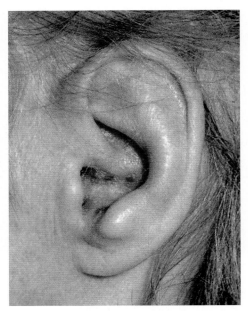

Figure H.9. Vesicles in the external ear canal in a case of geniculate herpes (Ramsay Hunt syndrome). (From Campbell WW. *DeJong's the Neurologic Examination.* 7th ed. Philadelphia, PA: Wolters Kluwer Health/Lippincott Williams & Wilkins Health; 2013, with permission.)

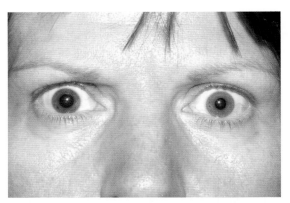

Figure H.10. A 35-year-old woman with different colored eyes since birth. The entire iris of the right eye is brown; the iris of the left eye is greenish brown. The left pupil is smaller than the right, which is consistent with the diagnosis of congenital Horner's syndrome. (From Ur RH. Heterochromia. *CMAJ* 2008;179:447–448, with permission. © CMAJ. This work is protected by copyright and the making of this copy was with the permission of Access Copyright. Any alteration of its content or further copying in any form whatsoever is strictly prohibited unless otherwise permitted by law.)

Hip abduction sign: A sign of hip adductor weakness causing hip abduction when the patient tries to arise from the ground, reported as evidence of LGMD with a sarcoglycan mutation.

Hip dip: The transient hip drop that occurs with pelvic girdle weakness as the patient steps onto a stool. The pelvic weakness interferes with the smooth transfer of weight from the trailing leg to the leading leg.[15]

Hip hike: The elevation of the hip during the swing phase characteristic of **circumduction gait**. See **gait disorders**.

Hippus (pupillary play, pupillary unrest, pupillary athetosis): The small-amplitude fluctuations in size under constant illumination often seen in normal pupils as a physiologic phenomenon. Hippus is of no clinical significance, even when pronounced. See **afferent pupillary defect**.

Hirschberg's sign: See **adductor reflex of the foot**.

Hirschberg's test: See **corneal light reflex test**.

Hirsutism: Abnormal, excessive hair growth, focal or diffuse. Polycystic ovary syndrome is the most common cause of hirsutism in women. Neurologically relevant disorders causing hirsutism include Cushing's disease, POEMS syndrome, ovarian tumors, adrenal tumors, fetal anticonvulsant syndrome, lysosomal storage disorders, hyperprolactinemia, and Flier's syndrome. Hirsutism is a common manifestation of porphyria, especially porphyria cutanea tarda (the most common porphyria), hereditary coproporphyria, and congenital erythropoetic porphyria. Hirsutism is a feature of several congenital dysmorphic disorders, such as Cornelia de Lange syndrome. It also occurs as a medication side effect; notable examples include phenytoin, valproate, cyclosporine, corticosteroids, and oral contraceptives. See **hypertrichosis**.

Hoffman's sign (reflex): A variant of the **finger flexor reflex**. The patient's relaxed hand is held with the wrist dorsiflexed and fingers partially flexed. With one hand, the examiner holds the partially extended middle finger between his index finger and thumb or between his index and middle fingers. With a sharp, forcible flick of the other thumb, the examiner nips or snaps the nail of the patient's middle finger, forcing the distal finger into sharp, sudden flexion followed by sudden release (Fig. H.11). The rebound of the distal phalanx stretches the finger flexors. If the

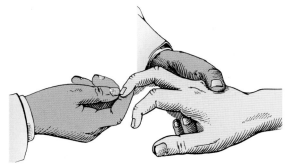

Figure H.11. Method of eliciting the Hoffman sign. (From Campbell WW. *DeJong's the Neurologic Examination*. 7th ed. Philadelphia, PA: Wolters Kluwer Health/Lippincott Williams & Wilkins Health; 2013, with permission.)

Hoffman sign is present, this is followed by flexion and adduction of the thumb and flexion of the index finger, and sometimes flexion of the other fingers as well. The sign is not necessarily pathologic and is often present to some degree in normal individuals; it is only of clinical significance when markedly active or very asymmetric. In the **Trömner sign**, the examiner holds the patient's partially extended middle finger, letting the hand dangle, and then, with the other hand, thumps or flicks the fingerpad (Fig. H.12). The response is the same as in the Hoffman. The two methods are equivalent, and either manner of testing may be used; both are sometimes referred to as Hoffman's sign. These signs are also classified as **frontal release signs**. See **pathologic reflexes, primitive reflexes.**

Hollenhorst plaque: A common cause of branch retinal artery occlusions and often associated with symptomatic carotid stenosis and amaurosis fugax (Fig. H.13). Three main types of retinal emboli have been identified: cholesterol (Hollenhorst plaque), fibrin-platelet, and calcific. The cholesterol emboli most often arise from the ipsilateral carotid and are yellow-orange in color and refractile. Fibrin-platelet emboli appear long, smooth, and white colored and are associated with carotid or cardiac thrombi. Calcific emboli are solid, white, nonrefractile plugs that usually arise from calcified cardiac valves or the aorta. Less commonly, retinal emboli may arise from atrial myxoma or other tumors, fat, septic emboli, or foreign substances.

Holmes (Stewart-Holmes) rebound test: See **checking reflex** and **rebound phenomenon.**

Holmes tremor: See **rubral tremor.**

Homonymous diplopia: See **crossed diplopia.**

Homonymous hemianopia: See **visual field defects.**

Hoover's (automatic walking) sign: A sign useful for evaluating suspected functional, nonorganic leg weakness (see **functional signs, functional weakness**).

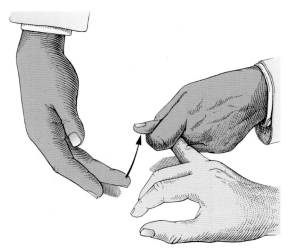

Figure H.12. Method of eliciting the Trömner sign. (From Campbell WW. *DeJong's the Neurologic Examination.* 7th ed. Philadelphia, PA: Wolters Kluwer Health/Lippincott Williams & Wilkins Health; 2013, with permission.)

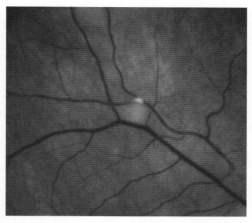

Figure H.13. Branch retinal artery occlusion with Hollenhorst plaque. (From Gerstenblith AT, Rabinowitz MP. *The Wills Eye Manual: Office and Emergency Room Diagnosis and Treatment of Eye Disease.* 6th ed. Philadelphia, PA: Wolters Kluwer Health/Lippincott Williams & Wilkins; 2012, with permission.)

When a normal supine patient flexes the thigh to lift one leg, there is a downward movement of the other leg. The extension countermovement of the opposite leg is a normal **associated movement**, since an extension movement of one leg normally accompanies flexion of the other leg when walking. Hoover's sign is absence of the expected associated movement. In organic leg weakness, the downward pressure of the contralateral heel occurs when the patient tries to raise the weak leg, and the examiner can feel the extension pressure by placing a hand beneath the heel that remains on the bed. Downward pressure is also present, to a lesser degree, in the weak leg as the patient raises the normal leg. In functional leg weakness, there is no downward pressure of the contralateral heel, but the extension movement of the "paralyzed" leg may be felt as the good leg is raised, proving it is not weak, although extension power is typically nil to direct testing.[16] Hoover's sign has two components: the absence of downward pressure of the sound leg when raising the weak leg and the presence of downward pressure of the weak leg, showing greater power than with direct testing, when raising the sound leg. The patient with functional weakness cannot suppress the normal associated extension movement of the bad leg when raising the good leg, and the absence of the associated movement of the good leg proves lack of effort when flexing the bad leg. Similarly, normally and with organic hemiparesis, if the patient presses down on the bed with the good leg, the opposite leg may flex slightly; this movement does not occur in nonorganic weakness. There is experimental evidence to support the utility of Hoover's sign in the diagnosis of functional weakness.[17] The sensitivity is 85%, the specificity 97%, the positive LR 30.7, and the negative LR 0.2.[5] See **abductor sign, Spinal Injuries Center test.**

Horizontal gaze palsy: See **gaze palsy.**

Horner's (Bernard-Horner) syndrome: Ocular sympathetic dysfunction causing ptosis, miosis, and anhidrosis (Fig. H.14). The ptosis is due to lack of sympathetic

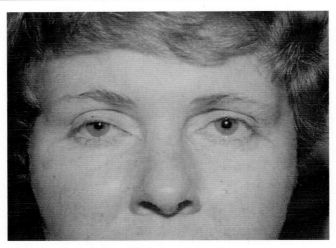

Figure H.14. A patient with a right Horner syndrome.

input to the accessory lid retractors (Müeller's muscle). The ptosis of the upper lid is only 1 to 3 mm and never as severe as with a complete CN III palsy, although it may simulate partial third nerve palsy. Horner's syndrome ptosis can be subtle and is often missed. The lower lid is frequently elevated 1 to 2 mm because of loss of the action of the lower lid accessory retractor that holds the lid down (inverse or upside down ptosis). The resulting narrowing of the palpebral fissure causes apparent **enophthalmos**. Since the fibers mediating facial sweating travel up the external carotid, lesions distal to the carotid bifurcation produce no facial **anhidrosis** except for perhaps a small area of medial forehead that is innervated by sympathetic fibers traveling with the internal carotid. A lesion proximal to the carotid bifurcation produces all components of Horner's syndrome (ptosis, miosis, and anhidrosis); a lesion distal to the bifurcation causes **oculosympathetic paresis** (Horner's syndrome minus facial anhidrosis). The effects on the eye of oculosympathetic paresis and Horner's syndrome are the same, and the terms are often used interchangeably. The small Horner's pupil dilates poorly in the dark (see Fig. A.5) and less quickly than normal (**dilation lag**). Other findings in Horner's syndrome include loss of the **ciliospinal reflex**, ocular hypotony, increased amplitude of accommodation and vasodilation in the affected distribution. **Heterochromia iridis** and other trophic changes of the head and face may result when Horner's syndrome is congenital or acquired early in life.

The causes of Horner's syndrome are legion and include the following: brainstem lesions (especially of the lateral medulla), cluster headache, internal carotid artery thrombosis or dissection, cavernous sinus disease, apical lung tumors, neck trauma, lower brachial plexus lesions, and other conditions.

Pseudo-Horner's syndrome refers to patients who have physiologic **anisocoria** causing **miosis** with incidental **ptosis** on the same side due to a completely unrelated condition, most often **levator dehiscence** or **dermatochalasis**, with the combination of those two findings simulating oculosympathetic paresis.[18] The rare condition of **reverse Horner's syndrome** (Pourfour du Petit syndrome) is unilateral mydriasis, sometimes with facial flushing and hyperhidrosis, due to transient sympathetic overactivity in the early stages of a lesion involving the sympathetic pathways to one eye.

Pharmacologic testing is occasionally done to help determine whether a miotic pupil is due to Horner's syndrome.[19] In about half the patients, the etiology is apparent from other signs and the history. In the other half, clinical localization is uncertain and pharmacologic testing may help determine the level of the lesion and guide further investigations.

Hoyne's sign: See **tripod sign.**

Hung-up reflex (Woltman's sign, delayed ankle jerks): Prolonged relaxation phase of a **deep tendon reflex**. Delayed reflexes are a classical finding of hypothyroidism, but may also occur in chorea when random involuntary agonist contraction interrupts the relaxation phase. Cold ankles cause a slowly relaxing reflex far more often than hypothyroidism. Some medications have been reported to cause delayed reflexes, especially beta blockers. In hypothyroidism, the slow relaxation phase has been attributed to a slowing in the reuptake of calcium into the sarcoplasmic reticulum, an energy-dependent process necessary for muscle relaxation.

Hutchinson's pupil: Dilated pupil due to oculomotor nerve compression as a result of uncal herniation. For detecting an intracerebral structural lesion in comatose patients, anisocoria of >1 mm has a sensitivity of 39%, specificity of 96%, and positive LR of 9.0.[5]

Hutchinson's sign: Involvement of the skin at the tip of the nose by the rash of herpes zoster (Fig. H.15). Vesicles in that location indicate involvement of the nasociliary branch of the trigeminal nerve and increase the likelihood of uveal tract inflammation and ocular damage.[20]

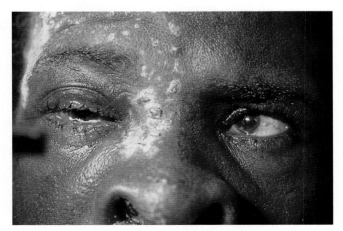

Figure H.15. *H. zoster* ophthalmicus with characteristic skin lesions affecting the dermatome of the first branch of the facial nerve. The tip of the nose is involved, a harbinger of ocular involvement (Hutchinson's sign). (From Tasman W, Jaeger E. *The Wills Eye Hospital Atlas of Clinical Ophthalmology.* 2nd ed. Philadelphia, PA: Wolters Kluwer Health/Lippincott Williams & Wilkins; 2001, with permission.)

Hutchinson's teeth: Notched teeth, a sign of congenital syphilis.

Hydrocephalus: A dilatation of the ventricular system that may occur because of obstruction of CSF flow, impaired resorption, or as a compensatory mechanism for loss of brain volume (hydrocephalus ex vacuo). Obstructive, or noncommunicating, hydrocephalus is due to blockage of the CSF circulation within the ventricular system. Communicating hydrocephalus is due to impaired circulation of the CSF after it leaves the ventricular system, such as from fibrosis and scarring of the basal cisterns because of meningitis, or impaired function of the arachnoid granulations from scarring due to previous SAH. Hydrocephalus that develops prior to suture closure often results in an enlarged, sometimes massive, head **(Fig. H.16)**. Lesser degrees of severity may produce **frontal bossing**. Normal pressure hydrocephalus refers to a spontaneously occurring form of communicating hydrocephalus featuring a clinical triad of dementia, a **gait disorder**, and urinary incontinence.

Hypalgesia: A decrease in pain sensation.

Hyperacusis: A hypersensitivity of hearing, seen most often in patients with peripheral facial palsy where the lesion is proximal to the takeoff of the branch to the stapedius, which produces an inability to dampen tympanic membrane oscillations, causing low tones to sound louder and higher. Hyperacusis may also occur as an epileptic aura, in migraine (where it is referred to phonophobia or sonophobia), in certain psychiatric conditions, and in drug-related disorders.

Hyperalgesia: See **allodynia.**

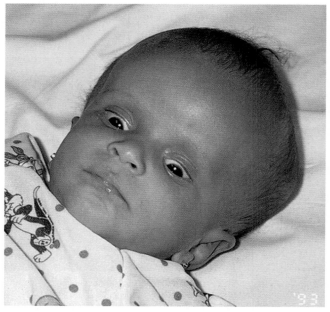

Figure H.16. Forced downgaze (setting sun sign) in a child with hydrocephalus and macrocephaly. (From Lippincott's Nursing Advisor, 2012.)

Hyperekplexia: Also known as startle disease or pathologic startle, refers to disorders characterized by an exaggerated startle response in the absence of other evidence of neurological disease. It is sometimes accompanied by **echolalia, echopraxia,** or **automatic obedience.** Hyperekplexia may be sporadic or hereditary. Colorful names have been used for variants of the condition described in different geographic regions (jumping Frenchmen of Maine, latah, miriachit). An excessive startle response may also occur in Creutzfeldt-Jakob disease, Tay-Sachs disease, stiff-person syndrome, and lipidoses. See Della Marca et al[21] for a video of a pathologic startle response.

Hyperextensible joints: See **hypermobile joints.**

Hyperextensible skin (cutis laxa): Overly stretchable skin (Fig. H.17). Hyperextensible skin is one of cardinal manifestations of Ehlers-Danlos syndrome (EDS) and pseudoxantoma elasticum (PXE), both of which may have neurologic features. EDS predisposes to aneurysm formation, arterial dissection, and carotid-cavernous fistula. Neurovascular disease in PXE is characterized by intracranial aneurysms and premature arterial occlusive disease. Patients develop accelerated atherosclerosis that can result in cerebrovascular disease and myocardial infarction at a young age.

EDS has been divided into at least 10 subtypes, all characterized by **hypermobile joints;** hyperextensible skin that is fragile with easy bruising and the formation of thin, tissue paper scars; and a predisposition to vascular disease.

PXE is a genetic disorder characterized by abnormal elastic tissue affecting primarily the skin, eyes, and cardiovascular systems. The characteristic skin findings are 2-to-5-mm yellow to orange papules that aggregate to form irregularly shaped plaques. The yellowish, papular lesions resemble **xanthomas** but are not lipid and are referred to as pseudoxanthomas. The skin texture resembles plucked chicken skin or Moroccan leather. The skin lesions tend to occur in the antecubital and

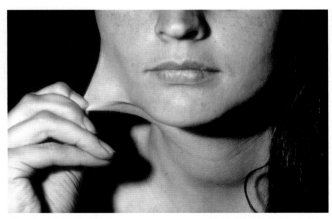

Figure H.17. Stretchy skin. Increased skin stretch in a patient with Ehlers-Danlos syndrome. (From Schaaf CP, Zschocke J, Potocki L. *Human Genetics: From Molecules to Medicine.* Philadelphia, PA: Wolters Kluwer Health/Lippincott Williams & Wilkins Health; 2012, with permission.)

popliteal fossae and involve the sides of the neck, axillae, periumbilical area, and the inner lower lip. As the disease progresses, lax, redundant skin folds appear over the involved areas. The characteristic eye finding is **angioid streaks**.

Hyperesthesia: Increased sensitivity to a sensory stimulus. If tactile hyperesthesia causes pain, then the terms *allodynia* and *hyperpathia* are used.

Hyperhidrosis: Sweating excessive for a given thermoregulatory or emotional stimulus; may be generalized or localized. Generalized hyperhidrosis may occur with many medical conditions causing sympathetic hyperactivity, with lymphoproliferative disorders and with syndromes associated with central autonomic hyperactivity, such as NMS and serotonin syndrome. Primary focal or essential hyperhidrosis affects the palms, soles, and axillae. Some patients develop areas of paroxysmal, focal, circumscribed hyperhidrosis, without other demonstrable abnormalities. Cold-induced sweating syndromes are rare genetic disorders. Compensatory hyperhidrosis occurs in Ross's syndrome, autonomic neuropathy, and at the segments above a spinal cord injury. **Gustatory sweating** and **lacrimal sweating** are due to aberrant nerve regeneration. Harlequin syndrome refers to unilateral facial flushing and sweating after exercise or heat exposure.

Hyperkinesia: Abnormal involuntary movements that occur in a host of neurologic conditions. The term may be applied to any form of increased movement and includes a range of conditions such as tremor, dyskinesias, chorea, athetosis, dystonia, grimacing, tics, myoclonic movements, and hemiballismus. They usually disappear in sleep. See **dyskinesias** (see Video D.2).

Hyperlordosis: An increase in the normal anterior spinal curvature in the lumbar and cervical segments. In some conditions, the lordosis in the lumbar region is dramatically accentuated (Fig. H.18). Any disorder that produces pelvic girdle weakness may cause a lumbar hyperlordosis, including myopathies, such as the muscular dystrophies, especially FSH dystrophy, and spinal muscular atrophy, especially SMA type III (Kugelberg-Welander disease). Other conditions that may cause lumbar hyperlordosis include stiff-person syndrome, HSP, generalized dystonia, and orthopedic conditions such as spondylolisthesis and hip flexor contractures.

Hypermetria: An error in judging the range of movement, causing overshoot; see **dysmetria**.

Hypermetric saccade: A saccadic movement that overshoots the target, requiring corrective saccades back in the opposite direction to acquire the target.

Hypermobile joints: Abnormal laxity of the joints, resulting in an ability to move beyond the normal range of motion without pain. Several conditions may cause abnormal joint hypermobility, and some have neurological relevance. Marfan's and Ehlers-Danlos syndromes are both prone to arterial dissections, cerebral aneurysms, as well as other neurological complications. Not all patients have an obviously Marfanoid habitus, but most have hypermobile joints on examination. Patients with joint hypermobility syndrome (JHS, benign joint hypermobility) are increasingly recognized as having a more complex and not necessarily so benign disorder that has some overlap with conditions often seen by neurologists.[22] They may have a chronic pain syndrome because of multiple unrecognized musculoskeletal strains and sprains related to the hypermobility that has been either misdiagnosed as fibromyalgia, or they have a chronic pain syndrome of some other similar origin related to the JHS. Dysautonomia may be associated with JHS, most

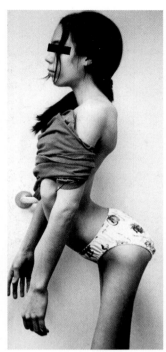

Figure H.18. Marked lumbar lordosis in a 15-year-old girl with FSH dystrophy. (From Weinstein SL, Flynn JM, eds. *Lovell and Winter's Pediatric Orthopaedics.* 7th ed. Philadelphia, PA: Wolters Kluwer Health/Lippincott Williams & Wilkins; 2014, with permission).

commonly taking the form of the postural orthostatic tachycardia syndrome, presenting to the neurologist with syncope. Ptosis, chronic low-back pain, and CTS also occur with increased frequency in this patient population.

Recognizing joint hypermobility is not difficult. The patients tend to have a tall and slender habitus. Telltale features include the ability to place the thumb flat against the volar forearm (thumb abduction sign), hyperextend the small finger past 90 degrees, and place the palms flat on the floor with the knees locked (**Fig. H.19**). The ability to thrust the thumb across the closed fist so that it protrudes past the ulnar border of the hand (Marfan's thumb sign) or overlap of the thumb and little finger when encircling the opposite wrist (Marfan's wrist sign) are also frequently present (**Fig. H.20**). **Arachnodactyly** (wingspan greater than height) and **hyperextensible skin** may also be present and begin to suggest a more serious disorder than JHS. The Beighton hypermobility score is widely used in assessing hypermobility of peripheral joints; a Beighton score of ≥ 4 is considered indicative of generalized hypermobility.[23]

Hyperopia and myopia: An abnormality of the ability of the eye to focus, due to a developmental imperfection resulting in an eyeball that is too short or too long.

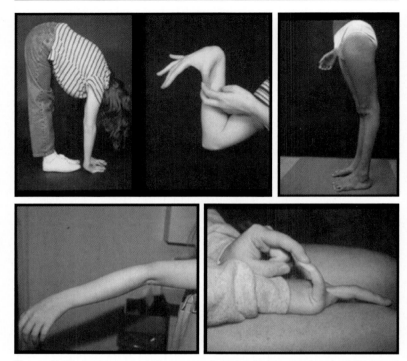

Figure H.19. Joint hypermobility as seen in Ehlers-Danlos syndrome: ability to put hands flat on the ground, thumb abduction sign, and hyperextension of fingers, elbows, and knees. (From McMillan JA, Oski FA. *Oski's Solution: Oski's Pediatrics: Principles and Practice.* 4th ed. Philadelphia, PA: Wolters Kluwer Health/Lippincott Williams & Wilkins; 2006, with permission.)

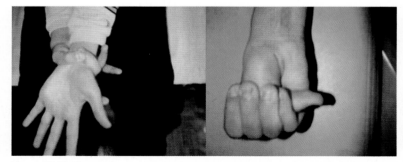

Figure H.20. The Marfan wrist and thumb signs. (From Cocco G. Images in cardiology: The "thumb and wrist sign" in Marfan syndrome. *Heart.* 2001;86:602, with permission.)

The **near point of accommodation** (NPA) is the closest point at which an object can be seen clearly. The **far point of accommodation** (FPA) is the distance at which a distant image is focused on the retina with no accommodative effort. A person with a perfectly normal eye (emmetropia) has an FPA of infinity, and distant objects are properly focused on the fovea. In hyperopia (farsightedness, hypermetropia), the eyeball is too short, the FPA is behind the eye, and accommodation can bring far objects into focus but may fail with near objects. In myopia (nearsightedness), the eyeball is too long or refractive power is excessive, the FPA falls in front of the fovea, and relaxation of accommodation can bring near objects into focus but fails for distant objects.

Hyperpathia: See **allodynia** and **hyperesthesia.**

Hyperpigmentation: Darkening of the skin. In Caucasians, hyperpigmentation may appear as a browning, or bronzing, similar to a suntan, due to excess melanin activity, or yellowish, due to hypercarotenemia. Browning is most often related to increased levels of ACTH, which is biochemically very similar to melanocyte-stimulating hormone (MSH) and can stimulate melanocytes to produce melanin. Some of the conditions with neurologic features or complications that are associated with increased ACTH production are adrenal insufficiency, as from Addison's disease or adrenoleukodystrophy; Nelson's syndrome; Cushing's disease, in which a pituitary tumor secretes ACTH; and ectopic ACTH production as a paraneoplastic syndrome. Other disorders associated with hyperpigmentation include hyperthyroidism, hemochromatosis (bronze diabetes), ataxia-telangiectasia, primary biliary cirrhosis, and Niemann-Pick disease. Some drugs may cause hyperpigmentation, including chemotherapeutic agents, aminoquinolines, oral contraceptives, heavy metals, and psychotropics. Hyperpigmentation is also a feature of several congenital and inherited disorders. Pathologic hyperpigmentation is not limited to sun-exposed areas and often involves the nasolabial folds and palmar creases, causing dark lines to stand out against the normal paleness.

Hypercarotenemia most often results from excessive vitamin A intake through the consumption of vegetables, especially carrots. Since vitamin A intoxication may cause pseudotumor cerebri, a yellowish skin tone in the appropriate clinical circumstances may provide a clue. Other conditions associated with a yellowish skin discoloration include hypothyroidism and porphyria.

Hyperphoria: See **strabismus.**

Hyperreflexia: See **deep tendon reflex.**

Hypertelorism: Widely spaced eyes; a very common anomaly defined as an increase in both the inner and outer intercanthal distances (Fig. H.21). It is often confused with telecanthus, an increase in the distance between the inner canthi with normally spaced outer canthi and a normal interpupillary distance (Fig. H.22). Hypertelorism is frequently confused with exotropia, epicanthal folds, widely spaced eyebrows, or a flat nasal bridge, all of which may cause a superficially similar appearance.

Hypertelorism occurs in many medical conditions; entities of particular neurologic importance include nasal **encephalocele, craniosynostosis** syndromes such as Apert's and Crouzon's, Hurler's syndrome, Andersen-Tawil syndrome, and septo-optic dysplasia.

Hypertonia: An increase in muscle tone, which comes in two common variants: **rigidity** and **spasticity.** Rigidity is hypertonia that occurs to more or less the same

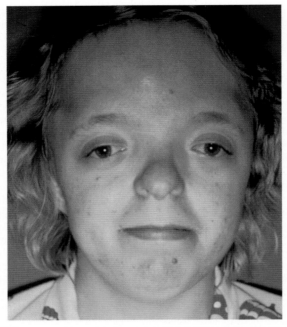

Figure H.21. Pronounced hypertelorism in Apert's syndrome. Note also the antimongoloid slanting of the palpebral fissures, exophthalmos, oxycephaly, and midfacial hypoplasia. (From Gold DH, Weingeist TA. *Color Atlas of the Eye in Systemic Disease*. Baltimore, MD: Wolters Kluwer Health/Lippincott Williams & Wilkins; 2001, with permission.)

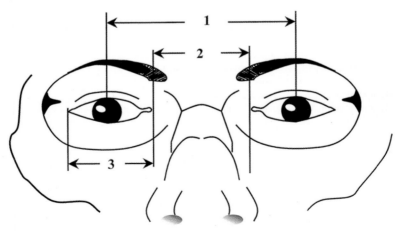

Figure H.22. Facial measurements. 1 = interpupillary distance (IPD); 2 = intercanthal distance (ICD); 3 = palpebral fissure length (PF). (From Barretto RL, Mathog RH. Orbital measurement in black and white populations. *Laryngoscope*. 1999;109(7, pt 1):1051–1054, with permission.)

degree throughout the range of motion of a limb and is independent of the speed of the movement. Spasticity is most marked near the middle of the range of motion and is more apparent with fast than with slow passive movement. Spastic hypertonia is typically associated with increased **deep tendon reflexes**, loss of **superficial reflexes**, and **pathologic reflexes**. Rigidity occurs primarily in extrapyramidal disorders; spasticity is a manifestation of dysfunction of the CST.

Hypertonia also occurs with disease of spinal cord interneurons, stiff-person syndrome, dystonia, and even with muscle disorders in continuous muscle fiber activity syndromes. Nonneurologic processes such as muscle fibrosis and contracture may be confused with hypertonia. **Paratonia** is a form of hypertonia with an involuntary increase in resistance during passive movement.

Hypertrichosis: An abnormal, excessive amount of hair. While not a neurological sign per se, hypertrichosis may constitute an important clue to the diagnosis of a number of conditions relevant to the neurologist, such as porphyria, acromegaly, plasmacytoma, osteosclerotic myeloma, POEMS syndrome, ataxia-telangiectasia, Hunter's syndrome, Hurler's syndrome, and MELAS. Hypertrichosis may also result from drugs.

Hypertropia: See **hirsutism** and **strabismus**.

Hypertrophy: See **muscle hypertrophy** and **nerve hypertrophy**.

Hyperventilation-induced nystagmus: Thirty seconds of hyperventilation may induce nystagmus in a number of central and peripheral conditions, including compensated peripheral vestibulopathy, perilymphatic fistula, acoustic neuroma, craniocervical junction lesions, and cerebellar degeneration.[10] Hyperventilation-induced nystagmus beating ipsilateral to a reduced caloric response, hearing impairment, or abnormal auditory brainstem responses suggests the presence of a CPA tumor **(Video Link H.4)**.[24]

Hypesthesia: A decrease in sensation, generally used to refer to tactile sensibility, hypalgesia being used to refer to a decrease in pain sensibility.

Hypokinesia: See **akinesia** and **bradykinesia**.

Hypomelanotic macule: The typical skin lesions of tuberous sclerosis. They are seen in 90% of patients and are the earliest and most common sign, usually present at birth or during the first year. They are white, elongated, tapered at one end and round at the other, resembling the leaf of a mountain ash tree and are referred to as ash leaf spots **(Fig. H.23)**. See **adenoma sebaceum, periungual fibroma, poliosis, shagreen patch**.

Hypometria: An error in judging the range of movement, causing undershoot; see **dysmetria**.

Hypometric saccade: A saccadic movement that undershoots the target, requiring corrective saccades in the same direction to acquire the target.

Hypomimia: See **masked facies**.

Hypophonia: A low, soft voice, one of the characteristic features of **parkinsonism**. The voice is monotonous and whispery because of **bradykinesia** and **rigidity** affecting the vocal cords and pharyngeal muscles. In early PD, the voice lacks the normal variations of pitch and volume and fatigues quickly. As the disease advances, the patients have difficulty initiating speech and the voice becomes progressively softer and more monotonous. Patients with hypophonia often have great difficulty making themselves understood.

Hyporeflexia: See **deep tendon reflex**.

Figure H.23. A hypomelanotic macule (ash leaf spot) in a patient with tuberous sclerosis.

Hypotelorism: Narrowly spaced eyes. May occur as a feature of hereditary neuralgic amyotrophy and in some developmental abnormalities of the brain (Fig. H.24).[25]

Hypotonia: A decrease in muscle tone. Hypotonia occurs in two primary settings in the adult: myopathies and cerebellar disease. When hypotonia is due to disease of the motor unit, there is invariably some degree of accompanying weakness. Cerebellar hypotonia is not associated with weakness and the reflexes are not lost, although they may be pendular; there are no pathologic reflexes. In a series of 444 patients with unilateral cerebellar lesions, mostly tumors, ipsilateral hypotonia was present in 76%.[5] The hypotonicity in cerebellar disease is never as severe

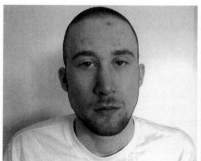 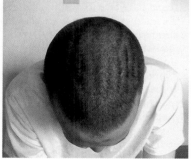

Figure H.24. Hypotelorism and prominent scalp ruggae in a patient with hereditary neuralgic amyotrophy. (From Jeannet PY, Watts GD, Bird TD, Chance PF. Craniofacial and cutaneous findings expand the phenotype of hereditary neuralgic amyotrophy. *Neurology.* 2001;57:1963–1968, with permission.)

as that which occurs with disease of the lower motor neuron. Tone may also be decreased when disease affects the muscle spindle afferent system. Tabes dorsalis affects proprioceptive fibers in the posterior root and may cause muscle hypotonia with **hypermobile joints**. Hypotonia may occur with some lesions of the parietal lobe, probably due to disturbances of sensation. Hypotonia is a common feature in Sydenham's chorea.

On examination, hypotonia may be detected in several ways. In the **arm dropping test,** the dropping is more abrupt than normal (**Bechterew's sign**). With the **shoulder shaking test** and the **pendulum test**, hypotonic limbs swing more than normal. Pendular knee jerks (see **knee reflex**) are caused by muscle hypotonicity and the lack of normal checking of the reflex response. Hypotonicity may cause the outstretched hands to assume a characteristic posture (**spooning**).

Hypotropia: See **strabismus.**

Hysterical gait: See **gait disorders.**

Hysterical signs: See **functional signs.**

Video Links

H.1. The elusive L5 reflex. (From Perloff MD, Leroy AM, Ensrud ER. Teaching video neuroimages: the elusive L5 reflex. *Neurology.* 2010;75:e50.) Available at: http://www.neurology.org/content/suppl/2010/09/12/75.11.e50.DC1/Video_1.mov

H.2. The elusive L5 reflex. (From Perloff MD, Leroy AM, Ensrud ER. Teaching video neuroimages: the elusive L5 reflex. *Neurology.* 2010;75:e50.) Available at: http://www.neurology.org/content/suppl/2010/09/12/75.11.e50.DC1/Video_2.mov

H.3. Abnormal head impulse test with a very obvious catch-up saccade, as well as an abnormal Unterberger-Fukuda stepping test in a patient with vestibular neuritis. (From Bassani R. Teaching video neuroimages: vestibular neuritis: basic elements for clinical and instrumental diagnosis. *Neurology.* 2011;76:e71.) Available at: http://www.neurology.org/content/suppl/2011/04/03/76.14.e71.DC1/Video_1.mov

H.4. Hyperventilation for 30 seconds induces leftward, downward, and counterclockwise nystagmus. (From Choi KD, Cho HJ, Koo JW, et al. Hyperventilation-induced nystagmus in vestibular schwannoma. *Neurology.* 2005;64:2062.) Available at: http://www.neurology.org/content/suppl/2005/06/11/64.12.2062.DC1/Video.mov

References

1. Yamada S, Won DJ. What is the true tethered cord syndrome? *Childs Nerv Syst.* 2007;23:371–375.
2. Schrier JC, Verheyen CC, Louwerens JW. Definitions of hammer toe and claw toe: an evaluation of the literature. *J Am Podiatr Med Assoc.* 2009;99:194–197.
3. Perloff MD, Leroy AM, Ensrud ER. Teaching video neuroimages: the elusive L5 reflex. *Neurology.* 2010;75:e50.
4. Marin R, Dillingham TR, Chang A, et al. Extensor digitorum brevis reflex in normals and patients with radiculopathies. *Muscle Nerve.* 1995;18:52–59.
5. McGee S. *Evidence Based Physical Diagnosis.* 3rd ed. Philadelphia, PA: Elsevier/Saunders; 2012.
6. Jensen OH. The medial hamstring reflex in the level-diagnosis of a lumbar disc herniation. *Clin Rheumatol.* 1987;6:570–574.
7. Wijdicks EF, Bamlet WR, Maramattom BV, et al. Validation of a new coma scale: The FOUR score. *Ann Neurol.* 2005;58:585–593.
8. Kattah JC, Talkad AV, Wang DZ, et al. HINTS to diagnose stroke in the acute vestibular syndrome: three-step bedside oculomotor examination more sensitive than early MRI diffusion-weighted imaging. *Stroke.* 2009;40:3504–3510.
9. Bassani R. Teaching video neuroimages: vestibular neuritis: basic elements for clinical and instrumental diagnosis. *Neurology.* 2011;76:e71.
10. Huh YE, Kim JS. Bedside evaluation of dizzy patients. *J Clin Neurol.* 2013;9:203–213.
11. Mulliken JB, Burrows PE, Fishman SJ. *Mulliken & Young's Vascular Anomalies: Hemangiomas and Malformations.* 2nd ed. Oxford: Oxford University Press; 2013.
12. Bartolomeo P, Bachoud-Levi AC, Thiebaut de, SM. The anatomy of cerebral achromatopsia: a reappraisal and comparison of two case reports. *Cortex.* 2014;56:138–144.

13. Hawley JS, Weiner WJ. Hemiballismus: current concepts and review. *Parkinsonism Relat Disord.* 2012;18:125–129.
14. Diesenhouse MC, Palay DA, Newman NJ, et al. Acquired heterochromia with horner syndrome in two adults. *Ophthalmology.* 1992;99:1815–1817.
15. Brooke MH. *A Clinician's View of Neuromuscular Disease.* 2nd ed. Baltimore, MD: Williams & Wilkins; 1986.
16. Lanska DJ. Functional weakness and sensory loss. *Semin Neurol.* 2006;26:297–309.
17. Stone J, Zeman A, Sharpe M. Functional weakness and sensory disturbance. *J Neurol Neurosurg Psychiatry.* 2002;73:241–245.
18. Martin TJ. Horner's syndrome, Pseudo-Horner's syndrome, and simple anisocoria. *Curr Neurol Neurosci Rep.* 2007;7:397–406.
19. Shin RK, Cheek AG. Teaching neuroimages: positive apraclonidine test in Horner syndrome. *Neurology.* 2011;76:e100.
20. Murrell GL, Hayes BH. Hutchinson sign and herpes zoster. *Otolaryngol Head Neck Surg.* 2007;136:313–314.
21. Della MG, Restuccia D, Mariotti P, et al. Pathologic startle following brainstem lesion. *Neurology.* 2007;68:437.
22. Fikree A, Aziz Q, Grahame R. Joint hypermobility syndrome. *Rheum Dis Clin North Am.* 2013;39:419–430.
23. Smits-Engelsman B, Klerks M, Kirby A. Beighton score: a valid measure for generalized hypermobility in children. *J Pediatr.* 2011;158:119–123.
24. Choi KD, Cho HJ, Koo JW, et al. Hyperventilation-induced nystagmus in vestibular schwannoma. *Neurology.* 2005;64:2062.
25. Jeannet PY, Watts GD, Bird TD, et al. Craniofacial and cutaneous findings expand the phenotype of hereditary neuralgic amyotrophy. *Neurology.* 2001;57:1963–1968.

Ice pack test: A procedure useful in the evaluation of suspected MG. Neuromuscular transmission improves with decreased temperature, and ptosis or ophthalmoparesis due to MG often improves with brief placement of an ice pack on the eye (Fig. I.1A and B). The ice pack test has high sensitivity and specificity in distinguishing ptosis due to MG from lid changes due to such things as **dermatochalasis** and **levator dehiscence**.[1] Studies have shown improvement in ptosis with the ice pack test with a sensitivity of 77% to 96%, a specificity of 83% to 98%, a positive LR of 19.3, and a negative LR of 0.2.[2] Improvement of diplopia and ophthalmoparesis with the ice pack test has a sensitivity of 97%, a specificity of 97%, a positive LR of 31.0, and a negative LR of 0.03.[2] Having the patient simply rest with eyes closed (see **rest test**) may also cause improvement, but less so than an ice pack. When the patient is symptomatic but the examination is normal or equivocal, application of a warm pack may bring out ptosis, but the warm pack test is less useful than the cold pack test (Fig. I.1C and D). The cold and warm pack tests are especially useful when edrophonium testing may be risky.

Ice water calorics: See **caloric tests**.

Ichthyosis: A dermatologic condition causing dryness, roughness, and scaliness of the skin that is persistent and diffuse (Fig. I.2). Ichthyosis may occur in several disorders with prominent neurologic features, including Refsum's disease,

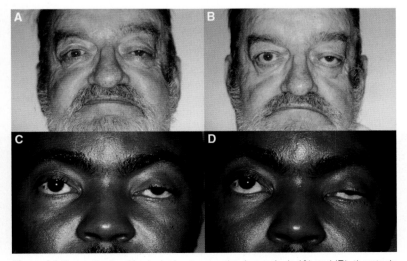

Figure I.1. Two patients with ptosis due to myasthenia gravis. In (**A**) and (**B**), the ptosis improved after application of an ice pack; in (**C**) and (**D**), the ptosis worsened after the application of a warm pack.

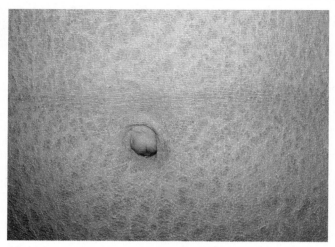

Figure I.2. Ichthyosis with typical dark polygonal scales. (From Burkhart CN, Morrell D. *VisualDx. Essential Pediatric Dermatology.* Philadelphia, PA: Wolters Kluwer Health/ Lippincott Williams & Wilkins; 2010, with permission.)

Sjögren-Larson syndrome, HSP, multiple sulfatase deficiency, and Chanarin-Dorfman syndrome.

Ideational apraxia: An inability to perform the entire sequence of a complex motor act properly despite preserved ability to carry out the individual components.[3] The patient may perform each step correctly, but in attempting the entire sequence omits steps or gets the steps out of order. There is an inability to correctly sequence a series of acts leading to a goal. Ideational apraxia involves an impairment in conceptualizing the overall goal of the activity or an inability to plan the series of steps. For instance, in showing how to drive a car, the patient might try to put the car in drive before starting the engine. When asked to demonstrate how to mail a letter, the patient may seal the envelope before inserting the letter, or mail the letter before affixing the stamp. Ideational apraxia may occur with damage to the left posterior temporoparietal junction or in patients with generalized cognitive impairment. In daily life, patients with ideational apraxia may perform tasks out of sequence. In one reported case, a woman trying to light a gas stove first struck the match, then filled the kettle, then turned on the gas, causing a minor explosion. See **apraxia, buccofacial apraxia, ideational apraxia, conceptual apraxia, conduction apraxia, constructional apraxia, dissociation apraxia, dressing apraxia.**[3]

Ideomotor apraxia: An **apraxia** in which the patient is unable to perform a complex command (e.g., salute, wave goodbye, snap the fingers, make a fist, show how to hitchhike, show V for victory) with the involved extremity, sometimes with either extremity.[3] As with other forms of apraxia, the deficit occurs in the absence of any weakness, sensory loss or other deficit in a patient who is alert and comprehends the task. The patient may be unable to pantomime how to use common implements (e.g., hammer, toothbrush, comb) or how to kick or throw a ball. She may substitute a hand or finger for the imagined object (see **body part as object).** The responsible lesion apparently causes a disconnection between the language or visual centers that understand the command and the motor areas tasked with carrying it out. Ideomotor ataxia is probably the most common form of apraxia and is present in as many as 40% of aphasic patients if correctly tested, but it frequently goes undetected. See **apraxia, buccofacial apraxia, ideational apraxia, conceptual apraxia, conduction apraxia, constructional apraxia, dissociation apraxia, dressing apraxia.**

Idioglossia: Imperfect articulation with utterance of meaningless sounds; the individual may speak with a vocabulary all his own. Idioglossia occurs in patients with partial deafness, aphasia, and congenital word deafness.

Idiomuscular contraction: A brief and usually feeble contraction of a muscle belly after it is tapped with a percussion hammer, causing a slight depression directly at the site the muscle was struck. The idiomuscular contraction is not related to the **deep tendon reflex** and occurs even when the DTR is absent and is different from **myoedema.** The idiomuscular contraction causes a slight depression, myoedema a rounding up.

Imitation behavior: Involuntary imitation of the examiner's gestures, even if specifically told to refrain, a form of **echopraxia.** Patients are not able to inhibit the response. Imitation behavior is a sign of frontal lobe damage and is related to **utilization behavior.** Mild imitation behavior might be elicited during the interview: the examiner rubs her nose; the patient does likewise. With severe imitation behavior, the patient might imitate the examiner's gesture while repeating the instructions not to do so. Behavior of this severity has been termed obstinate imitation behavior and may be more specific for FTD. Imitation and utilization behavior are examples of **defective response inhibition,** or **environmental dependency,** similar to **echolalia** and **echopraxia.**[4] The ability to test such **executive functions** at the bedside is very useful when a condition such as FTD is suspected. Other useful bedside executive tests include word-list generation (especially F words), the **Go/No-Go test,** the **antisaccade test,** the **applause sign,** and the **fist-edge-palm test.**

Impersistence: An inability to continue performing a task or to sustain an activity. A patient asked to cross out all of the A's on a written sheet or bisect lines randomly placed on a page may fail to complete the task. Motor impersistence is the inability to sustain motor acts. The patient is unable to sustain an activity, such as keeping the eyes closed, the hand raised, or the tongue protruded. Lesions of the right hemisphere are more likely to cause impersistence. Motor impersistence frequently accompanies chorea in disorders such as HD, and signs such as **trombone tongue** and **milkmaid grip** are due to both acting in concert. Impersistence is the opposite of perseveration.

Impingement sign: See **shoulder examination tests.**

Inattention: See **attentional deficits.**

Intention tremor: A form of **action tremor** seen primarily in cerebellar disease (see Video C.3). The tremor appears when precision is required to touch a target, as in the **finger-to-nose** or toe-to-finger test. It progressively worsens during the movement. Approaching the target causes the limb to shake, usually side-to-side perpendicular to the line of travel, and the amplitude of the oscillation increases toward the end of the movement. The intention tremor of multiple sclerosis and cerebellar disease is usually of medium amplitude and may vary in degree from mild to severe; it may be coarse and irregular, especially when associated with other signs of ataxia. Studies of patients with a unilateral cerebellar hemisphere lesion show that intention tremor was present in approximately 30%.[5]

Interlocking finger test: A quick, simple screen for parietal lobe dysfunction in which the patient is asked to imitate a standardized set of four interlocking finger figures **(Fig. I.3)**.[6]

Intermanual conflict: See **alien hand** and **anarchic hand.**

Internal anal sphincter reflex: See **anal reflex.**

Internal hamstring reflex: See **hamstring reflexes.**

Internuclear ophthalmoplegia (INO): An ocular motility disorder due to a lesion involving the medial longitudinal fasciculus (MLF). The primary function of the MLF is to coordinate lateral gaze by connecting the pontine paramedian reticular formation (PPRF), which lies near the CN VI nucleus in the pons, on one side with the nucleus of CN III on the opposite side in order to allow the two eyes to move synchronously. The MLF crosses in the pons, soon after beginning its ascent to the contralateral third nerve complex.

Lesions of the MLF disrupt communication between the two nuclei, causing an INO **(Fig. I.4**; see Video D.1). The contralateral medial rectus receives no signal to contract when the PPRF and sixth nerve nucleus act to initiate lateral gaze. As a result, gaze to one side results in abduction of the ipsilateral eye, but no adduction of its fellow. Typically the abducting eye has nystagmus as well, which may be sustained or only a few beats. By convention, the INO is labeled by the side of the adduction failure; a right INO produces adduction failure of the right eye. Failure of the medial rectus to adduct is an isolated abnormality in the affected eye; normality of the lid and pupil distinguish an INO from a third nerve palsy. Some patients

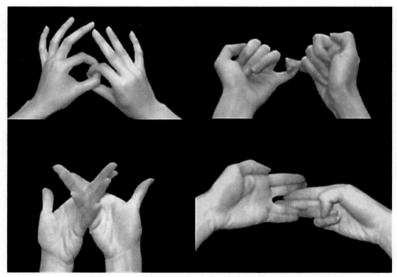

Figure I.3. The interlocking finger test. (From Moo LR, Slotnick SD, Tesoro MA, et al. Interlocking finger test: a bedside screen for parietal lobe dysfunction. *J Neurol Neurosurg Psychiatry.* 2003;74:530–532, with permission.)

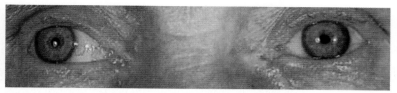

Figure I.4. An internuclear ophthalmoplegia. On gaze to the right, the left eye fails to adduct.

have total adduction failure, and some may have exotropia in primary gaze. Patients with bilateral INO and exotropia have the WEBINO syndrome (wall-eyed bilateral INO).[7] Those with a unilateral INO and exotropia have the WEMINO syndrome (wall-eyed monocular INO). An INO is commonly accompanied by vertical nystagmus, most commonly gaze-evoked upbeat.

The earliest detectable sign of an INO is slowness of adducting saccades compared with abducting saccades, demonstrated by rapid refixations or OKNs. Many brainstem lesions can cause an INO, but the common conditions are MS and brainstem stroke. INOs due to MS are usually bilateral and seen in young patients; those due to brainstem vascular disease are more often unilateral and seen in older patients. In a series of 410 patients, more than one-quarter had a cause other than demyelination or simple ischemia.[8] Etiologies were infarction in 38%, MS in 34% and unusual causes in 28%. The unusual causes included trauma, tentorial herniation, infection, tumor, iatrogenic injury, hemorrhage, vasculitis, and miscellaneous. The INO was unilateral in 87% of the infarct cases and bilateral in 73% of the MS cases.

Despite impaired adduction on horizontal gaze, some patients with an INO are still able to converge, and INOs have been divided into those with and without preservation of convergence. The convergence centers are in the midbrain. When adduction on convergence is impaired, the INO may be classified as rostral (anterior), and when convergence is preserved, the INO may be classified as caudal (posterior). However, many normal individuals have impaired convergence, and the proposed localizing value of convergence ability has not been borne out.

Conditions such as MG, Wernicke's encephalopathy, thyroid eye disease, GBS, Miller Fisher syndrome, or partial third nerve palsy can cause a "pseudo-INO." In MG, medial rectus muscle involvement is common and often disproportionately severe, and may lead to a myasthenic pseudo-INO, in which the ocular motility disturbance closely mimics an INO due to a lesion of the MLF **(Video I.1)**.

Since the MLF fibers decussate just after their origin, a medial pontine lesion can affect both the PPRF on one side and the MLF crossing from the contralateral side. Because of the ipsilateral lesion, the patient has a gaze palsy to the same side. Because of the MLF lesion, the patient has an INO on the same side. A lesion of the right pons can then cause a right gaze palsy with a superimposed right INO, which results in complete horizontal gaze palsy to the right and inability to adduct the right eye on left gaze ("half a gaze palsy" to the left). The only eye movement possible is abduction of the left eye. Fisher named this constellation of findings the "one-and-a-half syndrome" **(Video Link I.1)**.[9] The most common causes are infarction and demyelinating disease. Paralytic pontine exotropia refers to patients who have exotropia in primary position because of the preserved abduction in the contralateral eye.[10]

Inverse jaw winking (reverse jaw winking, inverse [reverse] Marcus Gunn phenomenon, Marin Amat sign): Automatic closure of one eye on opening the mouth. It occurs primarily in patients who have had a peripheral facial paralysis, usually Bell's palsy, and is probably an intrafacial **synkinesis** due to aberrant re-innervation between the platysma and the orbicularis oculi. A proposed alternative explanation is a trigemino-facial–**associated movement**. However, its almost universal association with peripheral facial paralysis suggests a synkinesis. Some sources confuse inverse jaw winking with the **corneomandibular reflex**; they are quite different responses both in manifestations and in implications.

Inverse Marcus Gunn phenomenon: See **inverse jaw winking.**

Inverse ocular bobbing: See **ocular bobbing.**

Inverse ptosis: See **Horner's syndrome.**

Inversion of optokinetic nystagmus: A sign of congenital nystagmus; see **nystagmus.**

Inverted knee reflex: See **inverted reflexes.**

Inverted radial periosteal (supinator) reflex: See **inverted reflexes.**

Inverted (paradoxic, indirect) reflexes: Unexpected and unusual responses on percussion of a tendon. When reflexes are very active, responses may occur from muscles that have not been directly stretched, even in normal patients. The response may involve adjacent or even contralateral muscles, as in the **crossed adductor** response. It is normal for percussion of the brachioradialis tendon to also cause slight finger flexion as well as biceps contraction in some patients. This is referred to as **spread**, or irradiation, of reflexes.

Inverted reflexes are responses more bizarre than simple spread. The term *inversion* was first used by Babinski in describing "inversion of the radial reflex."[11,12] *Paradoxical* or *perverted* might be better terms but *inverted* is firmly entrenched, although Robert Wartenberg disliked the term.[12] These responses are most often seen when the segmental reflex is absent or impaired, and there is also underlying hyperreflexia lowering the threshold for activation of the antagonist muscle. These responses have also been referred to as "indirect" reflexes because the reflex contraction occurs without direct stretch of the muscle involved. In some instances, the indirect response occurs in the absence of any direct reflex, whereas in other instances both the direct reflex and one or more indirect reflexes occur together.

The bulk of the evidence suggests these inverted and paradoxical reflexes are mediated by vibration in the periphery. The possibility of a transmitted mechanical vibration to the abnormally active muscle was first proposed in 1881.[13,14] Sherrington offered two explanations for these responses: a central mechanism related to central hyperexcitability with spread of the afferent volley to nearby motor neuron pools, and a peripheral mechanism related to direct activation of the muscles involved. He favored a peripheral mechanism mediated by vibration.[11] Some have proposed that indirect reflexes occur commonly but are not obvious because the direct reflexes are more active.

There are many examples of these inverted, perverted, or paradoxical reflexes: contraction of the finger flexors on percussion of the distal radius (inverted brachioradialis reflex), contraction of the biceps on eliciting the triceps reflex (paradoxical triceps jerk), contraction of the hamstring on eliciting the knee reflex (inverted knee jerk), contraction of the hamstring on eliciting the ankle reflex, and contraction of the adductors or quadriceps on eliciting the contralateral knee reflex. Multiple ipsilateral, or even contralateral, upper extremity responses may occur with percussion of the pectoralis major tendon or over the distal clavicle (**clavicle reflex**).

A study by Lance and De Gail using limb ischemia and local anesthetic block concluded that percussion initiates a vibration wave that is transmitted to other muscles, activating their muscle spindles and producing a reflex contraction.[14] Conversely, Estanol and Marin concluded the mechanism was central hyperexcitability.[11] A study using H-reflexes concluded the mechanism of the inverted brachioradialis reflex was peripheral rather than central.[15] The debate over central versus peripheral mechanisms may be a false dichotomy, as both are likely involved. These responses occur most commonly in the face of segmental central hyperexcitability combined with impairment of the local reflex arc, such as an inverted brachioradialis reflex in cervical spondylotic radiculomyelopathy.

The tonic vibration reflex has been investigated primarily in relation to the electrophysiologic H-reflex. Studies have shown that muscle vibration is a potent stimulus for spindle sensory endings. In humans, muscle vibration at a frequency of 100 Hz and an amplitude of 1 mm is adequate to activate virtually all the spindle primary endings within a muscle.[16] Muscle vibration causes presynaptic suppression of the monosynaptic reflex of the muscle vibrated, i.e., the agonist. Given the normal neurophysiology of reciprocal inhibition, the vibration induced by the percussion of the reflex hammer could activate antagonist spindles whose gain has been increased because of CST dysfunction, setting the stage for observing unusual reflex responses.

The easiest paradoxical reflexes to understand are the inverted triceps jerk and the inverted knee jerk, which are truly "inverted" because the response is the opposite of that expected: flexion of the elbow or knee with percussion of the triceps or patellar tendon. The paradoxical triceps reflex was first described by Souques in 1911.[12] It appears when the afferent arc of the triceps reflex is damaged, as in C7 or C8 radiculopathy, particularly when accompanied by an element of spasticity.[17] Care must be taken not to strike too distally; a blow delivered over the olecranon may cause the elbow to flex because of the biomechanics and force vectors involved or possibly because of inadvertent stretch of the biceps, simulating an inverted triceps reflex when one is not actually present. This response has been referred to as the **olecranon reflex**, but is more of a technical error in the point of the strike than a true reflex.

With an inverted knee jerk, there is knee flexion instead of extension. Lance referred to this response as an indirect hamstring reflex.[14] It was first described by Berger in 1879, but is not widely recognized.[12] Boyle reported two cases with inversion of the patellar reflex caused by lumbosacral spinal cord lesions and suggested the finding had the same localizing value for the lumbar cord as the inverted supinator jerk for the cervical cord.[18]

The inverted triceps and knee reflexes are straightforward: the response is the opposite of that expected. Other "inverted" reflexes are related to activation of muscles other than the antagonist. In the presence of spasticity and hyperreflexia, reflex contraction of the biceps or brachioradialis may be accompanied by pronounced flexion of the fingers and adduction of the thumb. The inverted brachioradialis reflex (often referred to as an inverted radial periosteal or inverted supinator reflex) does not result in true inversion, i.e., elbow extension, but instead produces a perverted or aberrant response with finger flexion, perhaps because the vibration wave activates the **finger flexor reflex** arc.

In the paradoxical ankle reflex, plantar flexion of the foot is produced by tapping the anterior aspect of the ankle in patients with hyperreflexia. The ankle reflex is not necessarily depressed, as with other inverted or perverted reflexes, and the response is the normal one, but is due to spread of the reflexogenic zone. Vibration transmitted to the gastrosoleus has been invoked as an explanation.

Inverted (paradoxical) triceps reflex: See **inverted reflexes.**

Iridoplegia: Pupillary paralysis. Complete iridoplegia produces a dilated, fixed pupil (Fig. I.5). Iridoplegia usually occurs as a feature of CN III palsy (see **Hutchinson's pupil**). Isolated iridoplegia may occur because of defective parasympathetic innervation or to the accidental or deliberate instillation of an anticholinergic agent, such as atropine, in the eye. In pharmacologic blockade, the pupil fails to constrict to pilocarpine, permitting rapid distinction between these two possibilities.[19]

Iritis/uveitis: Inflammation of the iris or the uveal tract (iris, ciliary body, and choroid). The anterior uvea is the iris and ciliary body; the posterior uvea is the choroid. Anterior uveitis is essentially synonymous with iritis. Iritis presents as a red eye, which must be distinguished from other causes of red eye, such as keratitis, conjunctivitis, episcleritis, and glaucoma. Features suggesting iritis or uveitis are pain, inflammation primarily at the limbus (limbitis), and a constricted pupil (Fig. I.6). A ciliary flush is diffuse erythema in a circumcorneal distribution.

Some of the conditions with neurologic features or complications in which iritis or uveitis may occur include Lyme disease, Rocky Mountain spotted fever, syphilis, tuberculosis, Whipple's disease, Behcet's disease, ankylosing spondylitis, MS, sarcoidosis, Sjögren's syndrome, SLE, vasculitis, and Vogt-Koyanagi-Harada syndrome. In a series of 236 consecutive patients with uveitis, the most frequently diagnosed systemic diseases were Reiter's syndrome, ankylosing spondylitis, Sjögren's syndrome, and sarcoidosis.[20] These diagnoses were usually not known prior to referral. Of patients with anterior uveitis, 53% had a causally related systemic illness; only 17% of patients with posterior uveitis and 22% of patients with chorioretinitis had an associated systemic disease.

Irradiation of reflexes: See **spread of reflexes.**

Isolated gait ignition failure: See **gait disorders.**

Isolation of the speech area (mixed transcortical aphasia, isolation aphasia): An **aphasia** syndrome in which the posterior inferior frontal (Broca's) and the posterior superior temporal (Wernicke's) areas and the connecting arcuate fasciculus are intact, but the surrounding brain is damaged. The patients are aphasic but have a paradoxical preservation of the ability to repeat. The isolation syndrome is one of the **transcortical aphasias**, in which the perisylvian language areas are preserved

Figure I.5. Iridoplegia from instillation of mydriatic drops.

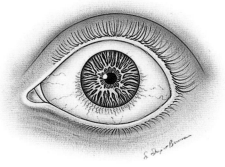

Figure I.6. A depiction of the appearance of acute iritis. The inflammation is most intense at the limbus. (From Bickley LS, Szilagyi P. *Bates' Guide to Physical Examination and History Taking*. 8th ed. Philadelphia, PA: Wolters Kluwer Health/Lippincott Williams & Wilkins; 2003, with permission.)

but disconnected from the rest of the brain. Isolation of the speech area is the most severe form. The entire perisylvian language complex is separated from the rest of the brain, rendering the patients nonfluent in spontaneous speech and unable to comprehend, but curiously able to repeat. Repetition can be so well preserved that the patients display **echolalia**, repeating everything they hear. The usual etiology is a border zone infarction.

Video Link

I.1. A patient with the one-and-a-half syndrome. (From the Shirley H. Wray Neuro-ophthalmology Collection, Neuro-ophthalmology Virtual Education Library [NOVEL], University of Utah.) Available at: http://stream.utah.edu/m/dp/frame.php?f=ae16674c857f0555181

References

1. Fakiri MO, Tavy DL, Hama-Amin AD, et al. Accuracy of the ice test in the diagnosis of myasthenia gravis in patients with ptosis. *Muscle Nerve*. 2013;48:902–904.
2. McGee, S. *Evidence Based Physical Diagnosis*. 3rd ed. Philadelphia, PA: Elsevier/Saunders; 2012.
3. Foundas AL. Apraxia: neural mechanisms and functional recovery. *Handb Clin Neurol*. 2013;110:335–345.
4. Besnard J, Allain P, Aubin G, et al. A contribution to the study of environmental dependency phenomena: the social hypothesis. *Neuropsychologia*. 2011;49:3279–3294.
5. Dennis M, Bowen WT, Cho L. *Mechanisms of Clinical Signs*. Sydney, Australia: Churchill Livingstone; 2012.
6. Moo LR, Slotnick SD, Tesoro MA, et al. Interlocking finger test: a bedside screen for parietal lobe dysfunction. *J Neurol Neurosurg Psychiatry*. 2003;74:530–532.
7. Sakamoto Y, Kimura K, Iguchi Y, et al. A small pontine infarct on DWI as a lesion responsible for wall-eyed bilateral internuclear ophthalmoplegia syndrome. *Neurol Sci*. 2012;33:121–123.
8. Keane JR. Internuclear ophthalmoplegia: unusual causes in 114 of 410 patients. *Arch Neurol*. 2005;62:714–717.
9. Wall M, Wray SH. The one-and-a-half syndrome—a unilateral disorder of the pontine tegmentum: a study of 20 cases and review of the literature. *Neurology*. 1983;33:971–980.
10. Sharpe JA, Rosenberg MA, Hoyt WF, et al. Paralytic pontine exotropia. A sign of acute unilateral pontine gaze palsy and internuclear ophthalmoplegia. *Neurology*. 1974;24:1076–1081.
11. Estanol BV, Marin OS. Mechanism of the inverted supinator reflex. A clinical and neurophysiological study. *J Neurol Neurosurg Psychiatry*. 1976;39:905–908.

12. Wartenberg R. *The Examination of Reflexes.* Chicago: Year Book Publishers; 1945.
13. Lance JW. The mechanism of reflex irradiation. *Proc Aust Assoc Neurol.* 1965;3:77–81.
14. Lance JW, DeGail P. Spread of phasic muscle reflexes in normal and spastic subjects. *J Neurol Neurosurg Psychiatry.* 1965;28:328–334.
15. Teasdall RD, Magladery JW. Brachioradialis reflex and contraction of forearm flexors. An electromyographic study. *Arch Neurol.* 1974;30:94–95.
16. Latash MH. *Neurophysiological Basis of Movement.* 2nd ed. Champaign, IL: Human Kinetics; 2008.
17. Kochar DK, Agarwal N, Sharma BV, et al. Paradoxical triceps jerk, a neglected localising sign in clinical neurology. *Neurol India.* 2001;49:213.
18. Boyle RS, Shakir RA, Weir AI, et al. Inverted knee jerk: a neglected localising sign in spinal cord disease. *J Neurol Neurosurg Psychiatry.* 1979;42:1005–1007.
19. Thompson HS, Newsome DA, Loewenfeld IE. The fixed dilated pupil. Sudden iridoplegia or mydriatic drops? A simple diagnostic test. *Arch Ophthalmol.* 1971;86:21–27.
20. Rosenbaum JT. Uveitis. An internist's view. *Arch Intern Med.* 1989;149:1173–1176.

Jackson's compression test: See **Spurling's maneuver.**

Jargon aphasia: Speech rendered unintelligible by paraphasias and neologisms, also described as word salad.

Jaw deviation: Movement of the mandible to one side on opening. Unilateral trigeminal motor weakness causes deviation of the jaw toward the weak side on opening, due to the unopposed action of the contralateral lateral pterygoid. The jaw deviates toward the weak side (see **Fig. J.1**). Whether this is toward or away from the lesion depends on the specifics of the lesion. Careful observation of jaw opening is often the earliest clue to the presence of an abnormality. It is occasionally difficult to be certain whether the jaw is deviating or not. The relationship of the midline notch between the upper and lower incisor teeth is a more reliable indicator than lip movement. The tip of the nose and the interincisural notches should line up. A straightedge against the lips can help detect deviation. Another useful technique is to draw a vertical line across the midline upper and lower lips using a felt-tip marker. Failure of the two vertical marks to match when the jaw is opened indicates deviation. With unilateral weakness, on moving the jaw from side to side the patient is unable to move the jaw contralaterally. With facial weakness, there may be apparent deviation of the jaw, and of the tongue, because of the facial asymmetry. Holding up the weak side manually sometimes eliminates the pseudodeviation.

Other techniques for examining trigeminal motor function include having the patient protrude and retract the jaw, noting any tendency toward deviation; and having the patient bite on tongue depressors with the molar teeth, comparing the impressions on the two sides and comparing the difficulty of extracting a tongue depressor held in the molar teeth on each side.

Unilateral weakness of CN V–innervated muscles generally signifies a lesion involving the brainstem, Gasserian ganglion, or the motor root of CN V at the base of the skull. Severe bilateral weakness of the muscles of mastication with inability to close the mouth (dangling jaw) suggests motor neuron disease, a neuromuscular

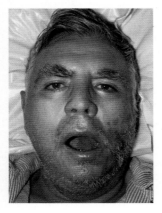

Figure J.1. A patient with *H. zoster* of the mandibular division on the left involving the motor root, producing weakness of the pterygoids, and causing deviation of the jaw to the left. The herpetic rash is in the distribution of CN V_3. (From Campbell WW. *DeJong's the Neurologic Examination.* 7th ed. Philadelphia, PA: Wolters Kluwer Health/Lippincott Williams & Wilkins Health; 2013, with permission.)

transmission disorder, or a myopathy. With significant atrophy of one masseter, a flattening of the jowl on the involved side may be apparent. Temporalis atrophy may cause a hollowing of the temple. Because of bilateral innervation, unilateral UMN lesions rarely cause significant impairment of trigeminal motor function, although there may be mild, transitory unilateral weakness.

Jaw (masseter, mandibular) reflex: Contraction of the jaw closure muscles in response to a stretch stimulus. The reflex is elicited by placing an index finger or thumb over the middle of the patient's chin, holding the mouth open about midway with the jaw relaxed, then tapping the finger with the reflex hammer. The response is an upward jerk of the mandible. Other methods to elicit the reflex include tapping the chin directly and placing a tongue blade over the tongue or the lower incisor teeth and tapping the protruding end. All of these cause a bilateral response. A unilateral response may sometimes be elicited by tapping the angle of the jaw or by placing a tongue blade over the lower molar teeth along one side and tapping the protruding end.

In normal individuals, the jaw jerk is minimally active or absent. Its greatest use is in distinguishing limb hyperreflexia due to a cervical spine lesion (where the jaw jerk is normal) from a state of generalized hyperreflexia (where the jaw jerk is increased along with all of the other reflexes). The reflex is exaggerated with lesions affecting the corticobulbar pathways above the motor nucleus, especially if bilateral, as in pseudobulbar palsy or ALS. The reflex may be unilaterally depressed in lesions involving the reflex arc **(Video Link J.1)**.

Jaw winking: An aberrant innervation syndrome that occurs when there is congenital ptosis associated with abnormal communication between CN V and the levator palpebrae, causing the ptotic lid to open and sometimes retract with jaw movement **(Video J.1)**. When the jaw opens or moves laterally the lid pops open, and when the jaw closes the lid winks closed. Jaw winking is considered a trigemino-oculomotor synkinesis due to misdirection of proprioceptive impulses from the pterygoid muscles to the oculomotor nucleus and occurs in 2% to 13% of patients with congenital ptosis.[1] In **inverse jaw winking**, the lid closes on opening the mouth.

Jendrassik's maneuver: See **reflex reinforcement**.

Jerk nystagmus: See **nystagmus**.

Jolly's sign: A posture seen in patients with a transverse myelopathy at the C7 spinal level. There is paralysis of the triceps and the extensors of the wrist and fingers, and the patient holds the shoulder abducted with the elbow flexed, usually with flexion of the wrist and fingers. This position, if unilateral, is referred to as Jolly's sign, and if bilateral either Bradborn's or Thorburn's sign. The **bodybuilder sign** is similar, probably identical.[2]

Junctional scotoma: See **scotoma**.

Video Link

J.1. Hyperactive jaw reflex in a patient with ALS and pseudobulbar palsy. Available at: http://www.youtube.com/watch?v=ctFvOasAKo0

References

1. Carman KB, Ozkan S, Yakut A, et al. Marcus Gunn jaw winking synkinesis: report of two cases. *BMJ Case Rep.* Jan 23, 2013.
2. Espinosa PS, Berger JR. Acute central cord syndrome with bodybuilder sign. *Clin Neurol Neurosurg.* 2007;109:354–356.

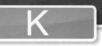

Kayser-Fleischer rings: Bands of yellowish-orange, brown, or green-brown discoloration 1 to 3 mm wide around the rim of the cornea seen in patients with Wilson's disease (Fig. K.1). The rings are seen more easily in light-eyed individuals. KF rings are due to copper deposition in the posterior stroma of the cornea and in Descemet's membrane. They are essentially always present in patients with neurological involvement, but may not be visible without a slit lamp.[1] Rarely, the disease presents without the rings.[2] Other conditions that may cause KF rings are primary biliary cirrhosis, multiple myeloma, and chronic active liver disease.

Keratoconjunctivitis sicca: See **xerophthalmia.**

Kernig's sign: One of the **meningeal signs.** There is some variability in the descriptions of how to elicit Kernig's sign. The most common method is to flex the hip and knee to right angles and then attempt to passively extend the knee (Fig. K.2). This movement produces pain, resistance, and inability to fully extend the knee. Kernig described an involuntary flexion at the knee when the examiner attempted to flex the hip with the knee extended. There is some overlap between Kernig's sign and the **straight leg-raising test.** The technique is similar, but the SLR is used to check for root irritation in lumbosacral radiculopathy. Both Kernig's sign and SLR are positive in meningitis because of diffuse inflammation of the nerve roots and meninges and positive with acute lumbosacral radiculopathy because of focal

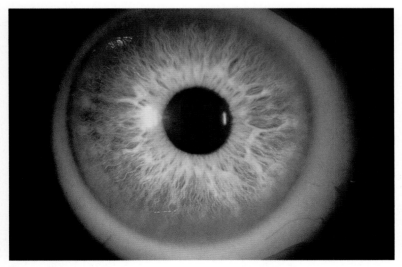

Figure K.1. Copper deposits in Descemet's membrane producing the brownish Kayser-Fleischer ring in Wilson's disease. (From Chern KC, Saidel MA. *Ophthalmology Review Manual.* 2nd ed. Philadelphia, PA: Wolters Kluwer Health/Lippincott Williams & Wilkins; 2012, with permission.)

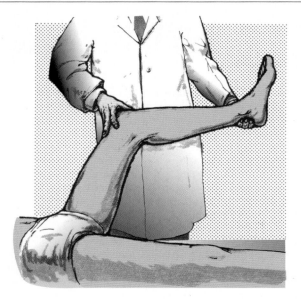

Figure K.2. Method of eliciting Kernig's sign. (From Campbell WW. *DeJong's the Neurologic Examination.* 7th ed. Philadelphia, PA: Wolters Kluwer Health/Lippincott Williams & Wilkins; 2013, with permission.)

inflammation of the affected root. In radiculopathy the signs are usually unilateral, but in meningitis they are bilateral. Hemiparesis may cause attenuation of Kernig's sign.[3] See **Brudzinski's neck sign.**

Kinetic tremor: See **tremor.**

Kinky hair: A peculiar appearance of the hair, seen most often in Menkes kinky hair disease and in giant axonal neuropathy **(Figs. K.3 and K.4)**. Patients have pili torti, with fine, brittle, tightly curled hair. Menkes is an X-linked disorder of copper metabolism that affects the CNS and connective tissue. Giant axonal neuropathy is an autosomal recessive multisystem disorder that affects intermediate filaments in the peripheral and central nervous systems. Kinky hair may also occur in arginosuccinic aciduria.

Kippdeviationen: See **saccadic intrusions.**

Klippel-Feil (or Weil) sign: Involuntary flexion, opposition, and adduction of the thumb on passive extension of the fingers when there is some degree of contracture in flexion; an upper extremity sign of CST dysfunction. See **pathologic reflexes.**

Knee (patellar or quadriceps) reflex: A contraction of the quadriceps femoris muscle, with resulting extension of the knee, in response to percussion of the patellar tendon (see Video B.4). The reflex is mediated by the femoral nerve (L2–L4).

The knee jerk can be elicited in various ways in addition to the usual method of having the patient sit on an examination table. The patient may sit in a chair with the knees slightly extended and the heels resting on the floor **(Fig. K.5)**. If the patient is lying in bed, the examiner should partially flex the knee by placing one hand beneath it and then tap the tendon **(Fig. K.6)**. Another technique is having

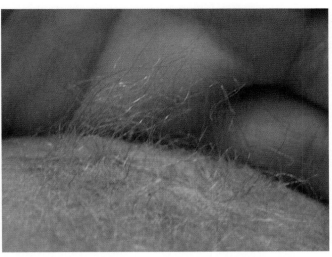

Figure K.3. Scalp hair in Menkes disease. The hair is sparse, short, thin, fragile, and light-colored, with a steel-wool appearance. (From Seshadri R, Bindu PS, Gupta AK. Teaching neuroimages: Menkes kinky hair syndrome. *Neurology.* 2013;81:e12–e13, with permission.)

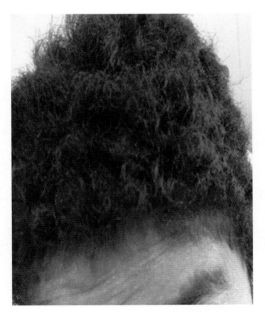

Figure K.4. Kinky hair in giant axonal neuropathy. (From Israni A, Chakrabarty B, Gulati S, et al. Giant axonal neuropathy: a clinicoradiopathologic diagnosis. *Neurology.* 2014;82:816–817, with permission.)

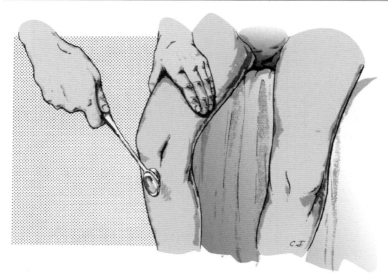

Figure K.5. Method of obtaining the knee reflex with the patient seated. (From Campbell WW. *DeJong's the Neurologic Examination.* 7th ed. Philadelphia, PA: Wolters Kluwer Health/Lippincott Williams & Wilkins; 2013, with permission.)

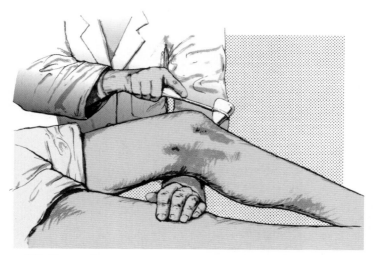

Figure K.6. Method of obtaining the knee reflex with the patient recumbent. (From Campbell WW. *DeJong's the Neurologic Examination.* 7th ed. Philadelphia, PA: Wolters Kluwer Health/Lippincott Williams & Wilkins; 2013, with permission.)

the patient sit with one leg crossed over the other and tapping the patellar tendon of the uppermost leg, but this method does not facilitate side-to-side comparison. By placing one hand over the muscle, the examiner can palpate the contraction as well as observe the rapidity and range of response, which may help in judging the latency between the time of the stimulus and the response (Video Link K.1).

If there is reflex **spread**, extension of the knee may be accompanied by adduction of the hip, which on occasion is bilateral, or there may be bilateral knee extension. If the reflex is exaggerated, the response may be obtained not only by tapping the tendon in the usual spot, but also just above the patella (see **suprapatellar reflex**). Marked exaggeration of the patellar reflex may be accompanied by patellar **clonus**. An **inverted reflex** results in contraction of the hamstrings and flexion of the knee.

Pendular knee reflexes, an increased number of back-and-forth swings after percussion of the tendon, may indicate hypotonia. The original definition of more than three swings is suspect, as many normal individuals have this finding.[4] In a series of 444 patients with unilateral cerebellar lesions, mostly tumors, a pendular knee jerk was present in 37%.[5]

Kyphosis: A spinal curvature with an abnormally increased posterior convex angulation leading to a rounding or hunchback deformity. Kyphosis often occurs in the thoracic spine as a result of osteoporosis in elderly women, leading to the "dowager hump" deformity. Kyphosis may also occur because of trauma, tumor, ankylosing spondylitis, Scheuermann's disease, and other conditions. Kyphoscoliosis is present when **scoliosis** and kyphosis are both present.

Video Link

K.1. How to elicit the knee reflex. (From Stanford Medicine 25, An Initiative to Revive the Culture of Bedside Medicine.) Available at: http://stanfordmedicine25.stanford.edu/the25/tendon.html

References

1. Taly AB, Meenakshi-Sundaram S, Sinha S, et al. Wilson disease: description of 282 patients evaluated over 3 decades. *Medicine (Baltimore)*. 2007;86:112–121.
2. Demirkiran M, Jankovic J, Lewis RA, et al. Neurologic presentation of Wilson disease without Kayser-Fleischer rings. *Neurology*. 1996;46:1040–1043.
3. Krasnianski M, Tacik P, Muller T, et al. Attenuation of Kernig's sign by concomitant hemiparesis: forgotten aspects of a well known clinical test. *J Neurol Neurosurg Psychiatry*. 2007;78:1413–1414.
4. Pickett JB, Tatum EJ. Pendular knee reflexes: a reliable sign of hypotonia? *Lancet*. 1984;2:236–237.
5. McGee S. *Evidence Based Physical Diagnosis*. 3rd ed. Philadelphia, PA: Elsevier/Saunders; 2012.

L

La belle indifference: A calm, inappropriately cavalier attitude regarding serious physical symptoms, characteristic of patients with conversion disorder or functional, nonorganic conditions (see **functional signs**). The patient seems unconcerned about a major neurologic deficit. The calmness is limited to the physical symptom, not the rest of the patient's life, which is typically chaotic. Patients who are depressed, stoic, parkinsonian, or simply unaware of the seriousness of the situation may show similar unconcern, which may lead the unwary to a misdiagnosis of a functional disorder.

In fact, la belle indifference discriminates poorly between functional and organic disease. A systematic review found that although the quality of the published studies was poor, the median frequency of la belle indifference was 21% in patients with conversion symptoms and 29% in patients with organic disease and suggested that la belle indifference should be abandoned as a clinical sign until both its definition and utility have been clarified.[1,2]

Lacrimal reflex: Tearing, usually bilateral, caused by stimulating the cornea.

Lacrimal sweating: Sweating in the medial supraorbital region, presumably due to aberrant reinnervation after damage to sudomotor fibers travelling with branches of the internal carotid artery, with sprouting of lacrimal parasympathetic fibers into the denervated sweat glands, causing facial sweating after ocular irritation.[3]

Lagophthalmos: Inability to close the eyelids completely, usually due to conditions causing weakness of the orbicularis oculi, such as facial nerve palsy or myopathy. When severe, lagophthalmos can lead to significant ocular complications.

Lalling (lallation, "baby talk"): A speech disorder in which the speech is childish, babbling, and characterized by a lack of precision in pronouncing certain consonants, especially the letters *r* and *l*. Lalling may occur because of hearing defects, or mental or physical retardation, or from psychogenic disorders. In lisping, the sibilants are imperfectly pronounced, and *th* is substituted for *s*; a similar defect in articulation may be associated with partial edentulism. Lalling and lisping are usually due to imperfect action of the articulatory apparatus (as in children), persistent faulty habits of articulation, imitation of faulty patterns of articulation, poor speech training, habit, or affectation.

Lambert's sign: The transient increase in strength after brief isometric exercise or repetitive muscle contraction in LEMS. The brief increase in strength is due to posttetanic potentiation and is a feature of presynaptic neuromuscular transmission disorders. The marked facilitation seen after brief isometric exercise or with rapid repetitive stimulation on repetitive nerve conduction studies is the electrodiagnostic corollary of the finding on examination. Although mentioned in the literature mostly in relation to grip strength, this finding can occur in any weak muscle. The postexercise facilitation may also cause a previously absent DTR to transiently reappear.

Lasègue sign: See **straight leg raising test.**

Latah: See **hyperekplexia.**

Latent nystagmus: A form of congenital **nystagmus** that occurs only when one eye is covered, causing jerk nystagmus with the fast component toward the uncovered eye. This may happen when the examiner blocks the patient's vision during ophthalmoscopic examination. The nystagmus disappears with binocular fixation. Latent nystagmus may exist in isolation or as a manifestation of typical congenital nystagmus.[4]

Lateral epicondylitis provocation tests: Maneuvers designed to elicit pain in patients with lateral epicondylitis (tennis elbow). Examination typically discloses tenderness to palpation over the lateral epicondyle, with maximal tenderness just distal to the epicondyle. With the elbow extended, supination (Mill's test) or extension (Cozen's sign) of the wrist against the examiner's resistance reproduces the pain (Fig. L.1). Forceful passive wrist flexion or pronation may stretch the inflamed region and also cause pain. In the chair raise test, the patient stands behind a chair, grasps the chair back with the hand pronated and the elbow extended, and tries to pick it up, reproducing the pain. The patient may also have pain with resisted middle finger extension, though this test was reported as a sign of radial tunnel syndrome, a dubious entity.

Lateral hamstring reflex: See **hamstring reflexes.**

Laterocollis: See **cervical dystonia.**

Lateropulsion: A tendency to sideways movement. Lateropulsion may involve the body, the limbs, or the eyes. It may occur in patients in the throes of acute vestibulopathy along with vertigo, nystagmus, and past pointing, which is due to lateropulsion of the limbs. It is a common manifestation of lateral medullary infarction and may be the sole manifestation.[5] When the patient is asked to look straight ahead and close the eyes, lateropulsion may occur as the intact, healthy labyrinth pushes

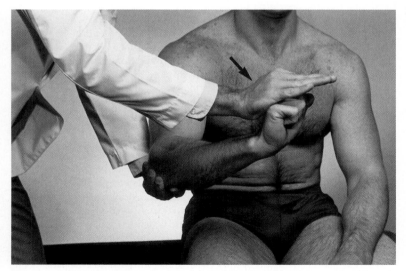

Figure L.1. Elicitation of lateral epicondylar pain by forceful wrist extension (Cozen's sign). (From Cipriano, JJ. *Photographic Manual of Regional Orthopedic and Neurological Tests.* 4th ed. Philadelphia, PA: Wolters Kluwer Health/Lippincott Williams & Wilkins; 2003, with permission.)

the eyes over, reflected by a series of corrective saccades back to primary position when the patient reopens the eyes. Saccadic lateropulsion, common in Wallenberg's syndrome, causes an undershoot of contralaterally directed saccades and an overshoot of ipsilaterally directed saccades.[6] When attempting to make a vertical saccade, an oblique or elliptical saccade may occur instead because lateropulsion interferes with the vector of movement.

Latissimus dorsi reflex: A DTR elicited by placing the examiner's fingers on the tendon of the latissimus dorsi near its insertion in the intertubercular groove of the humerus, with the patient prone and the arm abducted and in slight external rotation, then tapping with the reflex hammer.

This produces abduction and slight internal rotation of the shoulder. This reflex is mediated by the thoracodorsal nerve (C6–C8).

Lazarus sign: A spinal reflex movement seen in brain-dead patients, with bilateral arm flexion, shoulder adduction, raising of the arms, and crossing of the hands. Brain-dead patients can display impressive spontaneous and spinal reflex movements due to local spinal cord reflexes, which have become autonomous and are under no suprasegmental control. The Lazarus sign is dramatic. More common are finger jerks, undulating toe movements, facial myokymia, and the triple flexion response.[7,8] The neurological Lazarus sign is unrelated to the delayed return of spontaneous circulation after cessation of cardiopulmonary resuscitation, also referred to as the Lazarus phenomenon.

Lead line: A linear, purplish-black discoloration of the gums seen with severe lead toxicity. The line is about 1 mm from the gum margin and absent where there are missing teeth.

Lead pipe rigidity: See **rigidity.**

Leg drift (leg sign of Barré): One of the **subtle signs of hemiparesis,** but not as useful as many of the others and seldom done. Examination for leg drift may be done in two ways: (1) Have the prone patient attempt to maintain both knees flexed at about 45 degrees from horizontal with the feet slightly apart. When the knee flexors are weak on one side, as in a CST lesion, the involved leg will sink, gradually or rapidly. (2) Have the supine patient attempt to maintain both lower extremities flexed at the hip and extended at the knee, the legs at about a 45-degree angle off the bed, feet apart. This is a difficult callisthenic maneuver that not all patients can perform. If the hip flexors are mildly weak unilaterally, as in a CST lesion, the involved lower extremity will drift downward more rapidly than its fellow.

Lens dislocation (ectopia lentis): Displacement (subluxation) of the lens from its normal position. Lens dislocation typically causes profound visual impairment and is sometimes visible grossly or with a direct ophthalmoscope (Fig. L.2). It may be unilateral or bilateral, hereditary or sporadic. Lens dislocation is frequent in Marfan's syndrome (superiorly) and homocystinuria (inferiorly). It occurs as an uncommon feature in Ehlers-Danlos syndrome, Crouzon's syndrome, Refsum's disease, and Sturge-Weber syndrome. Bilaterally symmetric simple lens dislocation occurs as an autosomal dominant disorder.

Leri's sign: Flexion of the elbow when the examiner forcibly flexes the patient's fingers and wrist; there may also be adduction of the shoulder. This response is absent with lesions of the corticospinal system, and the absence is known as Leri's sign. Associated flexion at the elbow may be increased with frontal lobe lesions. See **pathologic reflexes.**

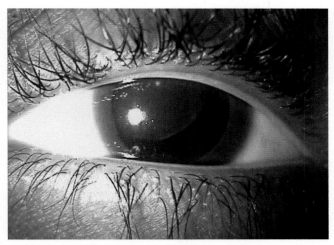

Figure L.2. Ectopia lentis with lens dislocation in the superonasal direction typically seen in Marfan's syndrome. (From Nelson LB. *Pediatric Ophthalmology*. Philadelphia, PA: Wolters Kluwer Health/Lippincott Williams & Wilkins; 2012, with permission.)

Letter (phonemic) fluency: The ability to name as many words as possible in 1 minute beginning with a particular letter; commonly used letters are F, A, and S. See **category fluency.**

Levator dehiscence: Detachment of the aponeurosis attaching the levator muscle to the tarsal plate that forms the eyelid, usually due to aging **(Figs. L.3 and L.4)**. Levator dehiscence may simulate **ptosis** (see **Horner's syndrome**). Trauma to the eyelid, as from contact lenses, may cause levator dehiscence in younger patients. Normally,

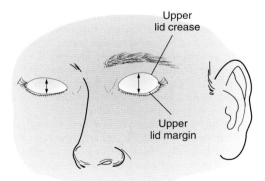

Figure L.3. Levator dehiscence-disinsertion on the left. The distance between the upper lid margin and the upper lid crease is increased compared to the normal right side. (From Campbell WW. *DeJong's the Neurologic Examination*. 7th ed. Philadelphia, PA: Wolters Kluwer Health/Lippincott Williams & Wilkins; 2013, with permission.)

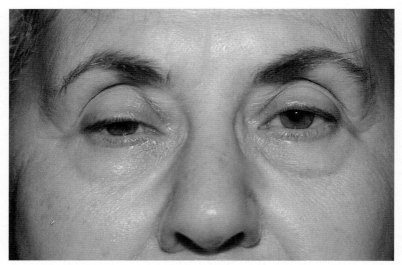

Figure L.4. Bilateral ptosis from dehiscence of the levator aponeurosis. Note the high, very defined upper eyelid crease. Levator function was 18 mm. (From Penne RB. *Oculoplastics.* 2nd ed. Philadelphia, PA: Wolters Kluwer Health/Lippincott Williams & Wilkins Health; 2012, with permission.)

with the eyelids gently closed, the upper lid margin lies 5 to 7 mm below the upper lid fold. An increase in this distance suggests levator dehiscence. **Dermatochalasis** can also simulate ptosis and may coexist with levator dehiscence.

Levitation: The spontaneous raising up of an extremity, most often the arm. Levitation can occur with a parietal lobe lesion of any sort (see **parietal updrift**), but has been reported particularly in CBD and in **alien hand** syndrome. It may also occur in PSP and occasionally as a manifestation of a posterior column lesion.

Lhermitte's sign: Sudden electric-like or painful sensations spreading down the body or into the back or extremities on flexion of the neck; more often a symptom than a sign. Seen most often because of involvement of the posterior columns in MS, but may occur with many other conditions involving the cervical cord, especially cervical spondylosis or large disc herniations **(Table L.1)**.[9] In MS, Lhermitte's sign may occur early in the disease when few other signs are present. A "reverse" Lhermitte's sign, with paresthesias radiating from the lower back upward, may occur in nitrous oxide myelopathy. See **Soto-Hall test.**

Lid lag (von Graefe sign): Eyelid retraction that worsens in down gaze, one of the cardinal eye signs of thyrotoxicosis. The pseudo-Graefe sign occurs with **aberrant reinnervation of CN III**. Aberrant innervation of the levator palpebrae superioris causes the upper lid to retract on down gaze because axons normally innervating the inferior rectus have regrown into the levator. Similarly, the lid may retract on adduction because of synkinesis between the medial rectus and the levator. See **eyelid retraction.**

Lid nystagmus: Eyelid jerking due to a slow down drift and an upward corrective movement. It may be associated with vertical nystagmus or occur in the absence of any coincident ocular nystagmus. Lid nystagmus is rare, may be evoked by

Table L.1. Conditions that May Cause Lhermitte's Sign/Symptom

Multiple sclerosis
Cervical spondylosis
Cervical disc herniation
Transverse myelitis
Traumatic myelopathy
Radiation myelopathy
Spinal cord tumor
Subacute combined degeneration
Atlanto-axial subluxation
Arachnoiditis
Chemotherapy myelopathy (cisplatin, docetaxel)
HIV myelopathy
Behcet's disease
Chiari malformation
Herpes zoster
SSRI discontinuation syndrome
Nitrous oxide abuse ("reverse")

convergence (**Pick's sign**) or horizontal conjugate gaze, and is usually accompanied by other eye signs such as ptosis and ophthalmoparesis. The most common type of lid nystagmus is associated with vertical nystagmus, with the lid movements synchronous but of greater amplitude than the eye movements. It has been reported in MS, Miller Fisher syndrome, cerebellar disease, lateral medullary infarction, and brainstem neoplasm **(Video Link L.1)**.[10]

Lid retraction: See **eyelid retraction.**

Lid twitch sign: See **Cogan's lid twitch sign.**

Lift-off test: See **shoulder examination tests.**

Light brightness comparison test: See **afferent pupillary defect.**

Light near dissociation: A disparity between the pupillary light and near reactions. The pupillary reaction to light is normally equal to or greater than the reaction to near. The reaction to near is often best brought out by having the patient fix on his own finger or thumb at a distance of 15 to 30 cm. This superimposes proprioceptive influences and will bring out the near reaction even in a blind person. The most common form of light near dissociation is a poor light response but good constriction with the near response; it is relatively common, and there are a number of causes. The converse, better reaction to light than to near, is rare. The classic cause of light near dissociation is neurosyphilis (the **Argyll Robertson pupil**), but many other conditions may cause it that are now more common **(Table L.2)**. Most of these lack the **miosis** and irregularity characteristic of Argyll Robertson pupils.

Lightning eye movements: See **opsoclonus.**

Limb kinetic apraxia: A dubious category of apraxia because these patients have difficulty with **fine motor control**, a loss of deftness, due to very mild lesions involving the CST impairing coordination and dexterity but not severe enough to cause detectable weakness. Impaired fine motor control is one of the **subtle signs of hemiparesis** (see Video F.4). Limb kinetic apraxia shares no features with the other forms of apraxia and is a misapplication of the concept. See **apraxia, buccofacial apraxia, ideational apraxia, conceptual apraxia, conduction apraxia, constructional apraxia, dissociation apraxia, dressing apraxia.**

Table L.2. Causes of Pupillary Light Near Dissociation

Neurosyphilis
Other lesions involving the dorsal rostral midbrain
Diabetic autonomic neuropathy (tabes diabetica)
Lyme disease
Chronic alcoholism
Chiasmal lesions (tabes pituitaria)
Myotonic muscular dystrophy
Amyloidosis
Adie's pupil
Aberrant regeneration of CN III
Neurosarcoidosis
Multiple sclerosis
Severe retinal or optic nerve disease

Limb placement test: See **paratonia.**

Lindner's (Lidner's) sign: See **straight leg raising test.**

Line bisection test: A test for visual (visuospatial) neglect that requires the patient to cross out lines on a sheet of paper with a vertical tick. The proportion and placement of lines left uncrossed relates to the severity of the neglect and localization of the lesion. Patients with multimodal hemineglect may fail to see the left half of the line. They bisect the right half, drawing their vertical line about one-quarter of the way down the line from the right. If lines are drawn all over the page, patients may fail to bisect any of the lines on the left.

Lipoma: See **hairy patch.**

Lippman's test: See **shoulder examination tests.**

Lisch nodules: Pigmented iris hamartomas (Fig. L.5). Lisch nodules are elevated, pale brown lesions that vary in appearance depending on the underlying color of the iris. They are highly suggestive of NF1, but may not appear until later childhood. The prevalence in patients with NF1 increases from birth to about 50% of 5-year-olds, 75% of 15-year-olds, and 95% to 100% of adults above the age of 30.

Lisping: See **lalling.**

Literal alexia: A inability to read individual letters but not necessarily words. The letters are apparently not perceived clearly or are confused with one another, e.g., *d* with *b*, and *g* with *q*; or the letters are perceived but their meaning lost. The paradoxical dissociation between word and letter reading may be due to a difference in the relative contributions of dorsal and ventral occipital structures to the reading process.[11]

Literal paraphasia: See **paraphasia.**

Litten's sign: The moving shadow caused by retraction of the lower intercostal spaces during inspiration; its absence is a sign of diaphragmatic weakness.

Little toe reflex of Puusepp: Tonic slow abduction of the little toe on plantar stimulation; seen in the same situations that cause **Babinski's plantar sign.** Occasionally, Puusepp's sign is present when great toe extension is absent and may be the only elicitable pyramidal sign.[12]

Livedo reticularis: A dermatologic condition that produces a network of erythematous, spidery streaks and discolorations on the trunk or extremities (Fig. L.6). While usually harmless, livedo reticularis may be of some interest to the neurologist.

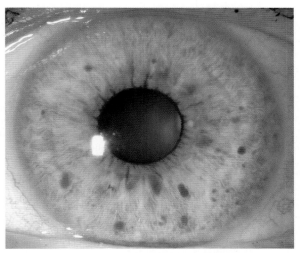

Figure L.5. Lisch nodules. (From Gerstenblith AT, Rabinowitz MP. *The Wills Eye Manual: Office and Emergency Room Diagnosis and Treatment of Eye Disease.* 6th ed. Philadelphia, PA: Wolters Kluwer Health/Lippincott Williams & Wilkins; 2012, with permission.)

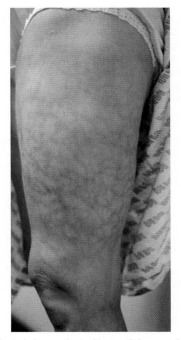

Figure L.6. Livedo reticularis in a patient with meralgia paresthetica.

It occurs in patients with Sneddon's syndrome, connective tissue disorders, hyperviscosity and hypercoagulable states, autoimmune disease, antiphospholipid syndrome, cryoglobulinemia, TTP, and systemic vasculitis and as a side effect of amantadine.[13] In up to 40% of patients with antiphospholipid syndrome, livedo reticularis is the first sign of the disorder.[14] In the figure, the livedo reticularis occurred in the distribution of the lateral femoral cutaneous nerve in a patient who presented with meralgia paresthetica.

Logopenia: An aphasic disorder characterized by a reduced rate of language output but with relatively preserved phrase length and syntax. This speech disturbance is seen in the logopenic variant of primary progressive aphasia, which is characterized by decreased spontaneous speech output with frequent word-finding pauses, phonologic paraphasias, and repetition deficits.[15]

Logorrhea: Excessive verbal output. The speech is well articulated and free of paraphasias or other evidence of aphasia but is circuitous and with minimal meaningful content. Logorrhea is abnormal and is seen in schizophrenia, mania, and confusional states. The line between pathologic logorrhea and tiresome loquaciousness, as in politicians, is not always clear. The term is also used to describe the verbal output in **Wernicke's aphasia**. In those patients, language function is severely impaired. The speech is replete with **paraphasias** and **neologisms** and associated with impaired comprehension.

Long tract signs: Abnormalities on neurologic examination reflecting dysfunction of the white matter tracts, such as the corticospinal and spinothalamic tracts, that run longitudinally for long distances in the brainstem and spinal cord. Examples would include CST signs, such as upper motor neuron **weakness**, hyperactive **deep tendon reflexes**, **clonus**, depressed **superficial reflexes**, **pathologic reflexes**, impaired **fine motor control**, loss of normal **associated movements** and the appearance of abnormal associated movements (the pyramidal syndrome, **Table L.3**), **posterior column signs,** and hemisensory loss. Long tract signs are common in disorders of white matter, such as MS.

Lordosis: Anterior spinal curvature. Loss of the normal lordosis is common in patients with acute low-back pain. An increase in the lordotic curve occurs in other conditions; see **hyperlordosis.**

Low hairline: A feature of congenital dysmorphic and hereditary disorders. A low frontal hairline occurs in acrocephalsyndactyly and fetal alcohol syndrome. A low occipital hairline occurs in Klippel-Feil syndrome and other congenital spine defects and may be a feature of Chiari malformation.

Table L.3. Clinical Signs of Corticospinal Tract Dysfunction

Pyramidal distribution weakness
Impaired fine motor control
Hyperactive deep tendon reflexes
Clonus
Depressed superficial reflexes
Hypertonicity (spasticity)
Pathologic reflexes
Loss of normal associated movements
Presence of abnormal associated movements

Lower motor neuron (LMN) signs: Abnormalities that reflect dysfunction of the anterior horn cells in the spinal cord or the motor neurons in the brain stem. The primary LMN signs are **atrophy**, **weakness**, **fasciculations**, and loss of reflexes. Patients with LMN disorders frequently experience cramps, as well as symptoms related to weakness of the specific muscles involved, such as dysarthria and dysphagia. The prototypical LMN disorder is motor neuron disease. In classical ALS, there are also **upper motor neuron signs**.

Luria manual sequencing task: See **fist-palm-side test.**

Lust's (peroneal) phenomenon: A sign of **tetany**; tapping over the common peroneal nerve as it winds around the neck of the fibula causes dorsiflexion and eversion of the foot. Like **Chvostek's sign**, this is essentially a motor Tinel's sign.

Lymphadenopathy: Enlargement of peripheral lymph nodes, localized or generalized. A great many diseases can cause lymphadenopathy. Some of the notable conditions with neurological manifestations include Whipple's disease, sarcoidosis, lymphoma, POEMS, brucellosis, Waldenstrom's macroglobulinemia, Castleman's disease, cat scratch disease, HIV infection, infectious mononucleosis, SLE, amyloidosis, secondary syphilis, and phenytoin pseudolymphoma.

Video Link

L.1. Eyelid nystagmus. (From the Robert B. Daroff Collection, Neuro-ophthalmology Virtual Education Library (NOVEL), University of Utah.) Available at: http://stream.utah.edu/m/dp/frame.php?f=41dd257795c88054698

References

1. Stone J, Smyth R, Carson A, et al. La belle indifference in conversion symptoms and hysteria: systematic review. *Br J Psychiatry.* 2006;188:204–209.
2. Donohue A, Harrington C. La belle indifference: medical myth or useful marker of psychiatric disease. *Med Health R I.* 2001;84:207–209.
3. van Weerden TW, Houtman WA, Schweitzer NM, et al. Lacrimal sweating in a patient with Reader's syndrome. *Clin Neurol Neurosurg.* 1979;81:119–121.
4. Brodsky MC, Tusa RJ. Latent nystagmus: vestibular nystagmus with a twist. *Arch Ophthalmol.* 2004;122:202–209.
5. Lee H, Sohn CH. Axial lateropulsion as a sole manifestation of lateral medullary infarction: a clinical variant related to rostral-dorsolateral lesion. *Neurol Res.* 2002;24:773–774.
6. Tilikete C, Koene A, Nighoghossian N, et al. Saccadic lateropulsion in Wallenberg syndrome: a window to access cerebellar control of saccades? *Exp Brain Res.* 2006;174:555–565.
7. Saposnik G, Maurino J, Saizar R, et al. Spontaneous and reflex movements in 107 patients with brain death. *Am J Med.* 2005;118:311–314.
8. Saposnik G, Bueri JA, Maurino J, et al. Spontaneous and reflex movements in brain death. *Neurology.* 2000;54:221–223.
9. Gemici C. Lhermitte's sign: review with special emphasis in oncology practice. *Crit Rev Oncol Hematol.* 2010;74:79–86.
10. Brodsky MC, Boop FA. Lid nystagmus as a sign of intrinsic midbrain disease. *J Neuroophthalmol.* 1995;15:236–240.
11. Sevush S, Heilman KM. A case of literal alexia: evidence for a disconnection syndrome. *Brain Lang.* 1984;22:92–108.
12. Tacik P, Krasnianski M, Zierz S. Puusepp's sign—clinical significance of a forgotten pyramidal sign. *Clin Neurol Neurosurg.* 2009;111:919–921.
13. Thornsberry LA, LoSicco KI, English JC III. The skin and hypercoagulable states. *J Am Acad Dermatol.* 2013;69:450–462.
14. Dennis M, Bowen WT, Cho L. *Mechanisms of Clinical Signs.* Sydney, Australia: Churchill Livingstone; 2012.
15. Harris JM, Gall C, Thompson JC, et al. Classification and pathology of primary progressive aphasia. *Neurology.* 2013;81:1832–1839.

Macewen's sign ("cracked pot" resonance): A tympanitic note on percussion of the skull in hydrocephalus and increased ICP in infants and children.

Macro square wave jerks: See **saccadic intrusions.**

Macrocephaly: Head enlargement, defined as more than two standard deviations above the mean. By this definition, 2.5% of the normal population has macrocephaly and most have no disease. The condition is often familial. Macrocephaly may occur in many conditions, such as hydrocephalus, megalencephaly, and conditions that cause thickening of the skull (see Fig. H.16). Megalencephaly is associated with a number of congenital, hereditary, and metabolic disorders.

Macroglossia: Enlargement of the tongue. Macroglossia may occur in amyloidosis, hypothyroidism, GM1 gangliosidosis, acid maltase deficiency, glycogen storage diseases, acromegaly, Down's syndrome, DMD, some forms of LGMD, ALS, neurofibromatosis, mucopolysaccharidosis, and with local conditions involving the tongue, such as angioma, hamartomas, and lymphoma. Acute tongue enlargement occurs in angioedema.

Macrographia: Abnormally large handwriting, seen in cerebellar disease, as opposed to the **micrographia** characteristic of PD.

Macrosaccadic oscillations: see **saccadic intrusions.**

Macular sparing: see **visual field defects.**

Macular star: A fine, stellate pattern of hard, yellow exudates surrounding the macula in a radiating pattern (Fig. M.1). A macular star may be seen in a number of

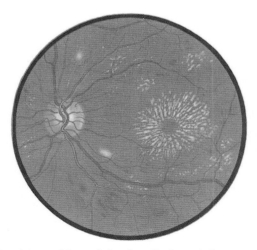

Figure M.1. Punctate exudates radiating from the fovea to form a macular star in a patient with hypertensive retinopathy. (From Michaelson IC. *Textbook of the Fundus of the Eye.* 3rd ed. Edinburgh, UK: Churchill Livingston; 1980, with permission.)

216

conditions, including hypertensive and diabetic retinopathy, neuroretinitis due to cat scratch disease and other infections, and in association with an optic neuropathy due to Lyme disease, sarcoidosis, or syphilis.

Maddox rod test: See **diplopia rules.**

Magnetic apraxia: A term used by Denny-Brown to refer to compulsive reaching, groping, and grasping, very similar to **utilization behavior**. It is common in patients with frontal lobe disease and in CBD and has been used to refer to the behavior of an **alien hand**. See **automatic responses, environmental dependency.**

Magnetic gait: See **gait disorders.**

Main en griffe: See **claw hand.**

Main d' accoucheur: See **Trousseau's sign.**

Main succulente: Edema and hyperhidrosis of the hand in syringomyelia, probably related to involvement of central autonomic pathways; may also occur in chronic regional pain syndrome.

Malar rash: See **dermatomyositis skin changes.**

Mandibular reflex: See **jaw jerk.**

Manifest latent nystagmus: See **nystagmus.**

Manual muscle testing: See **weakness, MRC scale.**

Marcus Gunn phenomenon: See **jaw winking.**

Marcus Gunn pupil: See **afferent pupillary defect.**

Marfan's thumb sign: See **hypermobile joints.**

Marfan's wrist sign: See **hypermobile joints.**

Marfanoid habitus: Patients who are tall and slender with long limbs (Fig. M.2). Conditions of particular neurologic significance associated with a Marfanoid habitus, in addition to Marfan's syndrome, include homocystinuria, Ehlers-Danlos syndrome, Klinefelter's syndrome, and multiple endocrine neoplasia, particularly types 2B and 3.[1]

Marie's paper test: A test of mental status and speech comprehension using a multistep command, such as "here is a piece of paper; tear it in three parts and place one on the table, give one to me, and keep one for yourself."

Marie-Foix sign: (1) A lower extremity **pathological reflex** seen in CST disease. Squeezing the toes or strongly plantar flexing the toes or foot causes extension of toes, especially the great toe, plus dorsiflexion of ankle and flexion at hip and knee (triple flexion); (2) an upper extremity pathological reflex also seen in CST lesions. Superficial stroking of the palm of the hand in the hypothenar region, or scratching the ulnar side of the palm, causes adduction and flexion of the thumb (as in **Wartenberg's sign**), sometimes with flexion of adjacent digits, more rarely with extension of little finger.

Marin Amat sign: See **inverse jaw winking.**

Mary Walker phenomenon (effect): An increase in ptosis or generalized muscle weakness after ischemic exercise in patients with MG. Dr. Walker, who also discovered anticholinesterases as a treatment for MG and was the first to report hypokalemia in familial periodic paralysis, used ischemic exercise of both forearms.[2] The effect may be due to the production of lactic acid with binding of calcium and a reduction in ionized and total serum calcium causing impaired neuromuscular transmission in the face of a marginal safety factor.[3] The effect is difficult to demonstrate, at least in patients with mild MG where the diagnosis is questionable.

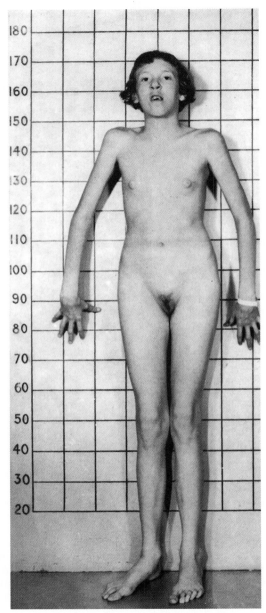

Figure M.2. Homocystinuria. Note the excessive height; long limbs; long, narrow feet; and mild anterior chest deformity. (From Koopman WJ, Moreland LW. *Arthritis and Allied Conditions A Textbook of Rheumatology.* 15th ed. Philadelphia, PA: Wolters Kluwer Health/Lippincott Williams & Wilkins; 2005, with permission.)

Masked facies: The lack of facial expressiveness seen in parkinsonism (see Video A.3). See **whistle-smile sign.**

Mass reflex: A response that occurs in patients with severe myelopathy after the stage of spinal shock. Stimulation below the level of the lesion causes a massive response, including not only leg flexion but also muscular contractions of the abdominal wall, often evacuation of the bladder and bowel, sweating, reflex erythema, pilomotor responses, and hypertension. The reflexogenic zone may extend to the bladder, and bladder distention may precipitate the entire reflex complex. Priapism and even ejaculation may be a part of the response.

Mayer's sign: An upper extremity sign of CST pathology. The patient's hand is held in the examiner's hand, palm up, fingers slightly bent and thumb in slight flexion and abduction. The examiner places slow but firm pressure on the proximal phalanges of the fingers, especially the third and fourth fingers, flexing them at the metacarpophalangeal joints and pressing them against the palm. Normally, this causes adduction and opposition of the thumb with flexion at the metacarpophalangeal joint and extension at the interphalangeal joint (finger-thumb reflex). Absence of this response is Mayer's sign. It is occasionally absent in normals, but the absence should be bilateral. The normal response may be difficult. See **pathologic reflexes.**

McArdle's sign: A reversible deterioration in gait and an increase in the degree of pyramidal weakness of the lower limbs produced by neck flexion and relieved by extension.[4] Presumably the motor equivalent of **Lhermitte's sign**, it occurs most often in MS, but can be seen with lesions anywhere from the foramen magnum to the thoracic level, including meningioma.

Medial epicondylitis provocation tests: Maneuvers designed to elicit pain in patients with medial epicondylitis (golfer's elbow). It is a common misconception that ulnar neuropathy at the elbow produces medial elbow pain. This is in fact not the case, but patients with medial epicondylitis are often referred for electrodiagnostic evaluation for suspected ulnar neuropathy. The common flexor tendon is a large tendon that arises from the medial epicondyle and serves as the origin of all the major flexor muscles of the forearm and hand. Similar to the lateral epicondylitis provocation tests, the patient either vigorously flexes the relevant muscle against resistance or the examiner passively stretches the muscle, in this case by extending the wrist, with the elbow also extended. Both maneuvers cause the tendon to pull against the involved structures and may produce local pain over the epicondyle.

Median nerve compression test: See **carpal tunnel syndrome provocative tests.**

Mees' lines: transverse white lines across the nails seen in arsenic intoxication (Fig. M.3). The lines appears several weeks after acute exposure and grow out slowly over several months. The lines are due to arsenic deposits in the nails and harvesting of the nails for arsenic assay can document the intoxication. Other conditions that may cause Mees' lines include thallium intoxication, heart failure, Hodgkin's disease, chemotherapy, carbon monoxide exposure, leprosy, and any severe systemic illness.

Memory: See **mental status examination.**

Menace (dazzle) reflex: Blink to threat. The examiner's hand or fingers are brought in rapidly from the side, as if to strike the patient or poke him in the eye. The patient may wince, draw back, or blink. The threatening movement should be deliberate enough to avoid stimulating the cornea with an induced air current. The reflex is useful in assessing the visual fields in obtunded patients and providing a very crude assessment of vision.

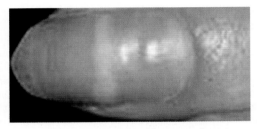

Figure M.3. Mees' lines. These are transverse lines, usually one per nail, with curves similar to the lunula, not the cuticle. The line often disappears if pressure is placed over the line. They emerge from under the proximal nail folds and grow out with the nails. Mees' lines occur with arsenic poisoning, thallium poisoning, and to a lesser extent other heavy metal poisoning. They may also follow any acute or severe illness.

Mendel-Bechterew reflex: See **dorsal foot response.**

Meningeal signs: Findings on physical examination indicating inflammation of the meninges. The various maneuvers used to elicit meningeal signs produce tension on inflamed and hypersensitive spinal nerve roots, and the resulting signs are postures, protective muscle contractions, or other movements that minimize the stretch and distortion of the meninges and roots. Patients with these signs are said to have meningismus. The most important meningeal sign is nuchal rigidity, which may range from mild to severe. Nuchal rigidity is the most widely recognized and frequently encountered meningeal sign, whether from infection or the presence of a foreign material, such as in subarachnoid hemorrhage, and the diagnosis is rarely made in its absence. In a review of 1,500 patients with either acute bacterial meningitis or SAH, nuchal rigidity was present in 84%.[5]

Normally the neck can be flexed, so that the chin rests on the chest, and rotated from side to side without difficulty. Nuchal rigidity primarily affects the extensor muscles, and the most prominent early finding in meningismus is resistance to passive neck flexion. The physician is unable to place the patient's chin on his chest, but can hyperextend the neck without difficulty; rotatory and lateral movements may also be preserved. With more severe nuchal rigidity, there may be resistance to extension and rotatory movements as well. When severe, nuchal rigidity progresses to head retraction and opisthotonos, the body assuming a wrestler's bridge or arc de cercle position, with the head thrust back and the trunk arched forward (**Fig. M.4**). To avoid spinal flexion, the patient with meningitis may sit in bed with the hands placed far behind, the head thrown back, the hips and knees flexed, and the back arched (Amoss's, Hoyne's, or tripod sign). In **Brudzinski's neck sign,** flexing the patient's neck results in flexion of the hips and knees bilaterally. **Kernig's sign** is pain, resistance, and inability to fully extend the knee after the hip and knee have been flexed to right angles. The Kernig and Brudzinski signs are less sensitive (61%) than is nuchal rigidity (84%) in acute bacterial meningitis or SAH.[5]

Other conditions may cause neck stiffness and rigidity. A common problem is to distinguish restricted neck motion due to cervical spondylosis or osteoarthritis from nuchal rigidity. Patients with osteoarthritis typically have difficulty with rotation and lateral bending of the neck; these motions are usually preserved in patients who have meningismus, unless the meningeal irritation is extremely severe.

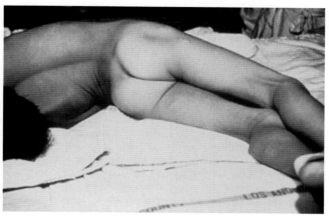

Figure M.4. Opisthotonos, in this case due to tetanus; the posture in severe meningismus is the same. (From Preston RR, Wilson TE. *Physiology*. Philadelphia, PA: Wolters Kluwer Health/Lippincott Williams & Wilkins; 2013, with permission.)

Restricted neck motion may also occur with retropharyngeal abscess, cervical lymphadenopathy, and neck trauma and as a nonspecific manifestation in severe systemic infections. Extrapyramidal disorders, particularly PSP, may also cause diffuse rigidity of the neck muscles. Meningeal signs may occur with increased spinal fluid pressure, and nuchal rigidity may be a manifestation of cerebellar tonsillar (foramen magnum) herniation.

Mental status examination: Testing used primarily to help determine if a patient has dementia or altered mental status. One possible organization of the mental status examination is shown in **Table M.1**.

Careful observation during history taking aids greatly in evaluating mental status. Observe the patient's general appearance, attitude, behavior, speech, posture, and facial expressions. A detailed MSE is in order if there is any complaint from the patient or family of memory difficulties, cognitive slippage, or a change in character, behavior, personality, or habits. The practitioner may devise a personally preferred MSE routine or use one of the many **cognitive screening instruments** available. The most widely used of these is the Folstein mini-mental state exam

Table M.1. One Possible Organization of the Mental Status Examination

Orientation
Attention and concentration
Fund of information
Language
Memory
Constructions
Calculation skills
Abstraction
Insight and judgment
Praxis

(MMSE; see Tables C.2 and C.3). Before making judgments about the patient's mental status, especially memory, the examiner should ensure that the patient is alert, cooperative, attentive, and has no language impairment. Mental status cannot be adequately evaluated in a patient who is not alert or is aphasic.

The formal MSE usually begins with an assessment of orientation. Normally, patients are referred to as "oriented times three" if they know their name, location, and the date. Some examiners assess insight or the awareness of the situation as a fourth dimension of orientation. The details of orientation are sometimes telling. The patient may know the day of the week but not the year. Orientation can be explored further when necessary by increasing or decreasing the difficulty level of the questions. Orientation questions can be used as a memory test for patients who are disoriented. If the patient is disoriented as to time and place, she may be told the day, the month, the year, the city, etc., and implored to try to remember the information. Failure to remember this information by a patient who is attentive and has registered it suggests a severe memory deficit. Occasionally patients cannot remember very basic information, such as the year, the city, or the name of the hospital, despite being repeatedly told, for more than a few seconds. In the presence of disease, orientation to time is impaired first, then orientation to place; only rarely is there disorientation to person.

Poor performance on complex tests of higher intellectual function cannot be attributed to cortical dysfunction if the patient is not attentive to the tasks. Defective attention taints all subsequent testing. Patients may appear grossly alert but are actually inattentive, distractible, and unable to concentrate. Patients with dementing illnesses are not typically inattentive until the cognitive deficits are severe. The possibility of a CNS toxic or metabolic disturbance should be considered when the patient is inattentive.

Having the patient signal whenever the letter *A* is heard from a string of random letters dictated by the examiner, or having the patient cross out all of the *A*'s on a written sheet may reveal a lack of attention or task impersistence. Serial 7s, forward **digit span**, and spelling *world* backward are popular tests of immediate attention. In the **line bisection test**, the patient is requested to bisect several lines randomly placed on a page. Another test of attention and concentration is a multistep task, such as **Marie's paper test**. Another multistep task might be, "Stand up, face the door, and hold out your arms." Attention has an important spatial component, and patients may fail to attend to one side of space; see **attentional deficits**.

Mental control or concentration is a higher-level function that requires the patient not only to attend to a complex task but also to marshal other intellectual resources, such as the ability to mentally manipulate items. Tests of attention, mental control, and working memory include serial 7s or 3s, spelling *world* backward (part of the MMSE), and saying the days of the week or months of the year in reverse. Most normal adults can recite the months of the year backward in less than 30 seconds. When underlying functions, e.g., calculation ability, are intact, defective mental control may indicate dorsolateral frontal lobe (executive) dysfunction, usually on the left.

Evaluation of language includes assessment of fluency, comprehension, naming, repetition, reading, and writing; see **aphasia**.

Memory has many facets and may be tested in different ways. Memory terminology is not used consistently, with different terms in use in general neurology and

Table M.2. The Three Stages of Memory

Memory Stage	Anatomy	Function and Terminology
First	Prefrontal lobe	Immediate Working
Second	Medial temporal lobe	Episodic Short-term Recent Declarative
Third	Lateral temporal and other cortical regions	Semantic Long-term Remote

in behavioral neurology **(Table M.2)**. A precise description of the task attempted is often more useful than describing the patient's "recent memory." The generally used classification includes immediate, short-term or recent, and long-term or remote memory. These correspond approximately to the terms working, episodic, and semantic memory used by behavioral neurologists and cognitive neuropsychologists. These designations attempt to reflect the neurophysiology of memory.

The first stage of memory—immediate or working memory—involves the circuits used to register, recall, and mentally manipulate transitory information. The prefrontal cortex mediates much of this function. This is a short-lived operation in which material is not actually committed to memory. Normal people can typically retain seven digits, a telephone number, in immediate memory. Retaining longer numbers, or *supraspan numbers*, and tasks such as reverse digit span, require more active memory processing. Working memory tends to decline with advancing age. Working memory also depends on executive function, the ability to remain focused on task despite distractions. The second stage of memory—short-term, recent, episodic, or declarative memory—involves retaining and recalling information or events for minutes to hours. The medial temporal lobe mediates much of this second stage of memory. The familiar test of the ability to recall three items after 5 minutes assesses episodic or short-term memory. The term episodic memory is also used to refer to the system involved in remembering particular episodes or experiences, such as the movie seen last weekend; episodic memory involves specific personal experiences. In the third stage, memories are consolidated and stored more permanently. The lateral temporal region and other cortical areas subserve this storage function. The fund of information stored in remote, long-term memory includes basic school facts, such as state capitals, past presidents, important dates, current events, and personal information, such as address, phone number, and the names of relatives. This long-term stage of memory is commonly referred to as semantic memory, a confusing term at best. Semantic memory includes generalized knowledge and factual information not related to memory of a specific thing or event, such as what a movie is. Semantic memory is distinct from personal long-term memory.

Digit span is a test of attention and immediate, working memory. Episodic (recent, short-term) memory is tested by giving the patient items to recall. The recall items may be simple objects, such as orange, umbrella, and automobile, or more complex, such as "John Brown, 42 Market St., Chicago." Some commonly used lists are apple, table, penny; hand, snow, telephone; city, nose, salt; and water,

M

chair, road. The items should be in different categories. After ensuring the patient has registered the items, proceed with other testing. After approximately 5 minutes, ask the patient to recall the items. Investigators have found considerable variability when using such three word lists; some normal subjects may recall zero or one word. Better tests for the bedside evaluation of memory are supraspan list learning tasks with delayed recall and recognition conditions. Assessing memory is frequently difficult in patients who work in very specialized fields and who have few outside interests. Patients with major cognitive impairment may still recall some deeply ingrained, overlearned memories, e.g., days of the week, months of the year, nursery rhymes, and jingles.

Patients with severe memory deficits may not only fail to recall the items, but also fail to recall being asked to recall. Some patients may fail to remember the items, but they can improve performance with hints or pick the items from a list. Patients who are able to remember items with cuing or by picking from a list are able to retain the information but not retrieve it. When cuing or picking do not improve performance, the defect is in retention. Patients with early dementing processes may have only a failure of retrieval. Another memory test is to ask the patient to remember the **Babcock sentence**. Normal patients can do this in three attempts.

Brain disease commonly causes impaired visuospatial abilities, and tests of construction are part of the mental status examination, e.g., drawing shapes, the **clock drawing test** or **Rey-Osterreith test.**

Ability to count and calculate may be evaluated by asking the patient to count forward or backward, to count coins, or to make change. Patients may be asked to select a certain amount from a handful of change presented by the examiner. Calculations may be more formally tested by having the patient perform simple arithmetic, either mentally or on paper. Basic calculations, such as 2 + 2, are often rote, overlearned items from early schooling; these test remote memory more than calculating ability. The average normal patient can perform mental calculations that involve two-digit operations and require simple carrying and borrowing. Another test is to ask the patient to sequentially double a number until failure. Simple mathematical problems may be presented. A commonly used calculation task is subtracting serial 7s from 100 (failing that, serial 3s). This function also requires attention and concentration. Counting to 20 is more of a remote memory test and counting backward from 20 more of an attentional task. There is little difference in calculating ability across age groups and little impairment in early AD. However, advancing disease dramatically alters calculation ability.

The ability to think abstractly is typically tested by asking the patient to describe similarities and differences, find analogies, and interpret proverbs and aphorisms. The patient may be asked how an apple and a banana, a car and an airplane, a watch and a ruler, or a poem and a statue are alike. She may be asked to tell the difference between a lie and a mistake, or between a cable and a chain. To test for the ability to find analogies, the patient might be asked: "Table is to leg as car is to what?" The patient may be unable to interpret a proverb, or may interpret it concretely or literally. The usefulness of proverb interpretation has been questioned. It seems many examiners are not precisely sure themselves what some of the proverbs mean. Bizarre, peculiar proverb interpretations may be given by patients with psychiatric disease, or by normal people not familiar with the idiomatic usage. Impaired abstraction occurs in many conditions, but is particularly common with frontal lobe disorders.

Common insight and judgment questions—such as asking the patient what she would do if she found a sealed, addressed, stamped letter on the sidewalk, or if she smelled smoke in a crowded theater—may be less useful than determining if the patient has insight into the illness and the implications of any functional impairment. Historical information from family members about the patient's actual judgment in real-life situations may be more enlightening than these artificial constructs. Patients with no concern about their illness have impaired judgment. Many neurological conditions may impair judgment, particularly processes that affect the orbitofrontal regions.

Executive function refers to high-level organization and execution of complex thoughts and behavior, which are primarily frontal lobe functions. Useful bedside executive tests include word-list generation, the **Go/No-Go test**, the **antisaccade test**, and the **fist-edge-palm test**. Word-list generation assesses **category fluency** and **letter fluency**. The Wisconsin card sort test provides a more formal frontal lobe assessment. **Perseveration** may occur with frontal lobe lesions. A common manifestation of frontal lobe dysfunction is **defective response inhibition** or **environmental dependency**. Other useful tests include **trail-making** and assessing for **utilization behavior** and **imitation behavior**.

Microcephepaly: A small head, defined as a head circumference of either two or three standard deviations below the mean for age and gender **(Fig. M.5)**. It is a clinical

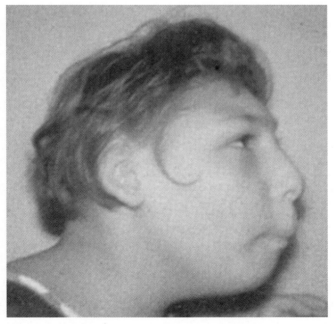

Figure M.5. Microcephaly. The face is of normal size, but the head is small with a sloping forehead. The scalp is redundant and furrowed. (From Orient JM, Sapira JD. *Sapira's Art & Science of Bedside Diagnosis*. 4th ed. Philadelphia, PA: Wolters Kluwer Health/Lippincott Williams & Wilkins; 2010, with permission.)

finding, not a disease, and there are many causes. Primary microcephaly is due to a mutation in one of the microcephalin genes. Secondary microcephaly develops after birth and predominantly reflects dendritic or white matter diseases. It occurs with many syndromes, such as Down's, Seckel's, William's, and cri-du-chat and with various inborn metabolic errors. It is important to distinguish microcephaly from **craniosynostosis**, which also causes a small head but is potentially treatable.

Micrognathia/micrognathism: An abnormally small chin. It occurs in a number of conditions and is present in many congenital dysmorphic syndromes. Conditions of particular neurologic relevance include Andersen-Tawil syndrome, Carpenter's syndrome, cleidocranial dysostosis, craniofacial dysostosis, Marfan's syndrome, Ehlers-Danlos syndrome, fetal alcohol syndrome, CMT with PMP-22 trisomy, and Möebius' syndrome.

Micrographia: Abnormally small handwriting, a classical sign of PD. On trying to sign her name, the script may begin at a normal size but very quickly becomes progressively smaller and more cramped, often ending as an illegible scrawl.

Microtia: Malformation of the external ear that may vary from barely discernible to total absence (anotia). It may occur as an isolated anomaly or part of a condition, such as Goldenhar's, Treacher-Collins, and first-arch syndromes. When microtia is seen in association with an ipsilateral facial paresis, it may indicate that the facial nerve lesion is congenital rather than acquired.

Midbrain tremor: See **rubral tremor.**

Midline splitting: A change in sensation precisely at the midline, characteristic of functional, nonorganic sensory loss. Midline splitting may also occur with thalamic lesions. See **functional signs, functional sensory signs, thalamic sensory loss.**

Milkmaid grip: Constant, small-amplitude movements of the fingers when the patient with chorea holds the examiner's finger in her fist. The twitches of individual fingers were thought to resemble milking movements. Motor **impersistence**—the inability to sustain a contraction—frequently accompanies chorea in disorders such as HD, and signs such as **trombone tongue** and milkmaid grip are due to both acting in concert.

Minicalorics: Instillation of small volumes, 2 to 10 cc, of an ice and water slush to assess vestibular function in dizzy patients. The latency to onset and the duration of the nystagmus elicited is compared on the two sides. A difference of more than 20% in nystagmus duration suggests a lesion on the side of the decreased response. Minicalorics have been compared to the classical caloric test procedures and determined to be a suitable procedure for bedside investigation of vestibular function outside the vestibular laboratory.[6]

Minipolymyoclonus (polyminimyoclonus): A term originally coined and used for decades to refer to fasciculations of small hand muscles in chronic anterior horn cell disease, particularly SMA, that cause small amplitude, subtle finger twitches, and are of course not real myoclonus. These **contraction fasciculations** involve enlarged motor units in conditions causing chronic denervation and are therefore capable of moving the finger joints. These movements do not occur in more rapidly evolving denervating disorders such as ALS.

Unfortunately, the term was later also applied to similar movements in patients with seizures and referred to as "minipolymyoclonus of central origin."[7]

Minor extensor toe signs: Alternate methods for eliciting the extensor plantar response in patients with lesions of the CST **(Table M.3)**. **Babinski's plantar sign** is

Table M.3. Minor Extensor Toe Signs, Alternate Methods for Eliciting the Toe Dorsiflexion in Lesions of the Corticospinal Tract

Sign	Stimulus
Gordon's sign	Squeezing of calf muscles
Schaefer's sign	Deep pressure on Achilles tendon
Bing's sign	Pricking dorsum of foot with a pin
Moniz's sign	Forceful passive plantar flexion at ankle
Throckmorton's sign	Percussing over dorsal aspect of metatarsophalangeal joint of great toe just medial to EHL tendon
Strumpell's phenomenon	Forceful pressure over anterior tibial region
Cornell's response	Scratching dorsum of foot along inner side of EHL tendon
Gonda's (Allen's) sign	Forceful downward stretching or snapping of either 2nd, 3rd or 4th toe; if response is difficult to obtain, flex toe slowly, press on nail, twist the toe, and hold it for a few seconds
Stransky's sign	Small toe forcibly abducted, then released
Allen's and Cleckley's signs	Sharp upward flick of 2nd toe or pressure applied to ball of toe
Szapiro's sign	Pressure against dorsum of 2nd through 5th toes, causing firm passive plantar flexion, while stimulating plantar surface of foot

EHL, extensor hallucis longus.

the mainstay of toe signs, and the most useful variation by far is the **Chaddock sign**; the **Oppenheim** is also sometimes useful. With severe CST disease, the threshold for eliciting an upgoing toe is lower and the reflexogenic zone wider, leading to many alternate methods of eliciting the response. These may occasionally be useful in cases where, for some reason, the plantar surface of the foot cannot be stimulated.

Minor's sign: A maneuver seen in lumbosacral radiculopathy. The patient rises from a seated position by supporting herself on the unaffected side, bending forward, avoiding weight bearing on the affected side, and placing one hand on the affected side of the back (Fig. M.6).

Miosis: A small pupil, by definition <2 mm in diameter. Common causes of acquired miosis include old age, hyperopia, alcohol abuse, and drug effects. Neurologically significant causes of miosis include neurosyphilis, diabetes, levodopa therapy, and **Horner's syndrome**. Acute, severe brainstem lesions, such as pontine hematoma, may cause bilaterally tiny, "pinpoint" pupils that still react. Thalamic lesions may produce small, reactive pupils (diencephalic pupils). Many ophthalmological conditions are associated with miosis, such as corneal or intraocular foreign bodies, trauma, iridocyclitis, chronic anterior segment ischemia, and an old **Adie's pupil**.

Mirror agnosia: A sign seen in dementia and parietal lobe lesions, causing a loss of the concept of a mirror and its use. The patient regards a reflected image in the mirror and thinks the object is inside the mirror. He may try to reach into the mirror to retrieve it. Many other mirror signs have been described, such as failure to recognize one's own image (autoprosopagnosia, see **prosopagnosia**).[8]

M

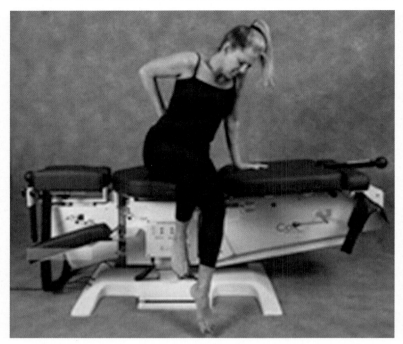

Figure M.6. Minor's sign. (From Cox JM. *Low Back Pain: Mechanism, Diagnosis, and Treatment.* 7th ed. Philadelphia, PA: Wolters Kluwer Health/Lippincott Williams & Wilkins; 2011, with permission.)

Mirror movements: A type of symmetric, contralateral **associated movement** seen commonly in the normal infant, where there is a tendency for movements of one limb to be accompanied by similar involuntary movements of the opposite limb; this disappears as coordination and muscle power are acquired. Mirror movements are usually benign and considered normal during infancy and early childhood. They usually diminish with time and rarely persist beyond 10 years of age. Some adults have benign persistent mirror movements **(Video Link M.1).**[9] These patients are usually otherwise healthy and have only relatively subtle mirroring generally precipitated by complex or effortful tasks.

Mirror movements may occur in patients with brain injuries, disturbances of cerebral development, and dysplasias of the upper portion of the spinal cord, such as Klippel-Feil syndrome; under such circumstances, there are usually associated abnormalities of motor function, tone, and reflexes. Mirror movements in Klippel-Feil syndrome are attributed to incomplete CST decussation.

In certain neurologic disorders, forceful voluntary movements of one limb may be accompanied by identical involuntary movements of the same limb on the other side (see **associated movements**). They are usually seen in the paretic limb when the normal limb is moved, although occasionally such movements may appear in the healthy limb on extreme attempts to move the affected extremity (especially in extrapyramidal disease). Imitation synkinesis by themselves have little localizing significance, occurring with lesions in various portions of the neuraxis. Their value in neurologic assessment is in conjunction with other findings.

Mirror test for functional visual loss: A test for nonorganic visual loss. A large mirror is used that fills most of the patient's field of view. As the mirror is tilted and moved the patient is unable to suppress the visual pursuit reflexes, proving vision is intact. See **visual acuity, sunglasses sign.**

Mirror writing: script in which the writing runs counter to normal, with individual letters reversed, so the writing is most easily read in a mirror. Healthy individuals may mirror write as a diversion but it is also associated with various focal brain lesions, most commonly involving the left hemisphere, and occasionally with diffuse cerebral disorders. Famous mirror writers included Leonardo da Vinci and Lewis Carroll.

Misdirection syndrome: See **aberrant regeneration.**

Misoplegia: hatred and rejection of paralyzed limbs; seen with right hemisphere lesions, see **anosognosia.**

Mitempfindung: Distant referral of cutaneous sensation. The experience of feeling a sensation at a site far away after scratching or touching an area of skin.[10]

Mitgehen: Facilitatory paratonia, the opposite of **gegenhalten,** see **paratonia.**

Moniz's sign: See **minor extensor toe signs.**

Monocular elevation deficiency (palsy): See **double elevator palsy.**

Monocular nystagmus: See **nystagmus.**

Monoparesis (monoplegia): Weakness of one extremity.

Monophasia: A retained speech fragment that an aphasic patient repeats over and over, also referred to as a recurring utterance, verbal stereotypy, verbal automatism, or verbigeration. The individual's vocabulary is limited to a single word, phrase, or sentence. Some monophasias are unusual and difficult to understand. One aphasic patient would say "Pontius Pilate" in response to any and all questions. Broca's original aphasic patient, M. Leborgne, was nicknamed "Tan" because that was the only word he could say. According to Critchley, Hughlings Jackson first became interested in aphasia when his family vacationed in a house where the aphasic landlady could utter only the neologistic stereotypy "watty." A patient may have several stereotypies in his repertoire, and preservation of stereotypic social responses ("hello," "fine") may trick the careless or rushed clinician into believing the patient is linguistically intact.

Moria: Silliness, inappropriate frivolity, and euphoria due to disinhibition, seen in patients with orbitofrontal lesions. See **witzelsucht.**

Motor extinction: Difficulty executing bilateral, simultaneous extremity movements with the extremity contralateral to a hemispheric lesion.

Motor impersistence: See **impersistence.**

Motor negativism: See **paratonia.**

Motor neglect: See **attentional deficits.**

Motor tics: Repetitive, stereotyped movements of a particular muscle group, such as squinting, forceful blinking, grimacing, shrugging or any number of similar habitual movements that occur in patients with the various tic disorders. Simple motor tics involve only one muscle group and consist of brief movements such as nose twitching and head jerking. Complex motor tics involve more complicated movements or a coordinated sequence of movements that are nonpurposeful such as facial contortions, or that appear to be purposeful such as hitting or touching, but actually serve no purpose.

Vocal or phonic tics are motor tics that involve the respiratory, laryngeal, and pharyngeal muscles that cause the patient to make sounds. Simple vocal tics include sounds such as grunting and throat clearing; complex vocal tics include syllables, phrases, and repetition of either the patient's own words (see **palilalia**) or the words of others (see **echolalia**).

Motor Tinel's sign: Twitching of a muscle, detected visually or by EMG, produced by tapping over the nerve that innervates it. The best and most obvious example is **Chvostek's sign**. The Lust phenomenon is another example (see **tetany**).The motor Tinel's sign has been reported as evidence of abnormal mechanosensitivity in entrapment neuropathies, but may also occur in normals.[11]

Mounding phenomenon: see **myoedema**.

MRC scale: A system for grading muscle strength, which was developed by the Medical Research Council in Britain in World War II to evaluate patients with peripheral nerve injuries **(Table M.4)**. The MRC scale has been widely applied to the evaluation of strength in general (see **weakness**). However, the scale is heavily weighted toward the evaluation of very weak muscles. In a severe peripheral nerve injury, improvement from grade 0 (no contraction) to grade 1 (a flicker) is highly significant, as it signals the beginning of reinnervation. A patient with a nerve injury who eventually recovers to grade 4 has had an excellent outcome. In contrast, a patient with polymyositis who is diffusely grade 4 has severe disease and is doing poorly. So the most commonly used strength grading scale has significant limitations when dealing with many patients.

The levels of the MRC scale are precisely defined, but not linear. It is a common error to believe the MRC grades are evenly spaced and that grade 5 is normal, grade 4 is minimal or mild weakness, grade 3 moderate weakness, grade 2 severe, and so forth. In fact, anything less than grade 5 denotes significant weakness. Grade 4 is moderate weakness, and anything less is severe weakness. A patient who is diffusely 4/5 does not have mild or equivocal weakness, but major and serious involvement. One must not confuse poor effort with weakness (see **collapsing weakness**). A muscle is graded by the maximal power demonstrated, even if it is only briefly.

The different levels of the MRC scale are so precisely defined that there is good interexaminer consistency once the fine points of proper positioning and other details are mastered. In clinical practice, the MRC scale is often expanded to include

Table M.4. The Medical Research Council Scale of Muscle Strength

0	No contraction
1	A flicher or trace of contraction
2	Active movement with gravity eliminated
3	Active movement against gravity
4−	Active movement against gravity and slight resistance
4	Active movement against gravity and moderate resistance
4+	Active movement against gravity and strong resistance
5	Normal power

From Campbell WW. *DeJong's the Neurologic Examination.* 7th ed. Philadelphia, PA: Wolters Kluwer Health/Lippincott Williams & Wilkins; 2013.

subgrades (e.g., 5–, 4+). The Medical Research Council eventually saw the need to include grades 4– and 4+. Mendell and Florence developed a formal modified MRC scale.[12] In general use, the subgrades are not so precisely defined and there is much less inter- and even intraexaminer consistency.

Muscle aplasia: Failure of a muscle to develop. Muscles that are congenitally absent or hypoplastic fairly commonly include the depressor anguli oris, the pectoralis major and minor, the trapezius, and the palmaris longus. Facial and extraocular muscle aplasia or hypoplasia occur in Möebius' and Duane's syndromes.

Congenital thenar hypoplasia, unilateral or bilateral, can occur as an isolated defect (Cavanagh's syndrome, Fig. M.7).[13] It may also be associated with cardiac defects (Holt-Oram syndrome) or eye and vascular abnormalities (Okihiro's syndrome). It is critical not to confuse congenital thenar hypoplasia from thenar atrophy due to median neuropathy.

Muscle hypertrophy: An increase in the bulk, or volume, of muscle tissues. It may result from excessive use of the muscles (physiologic hypertrophy) or occur on a pathologic basis. Persistent abnormal muscle contraction may cause hypertrophy. Patients with myotonia congenita have a diffuse muscularity without significant increase in strength (Fig. M.8). Patients with dystonia may develop hypertrophy of

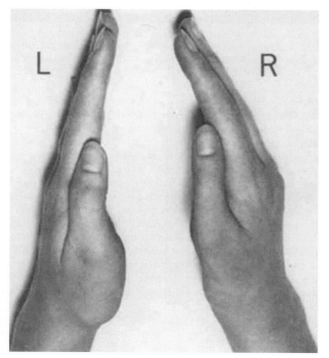

Figure M.7. Hypoplasia of the right thenar eminence. (From Cavanagh NP, Yates DA, Sutcliffe J. Thenar hypoplasia with associated radiologic abnormalities. *Muscle Nerve.* 1979;2:431–436, with permission.)

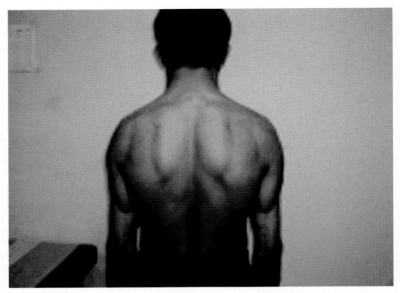

Figure M.8. Muscle hypertrophy in a patient with the recessive form of myotonia congenital (Becker's disease). The hypertrophy developed despite a sedentary lifestyle. (From Varkey B, Varkey L. Muscle hypertrophy in myotonia congenita. *J Neurol Neurosurg Psychiatry*. 2003;74:338, with permission.)

the abnormally active muscle. Muscular dystrophies, especially Duchenne's dystrophy, often cause **pseudohypertrophy** of muscle, with muscle enlargement, particularly **calf enlargement**, due to infiltration of the muscle (see Fig. C.2).

Muscle stretch reflex: See **deep tendon reflex.**

Mutism: A total inability to speak; usually the patient appears to make no attempt to speak or make sounds. Mutism is usually of psychogenic origin if present in an apparently otherwise normal patient, but may occur with lesions of the cerebrum, brainstem, and cerebellum. It is one of the frequent features of Foix-Chavany-Marie (bilateral anterior opercular) syndrome. Mutism may also be a feature of NMS. Selective (elective) mutism is a disorder of childhood characterized by a total lack of speech limited to certain situations—such as school—despite normal speech in other settings. Mutism may also occur in **catatonia**. With large, acute hemispheric lesions, mutism may occur initially but aphasia soon evolves. The cerebellar mutism syndrome consists of diminished speech progressing to mutism, emotional lability, and ataxia that may occur following resection of a posterior fossa tumor in children.

Myasthenic snarl: Poor elevation of the corners of the mouth when attempting to smile may result in a "vertical smile"; referred to as a myasthenic snarl or sneer (Fig. M.9).

Mydriasis: Pupillary dilation; pupils more than 6 mm in diameter are considered dilated. Common causes of bilateral mydriasis include anxiety, fear, pain, myopia, and drug effects. Persons with light irises have larger pupils than those with

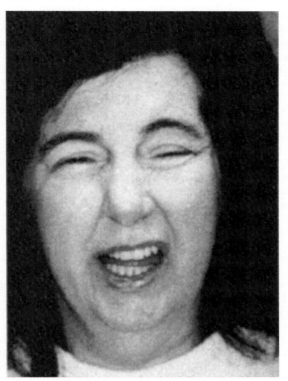

M

Figure M.9. The vertical myasthenic smile or snarl. (From Campbell WW. *DeJong's the Neurologic Examination.* 7th ed. Philadelphia, PA: Wolters Kluwer Health/Lippincott Williams & Wilkins; 2013, with permission.)

dark irises. Only severe, bilateral lesions of the retina or anterior visual pathways, enough to cause near blindness, will affect the resting pupil size. Neurologically significant bilateral mydriasis occurs in midbrain lesions, in comatose patients following cardiac arrest, in cerebral anoxia, and as a terminal condition. Bilateral mydriasis may also occur in botulism. Unilateral mydriasis is never due to isolated, unilateral visual loss; the reactivity of the normal eye and the consensual light reflex will ensure pupil size remains equal. Unilateral mydriasis can occur with local ocular trauma (traumatic iridoplegia). Both reverse **Horner's syndrome** and **springing pupil** may cause transient unilateral mydriasis, and periodic unilateral mydriasis has been reported in migraine and as an ictal phenomenon. Many drugs may cause pupillary dilation, particularly when instilled directly into the eye (**iridoplegia**). Mydriasis occurs as a manifestation of the toxidromes due to anticholinergics and to adrenergic agents, such as amphetamines, caffeine, cocaine, ephedrine, pseudoephedrine, phenylpropanolamine, and theophylline. Atropinic agents given during CPR may enlarge and fixate the pupils. Pilocarpine solution helps distinguish such pharmacologic pupillary blockade from mydriasis due to structural disease.[14]

Myelinated nerve fibers: See **pseudopapilledema.**

Myelomeningocele: A congenital malformation, most often affecting the lumbosacral spine, due to failure of the posterior neuropore to close normally. Myelomeningocele is the most severe manifestation of a spectrum of conditions referred to as dysraphism or neural tube defects. A mild defect of posterior neuropore closure results only in failure of normal fusion of the posterior arches of the lumbosacral vertebra. Patients are neurologically normal, and the defect is seen only on imaging studies (spina bifida occulta). Spina bifida occulta is quite common, affecting up to 10% of the population. In severe dysraphism, the posterior elements of the lumbosacral vertebra fail to develop, the spinal canal is open posteriorly, and the spinal cord and cauda equina are herniated dorsally into a sac that lies over the surface of the lower back. The patients have severe neurological deficits involving the lower extremities, bowel, and bladder. When the defect is less severe, the sac contains only meninges (meningocele).

The vast majority of myelomeningoceles occur posteriorly over the lumbosacral spine and present at birth with painfully obvious major clinical manifestations. But, as with **encephaloceles,** occasionally the herniation occurs anteriorly in either the cervical, thoracic, or lumbosacral region and is occult. The most common of these is the anterior sacral meningocele that usually presents as a presacral mass in adulthood, often associated with dysgenesis of the sacrum. The Currarino triad (Currarino's syndrome) is a sacral bony defect, anorectal malformation, and a presacral mass, most commonly an anterior sacral meningocele, that usually presents in infancy.

Myelopathy hand (Ono's hand, pseudopseudoulnar claw hand): A hand posture seen in patients with C8 radiculopathy, cervical spondylotic myelopathy or, most commonly, radiculomyelopathy. Patients have weakness of extension and adduction affecting primarily the small and ring fingers, causing the affected fingers to droop and abduct when the hand is held outstretched (see Fig. F.4). The hand position was originally described by Ono, who recognized the association with spinal cord pathology and thought it reflected pyramidal tract involvement.[15] A later article described four patients with the same hand posture as a result of C8 radiculopathy; two as a result of spondylotic radiculomyelopathy.[16] This report emphasized the potential confusion with other causes of selective **finger drop,** such as partial posterior interosseous nerve palsy (the pseudoulnar claw hand). The identical sign is widely referred to as the **finger escape sign,** with little to no appreciation in the literature that these are the same. Myelopathy hand is instantly recognizable, fairly common, and highly suspicious for significant cervical spondylosis and radiculomyelopathy.

Myerson's sign: See **glabellar tap reflex.**

Myoclonus: A term used for several different motor phenomena. In general, myoclonus may be defined as single or repetitive, abrupt, brief, rapid, lightning-like, jerky, arrhythmic, asynergic, involuntary contractions involving portions of muscles, entire muscles, or groups of muscles **(Video Link M.2).**

Myoclonus most often affects entire muscles or muscle groups, producing clonic movements of the extremities that may be so violent as to cause an entire limb to be suddenly flung out or even throw the patient to the ground. Myoclonus may also be subtle, a quick flick of a finger or foot. Myoclonus is seen principally in the muscles of the extremities and trunk, but it may also involve the facial muscles, jaws, tongue, pharynx, and larynx **(Video M.1).** The involvement is often multifocal, diffuse, or widespread. Myoclonus may appear symmetrically on both sides of the body; such synchrony may be an attribute unique to myoclonus. The sudden, shock-like contractions usually appear in paroxysms at irregular intervals, during either the resting or active state, and may be activated by emotional, mental, tactile, visual, and auditory stimuli. An **exaggerated startle response** causing a massive whole-body myoclonic jerk occurs in some conditions.

Myoclonus has been classified in numerous ways, including positive versus negative; epileptic versus nonepileptic; stimulus sensitive (reflex) versus spontaneous; rhythmic versus arrhythmic; anatomically (peripheral, spinal, segmental, brainstem, or cortical); and etiologically (physiologic, essential, epileptic, and symptomatic). Asterixis may be viewed as negative myoclonus, the transient, unwanted, abnormal relaxation of a muscle group. As typically used, the term myoclonus refers to positive myoclonus—abnormal jerks. Cortical reflex myoclonus is focal myoclonus triggered by stimulation or movement of the affected part. The Lance-Adams syndrome of action myoclonus occurs with use of the involved limbs, usually as a sequel to cerebral anoxia **(Video Link M.3)**.

Myoclonic movements may occur in a variety of conditions. Physiologic myoclonus occurs in normals as sleep starts and hiccups. Myoclonus is frequently encountered in epilepsy, particularly in such conditions as West syndrome, juvenile myoclonic epilepsy, the progressive myoclonic epilepsies, Lafora body disease, Gaucher's disease, sialidosis, gangliosidoses, ceroid lipofuscinosis, and myoclonic epilepsy with ragged red fibers.

Myoclonus occurs without prominent seizures in a number of other conditions, including metabolic disorders, especially uremic and anoxic encephalopathy, subacute sclerosing panencephalitis, Creutzfeldt-Jakob disease, and Alzheimer's disease. Opsoclonus accompanied by myoclonus may occur as a postinfectious encephalopathy or as a paraneoplastic syndrome, especially due to occult neuroblastoma.

Myoclonus is sometimes benign and without serious significance and may even have a psychogenic basis. Benign forms of myoclonus include paroxysmal kinesigenic myoclonus, hereditary essential myoclonus, and paramyoclonus multiplex. Movements difficult to differentiate from myoclonus may be nonorganic. Myoclonus is typically arrhythmic and diffuse, but the term has also been applied to rhythmic and localized motor phenomena, such as **palatal myoclonus**.

Spinal myoclonus is spasmodic jerking limited to a few contiguous segments of the spinal cord, usually bilateral, symmetric and synchronous, although sometimes unilateral. The muscular contractions are usually rhythmic at a rate of 3 to 5 Hz and persist during sleep. Spinal myoclonus occurs with paraneoplastic, radiation, and HTLV-1 associated myelopathies, with Devic's disease, and in association with glutamic acid decarboxylase antibodies. Propriospinal myoclonus is a variant of spinal myoclonus that causes axial, nonrhythmic jerks involving several segments that may be spontaneous or stimulus sensitive, usually starting in the thoracic level and propagating slowly rostrally and caudally. See **belly dancers dyskinesia**.

Myoclonic Dystonia: see dystonia.

Myoedema (mounding phenomenon): A local muscle contracture induced by tapping the muscle directly, probably caused by the liberation of calcium ions from the sarcoplasmic reticulum by percussion. The percussion causes a stationary ridge or lump that persists for many seconds. In contrast to the dimple that sometimes occurs with **myotonia** or an **idiomuscular contraction**, myoedema causes a mounding up.

Its presence alone does not indicate a neuromuscular disorder, but the response may be exaggerated in some circumstances, most notably hypothyroid myopathy, cachexia, and rippling muscle disease. Myoedema is electrically silent on EMG.

Myokymia: Involuntary, spontaneous, localized, transient or persistent quivering movements that affect a few muscle bundles within a single muscle but usually are not extensive enough to cause movement at a joint. The movements are somewhat coarser, slower, and undulating ("worm-like"), usually more prolonged, and involve a wider local area than fasciculations. They typically are not affected by motion or position and persist during sleep.

Myokymia often occurs in normal individuals, causing focal twitching of a muscle, most commonly the orbicularis oculi. Such myokymia usually occurs in isolation, without evidence of an accompanying neurological disease; it is exacerbated by fatigue, anxiety, and caffeine.

Myokymia may be generalized or focal/segmental. Focal myokymia is much more common than generalized myokymia. **Facial myokymia** sometimes occurs in patients with MS or other lesions of the brainstem or cranial nerves. Focal limb myokymia is particularly characteristic of radiation damage to a nerve or plexus. Generalized myokymia (Isaac's syndrome, syndrome of continuous muscle fiber activity, neuromyotonia) causes generalized muscle stiffness and persistent contraction because of underlying continuous muscle fiber activity **(Video Link M.4).**[17]

Myopathic facies: The particular facial appearance of a patient with facial weakness due to myopathy. Some myopathies are particularly likely to involve the facial muscles, and myopathic facies are particularly typical of FSH and myotonic dystrophy. The eyelids droop but the eyes cannot be tightly closed. In FSH, the lips droop tonelessly, with an involuntary protrusion of the upper lip (**bouche de tapir**). On smiling, the risorius pulls at the angle of the mouth, but the zygomaticus is unable to elevate the lips and the smile is transverse. The facial appearance in myotonic dystrophy is characteristic (Fig. M.10).

Myopia: See **hyperopia and myopia.**

Myotatic reflex: See **deep tendon reflex.**

Myotonia: A disorder of the muscle membrane that can occur in many different conditions, causing a kind of sustained muscle contraction, an inability to relax. Tone is normal when the muscles are relaxed, but contraction produces a temporary involuntary tonic persistence of muscle contraction with slow relaxation. In grip myotonia, the patient has difficulty letting go of an object after gripping it strongly (**Video M.2**). Percussion myotonia is elicited by tapping on the muscle. Percussion over the thenar eminence produces a prolonged tonic abduction and opposition movement lasting several seconds, over which the patient has no control (**Video M.3**). Tapping over the extensor digitorum communis to the middle finger causes the finger to snap into extension, after which it slowly falls over a much longer period of time than normal. Percussion myotonia can also be elicited from other muscles. Percussion of a tongue blade placed transversely on edge across the tongue may produce a segmental myotonic contraction that constricts the tongue circumferentially: the napkin-ring sign (**Video Link M.5**). Eyelid myotonia may cause transient difficulty opening the eyes after a forceful contraction or transient lid retraction after looking up (**Video Link M.6**). Mild myotonia may only be detectable in the facial muscles or eyelids. Myotonia improves with repeated contractions, the warm-up phenomenon, and may worsen in the cold or

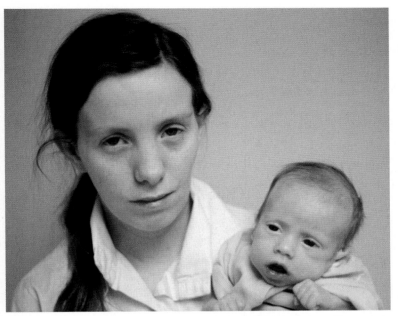

Figure M.10. Myopathic facies in a newly diagnosed young mother with myotonic dystrophy, holding her hypotonic infant, who has the congenital form. The mother has bilateral ptosis, hollowed temporalis, and a slack lower face. The infant has ptosis and the classic "tented upper lip."

M

after prolonged rest. **Paradoxical myotonia** is that which worsens after repetitive contraction. Myotonia is usually nonpainful and should not be confused with cramp, **spasticity**, **rigidity**, **dystonia**, or **myoedema**.

Myotonia occurs in myotonic dystrophy types 1 (DM1) and 2 (DM2, proximal myotonic myopathy) and in the sodium channelopathies (hyperkalemic periodic paralysis and paramyotonia congenita). The most common condition by far is DM1. DMD is the most prevalent muscular dystrophy in childhood; DM1 is the most prevalent dystrophy in adults. The different forms of myotonia congenita are associated with mutations in the chloride channel gene. The primary entities in the differential diagnosis of DM1 are DM2, myotonia congenita, paramyotonia congenita, Schwartz-Jampel syndrome, and drug-induced myotonia. The various conditions causing myotonia that are not DM1 or DM2 are sometimes referred to as the nondystrophic myotonias, channelopathies that cause myotonia but not the complications of DM1 or DM2. DM1 and DM2 cause muscle weakness and wasting; the nondystrophic myotonias are more likely to cause **muscle hypertrophy**.

Other conditions causing myotonia include Isaac's syndrome, chondrodystrophy, acid maltase, debrancher deficiency, and myotubular myopathy. Rippling muscle disease may cause prolonged muscle contraction similar to percussion myotonia. It is associated with rolling waves, or ripples, that spread laterally across the muscle after percussion or contraction **(Video Link M.7)**. The distribution of myotonia may vary in the different myotonic syndromes. In DM1, myotonia is most obvious in affected muscles and distal muscles; it may disappear as muscle atrophy sets in with disease progression. In DM2, the myotonia is typically less severe and more proximal.

Myriachit: See **hyperekplexia.**

Video Links

M.1. Some adults have benign persistent mirror movements. (From Lim EC, Seet RC. Through the looking glass: persistent mirror movements. *CMAJ.* 2007;176:619.) Available at: http://www.cmaj.ca/content/176/5/619/rel-suppl/0c155172ba9c032f/suppl/DC1

M.2. Myoclonus. (From Chan S, Turner MR, Young L, et al. Cephalosporin-induced myoclonus. *Neurology.* 2006;66:E20.) Available at: http://www.neurology.org/content/suppl/2006/03/20/66.6.E20.DC1/Video.mpg

M.3. A cardiorespiratory arrest survivor with action myoclonus induced by the mere intent to move. (From Espay AJ, Chen R. Myoclonus. *Mov Dis.* 2013;19(5):1264–1286.) Available at: http://journals.lww.com/continuum/pages/videogallery.aspx?videoId=81&autoPlay=true

M.4. Widespread myokymia. (From Chhibber S, Greenberg SA. Teaching video neuroimages: widespread clinical myokymia in chronic inflammatory demyelinating polyradiculoneuropathy. *Neurology.* 2011;77:e33.) Available at: http://www.neurology.org/content/suppl/2011/07/31/77.5.e33.DC1/Video1.mpg

M.5. Myotonia of the tongue. (From Wang ZJ, Huang XS. Images in clinical medicine. Myotonia of the tongue. *N Engl J Med.* 2011;365:e32.) Available at: http://www.nejm.org/doi/full/10.1056/NEJMicm1014605

M.6. Eye closure myotonia. (From Statland JM, Barohn RJ. Muscle channelopathies: the nondystrophic myotonias and periodic paralyses. *Musc Dis.* 2013;19(6):1598–1614.) Available at: http://journals.lww.com/continuum/pages/videogallery.aspx?videoId=107&autoPlay=true

M.7. Rippling muscle disease. Available at: https://www.youtube.com/watch?v=RicWrvozUsQ

References

1. Ramos-Levi AM, Diaz-Perez A, Sobrido MJ, et al. Axonal neuropathy, long limbs and bumpy tongue: think of MEN2B. *Muscle Nerve.* 2012;46:961–964.
2. Johnston JD. The contribution of Dr. Mary Walker towards myasthenia gravis and periodic paralysis whilst working in poor law hospitals in London. *J Hist Neurosci.* 2005;14:121–137.
3. Patten BM. A hypothesis to account for the Mary Walker phenomenon. *Ann Intern Med.* 1975;82:411–415.
4. O'Neill JH, Mills KR, Murray NM. McArdle's sign in multiple sclerosis. *J Neurol Neurosurg Psychiatry.* 1987;50:1691–1693.
5. McGee S. *Evidence Based Physical Diagnosis.* 3rd ed. Philadelphia, PA: Elsevier/Saunders; 2012.
6. Schmal F, Lubben B, Weiberg K, et al. The minimal ice water caloric test compared with established vestibular caloric test procedures. *J Vestib Res.* 2005;15:215–224.
7. Wilkins DE, Hallett M, Erba G. Primary generalised epileptic myoclonus: a frequent manifestation of minipolymyoclonus of central origin. *J Neurol Neurosurg Psychiatry.* 1985;48:506–516.
8. Ghika J, Dieguez S, Assal F, et al. Mirror behaviors in dementia: the many mirror signs. *Rev Med Suisse.* 2013;9:2095–2099.
9. Lim EC, Seet RC. Through the looking glass: persistent mirror movements. *CMAJ.* 2007;176:619.
10. Schott GD. Distant referral of cutaneous sensation (Mitempfindung). Observations on its normal and pathological occurrence. *Brain.* 1988;111:1187–1198.
11. Montagna P, Liguori R. The motor tinel sign: a useful sign in entrapment neuropathy? *Muscle Nerve.* 2000; 23:976–978.
12. Mendell JR, Florence J. Manual muscle testing. *Muscle Nerve.* 1990;13(suppl):S16–S20.
13. Sonel B, Senbil N, Yavus Gurer YK, et al. Cavanagh's syndrome (congenital thenar hypoplasia). *J Child Neurol.* 2002;17:51–54.
14. Thompson HS, Newsome DA, Loewenfeld IE. The fixed dilated pupil. Sudden iridoplegia or mydriatic drops? A simple diagnostic test. *Arch Ophthalmol.* 1971;86:21–27.
15. Ono K, Ebara S, Fuji T, et al. Myelopathy hand. New clinical signs of cervical cord damage. *J Bone Joint Surg Br.* 1987;69:215–219.
16. Campbell WW, Buschbacher R, Pridgeon RM, et al. Selective finger drop in cervical radiculopathy: the pseudopseudoulnar claw hand. *Muscle Nerve.* 1995;18:108–110.
17. Chhibber S, Greenberg SA. Teaching video neuroimages: widespread clinical myokymia in chronic inflammatory demyelinating polyradiculoneuropathy. *Neurology.* 2011;77:e33.

Naffziger's sign: (1) Occlusion of the jugular veins causing radicular symptoms in compressive radiculopathy; see **cervical radiculopathy signs, Bakody's sign, cervical distraction test, Viets' sign, upper limb tension test**. (2) Pressure in the supraclavicular fossa causing hand paresthesias in patients with TOS.

Naming: A complex and delicate language function often disturbed in patients with **aphasia**. Testing naming ability is an important part of the aphasia examination. Most aphasic patients have some difficulty with naming, but naming defects are nonspecific. In **anomic aphasia**, an inability to name is an isolated defect, but more often misnaming occurs as part of some other aphasic, or even nonaphasic, syndrome. Categories of naming often tested include confrontation naming, responsive naming, word-list generation, and body part naming.

In confrontation naming, the patient is asked to name simple objects such as a key, pencil, coin, or watch. When lost for the name of an object, the patient may describe it or tell its use. Frequently, the patient can name an object, such as a watch, but not the component parts. Another naming test is to have the patient point to something named by the examiner. Responsive naming uses audition rather than vision by asking the patient for nouns (e.g., "Where do teachers work?"), verbs (e.g., "What do you do with a cup?"), or adjectives (e.g., "How does sugar taste?").

A sensitive method of testing spontaneous naming ability is word-list generation. The patient is asked to name as many items as possible in a certain category, such as animals, in 1 minute (**category fluency**). Spontaneous naming ability depends on age and educational level. Normal patients should name a minimum of 12 items in a category; some adjustment may be necessary for poorly educated and older patients. Another measure of spontaneous naming is to ask the patient to list as many words as possible that begin with a certain letter, such as F, A, or S (letter fluency). For FAS, a person of average education should produce 12 or more words per letter in 1 minute, or 36 words with all three letters in 3 minutes. Poor word-list generation may also occur with dementia, depression, parkinsonism, and prefrontal lesions. Body part naming screens for **autotopagnosia**.

Nasal (sternutatory, sneeze) reflex: Wrinkling of the nose, eye closure, and often a forceful exhalation resembling a feeble sneeze after stimulation of the nasal mucosa with a wisp of cotton or a spear of tissue. The reflex is mediated by V_1, not by V_2, and a reflex center in the brainstem and upper spinal cord. The primary clinical utility is as a cross-check on the **corneal reflex**.

Nasal reflex of Bechterew: The nasal reflex elicited on one side, nasal tickle causes contraction of the ipsilateral facial muscles.

Nasal (hypernasal) speech (rhinolalia): Abnormal speech due to weakness of the soft palate or an inability to seal off the nasal from the oral cavity, referred to as velopharyngeal insufficiency. Voice sounds have an added abnormal resonance **(Audio N.1)**. There is special difficulty with the velar sounds, but labials and linguals are also affected because much of the air necessary for their production escapes through the nose. The speech resembles that of a patient with a cleft palate. Characteristically, *b* becomes *m*, *d* becomes *n*, and *k* becomes *ng*. Audible nasal air emission may occur with talking. ALS and MG are common causes of nasal speech. In MG, the voice may become more nasal, and dysarthria more severe, with prolonged talking. Nasal speech is often accompanied by other manifestations of bulbar weakness.

Nasolacrimal reflex: Tearing, usually bilateral, elicited by mechanical stimulation of the nasal mucosa, or by chemical stimulation using irritating substances such as ammonia.

Nasomental reflex: See **orbicularis oris reflex**.

Nasopalpebral reflex: See **orbicularis oculi reflex**.

Near point of accommodation: See **hyperopia and myopia** and **far point of accommodation**.

Near reflex (response): See **accommodation reflex**.

Near synkinetic triad: See **accommodation reflex**.

Negative myoclonus: Abrupt, brief involuntary movement due to the cessation of muscle activity by the agonist, causing transient, unwanted, abnormal relaxation of a muscle group. Four types of negative **myoclonus** have been recognized: **asterixis**, postural lapses, epileptic negative myoclonus and physiologic negative myoclonus.[1] Negative myoclonus involving trunk or leg muscles may result in an abrupt fall, a drop attack. Epileptic negative myoclonus is an interruption of tonic muscle activity synchronous with a cortical epileptic discharge. Physiologic negative myoclonus occurs in normal individuals, especially at sleep onset, but also after exercise or due to high anxiety.

Neglect: See **attentional deficits, anosognosia**.

Negro's sign: (1) In upper facial weakness, the eyeball on the paralyzed side deviates outward and elevates more than the normal one when the patient raises his eyes, akin to Bell's phenomenon. (2) cogwheel **rigidity**.

Neologisms: A type of **paraphasia** consisting of new, improvised words, usually meaningless, coined by the patient, that are often phonologic approximations of real words, usually heard in psychotic or aphasic patients.

Neologistic jargon: A type of jargon **aphasia** in which the speech consists largely of made-up, nonword **neologisms**.

Nerve hypertrophy: Enlargement of peripheral nerves. The enlargement may be palpable and sometimes visible. The greater auricular, superficial radial, ulnar at the elbow and peroneal at the knee are the sites where nerve enlargement is most commonly detected (Fig. N.1). Nerve hypertrophy is a classic finding in CMT type 1, aka the hypertrophic form of CMT disease, and CMT type 3 (Dejerine-Sottas disease). Enlarged nerves are common in lepromatous leprosy. Nerve hypertrophy may also occur in CIDP, Refsum's disease, and Lewis-Sumner syndrome.[2]

Neri's sign: (1) In acute lumbosacral radiculopathy, bending forward while standing causes the patient to flex the knee to avoid root stretch; also known as the knee-bending sign. (2) combined flexion of thigh and leg when the standing patient bends forward as far as possible. Normally, the knees remain extended; in CST lesions, the knee flexes. If the recumbent patient raises the legs alternately, the normal leg remains straight but the paretic leg flexes at the knee. Passively flexing the hip with the knee extended causes the knee to flex. See **Babinski's trunk-thigh sign**.

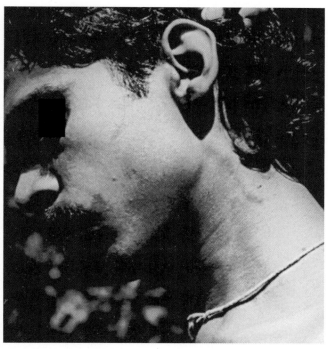

Figure N.1. Visible thickening of the great auricular nerve in leprosy. (From Gorbach SL, Bartlett JG, Blacklow NR. *Infectious Diseases*. 3rd ed. Philadelphia, PA: Wolters Kluwer Health/Lippincott Williams and Wilkins; 2004, with permission.)

Neurofibroma: A benign, slow-growing peripheral nerve tumor that occurs most frequently in NF1 **(Fig. N.2)**. Pathologically, the tumor consists of Schwann cells, perineurial-like cells, and fibroblasts. Neurofibromas occur as solitary or multiple lesions and can arise from any nerve; they most commonly involve skin, major nerve plexuses, and large nerve trunks **(plexiform neuroma)**. Multiple neuro-fibromas or a solitary, large plexiform neuroma is essentially diagnostic of NF1 **(Table N.1)**. Occasionally, a neurofibroma undergoes degeneration into a malig-nant peripheral nerve sheath tumor. Solitary cutaneous neurofibromas may occur in patients who do not have NF1; these do not carry the risk of sarcomatous de-generation. Pressure on a cutaneous neurofibroma can often cause it to disappear through what seems to be a defect in the skin (buttonhole sign).

Neuroma sign: See **Tinel's sign**.

Neuropathic arthropathy: See **Charcot joint**.

Neuropathic tremor: A coarse, 3- to 6-Hz, postural and kinetic tremor seen in pa-tients with peripheral neuropathy, probably related to deafferentation. Demyelinat-ing neuropathies are more likely to be associated with tremor.[3] See **finger-to-nose test**.

Nevus flammeus: See **port wine stain**.

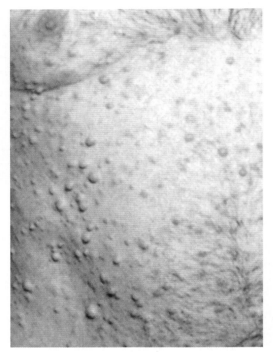

Figure N.2. Multiple cutaneous neurofibromas in a patient with NF1 (von Recklinghausen's disease). Other common features include café-au-lait spots, axillary freckling, and Lisch nodules. The disease has an increased frequency of benign and malignant tumors because of lack of protection from mutated neurofibromin, an antioncogene.

Table N.1. Diagnostic Criteria for Neurofibromatosis Type 1

- Six or more café-au-lait spots 1.5 cm or larger in postpubertal individuals, 0.5 cm or larger in prepubertal individuals
- Two or more neurofibromas of any type or one or more plexiform neurofibromas
- Freckling in the axilla or groin
- Optic glioma
- Two or more Lisch nodules
- A distinctive bony lesion, e.g., dysplasia of the sphenoid bone
- A first-degree relative with NF1

Nevus of Jadahsson: See **epidermal nevus.**

Nociceptive reflex of Riddoch and Buzzard: A mass reflex that may occur in patients with CST lesions. In spastic hemiplegia, the scratching, pricking, or pinching of the medial aspect of the upper extremity, the walls of the axilla, or the upper part of the chest results in mass upper-extremity movements, with abduction and external rotation of the shoulder, and flexion of the elbow, wrist, and finger joints.

In quadriplegia, especially due to a high cervical lesion, the same stimuli evokes an extensor response. The flexor response is most easily elicited by stimulation of the hand or forearm, whereas the extensor response is most easily initiated by a stimulus to the upper arm or axillary wall. These are postural reactions related to the reflexes of spinal automatism. See **pathologic reflexes**.

Nominal aphasia: See **anomia**.

Noncomitant (nonconcomitant) deviation: See **strabismus**.

Nonorganic signs: See **functional signs**.

Nuchal rigidity: See **meningeal signs**.

Nuchocephalic reflex: A **frontal release sign** or **primitive reflex** elicited by turning the patient's shoulders to the left and right with eyes closed.[4] Normally, the head turns in the direction of the shoulders after a very brief lag because of inhibition of the nuchocephalic reflex. In frontal lobe disease, loss of inhibition of the reflex causes the head to remain straight ahead as the shoulders turn. Disinhibition of the reflex becomes more common with advancing age, so it may also be considered an **age-related sign**.

Null point: See **congenital nystagmus**.

Numb cheek syndrome: Sensory loss in the distribution of the infraorbital nerve due to carcinomatous infiltration.[5] There is typically numbness of the anterior teeth and gums, which proves the lesion is at the infraorbital foramen and not intracranially. In the numb cheek-limp lower lid syndrome, there is accompanying lower eyelid or upper lip weakness due to involvement of distal facial nerve branches.[6]

Numb chin syndrome (Roger's sign): Sensory loss in the distribution of the mental nerve. The lesion may be at the mental foramen, at the base of the skull, or intracranially involving V_3. Numb chin syndrome is often associated with neoplasia, especially carcinoma of the breast.[7]

Nylen-Bárány maneuver: See **Dix-Hallpike maneuver**.

Nystagmus: A rhythmic, biphasic, involuntary jerking of the eyes. Nystagmus is a complex topic.[8-10] When faced with a patient with nystagmus or similar-appearing movements, the usual clinical exercises include the following two steps: (a) deciding if the nystagmus indicates neurologic pathology and (b) if so, whether the pathology is central or peripheral, and if central whether it has any localizing value **(Table N.2)**. Symptoms often associated with nystagmus are blurred vision, because of impaired foveation, and oscillopsia, an unsteadiness of the visual world.

A host of conditions can cause nystagmus, including ocular disease, drug effects, peripheral vestibular disease, and CNS disease. Schemes have classified nystagmus in many different ways. This discussion focuses on the types of nystagmus commonly encountered in neurologic practice and on the differentiation between nystagmus that likely signifies neurologic disease (neuropathologic) and that which does not (nonneuropathologic).

Nystagmus is classified in multiple ways: Pendular versus jerk; central versus peripheral; induced versus spontaneous; and physiologic versus pathologic. In pendular nystagmus, both phases have the same velocity. Nystagmus of ocular origin is often pendular. Pendular nystagmus only rarely signifies neurologic disease, but may occur with brainstem or cerebellar lesions, particularly in MS. Jerk nystagmus is classified by the direction of the fast phase. Alexander's law states that jerk nystagmus increases with gaze in the direction of the fast phase. First-degree nystagmus is present only with eccentric gaze. Second-degree nystagmus is present

Table N.2. Nystagmus with Localizing Significance

Nystagmus Type	Characteristics	Location of Pathology	Possible Disease or Condition
Upbeat nystagmus	Upbeating nystagmus in primary gaze	Cerebellar vermis (if nystagmus increases), or medulla (if it decreases) in upgaze	Cerebellar or medullary lesion; meningitis; Wernicke's encephalopathy; rarely drug intoxication
Downbeat nystagmus	Downbeating nystagmus in primary gaze, maximal in eccentric downgaze ("downbeat in the corners")	Cervico-medullary junction	Arnold-Chiari malformation; basilar invagination; MS; foramen magnum tumor; spinocerebellar degeneration; Wernicke's encephalopathy; vascular disease; rarely drug intoxication
Convergence-retraction nystagmus	Convergence motions and/or simultaneous retraction of globes back into the orbits	Rostral midbrain, pretectum, posterior commissure, posterior third ventricle	Mass lesions, especially pinealoma; vascular disease; upward transtentorial herniation
Rebound nystagmus	Horizontal nystagmus that briefly beats in the opposite direction on return to primary position	Cerebellum or cerebellar connections	MS; cerebellar or posterior fossa lesion
Periodic alternating nystagmus	Horizontal nystagmus that beats in one direction for 1–3 min, pauses, then beats in the other direction, cycling continuously	Brainstem or cerebellum	Craniocervical junction abnormality; MS; spinocerebellar degeneration; tumor; cryptococcosis; neurosyphilis; congenital drug effects
Seesaw nystagmus	Pendular nystagmus; one eye rises and intorts, the other falls and extorts; sometimes associated with bitemporal hemianopia	Anterior third ventricle, parasellar or optic chiasm region	Tumor, especially craniopharyngioma; head trauma; septo-optic dysplasia; congenital
Bruns' nystagmus	Large and coarse in one direction, fine in the opposite direction	Cerebellopontine angle	Tumor

in primary gaze and increases in intensity with gaze in the direction of the fast component. With third-degree nystagmus, the fast component continues to beat in the opposite direction even with gaze in the direction of the slow component. Dissociated nystagmus is different in the two eyes (e.g., the nystagmus in the abducting eye in INO).

Physiologic nystagmus. Types of physiologic nystagmus include end point, **optokinetic nystagmus** (OKN), and induced vestibular. Although these types of nystagmus are normal, they may be altered when disease is present in such a way as to assist in localization.

End-point nystagmus is fine, typically low-amplitude, irregular, and variably sustained nystagmus at the extremes of lateral gaze, especially with gaze eccentric enough to eliminate fixation by the adducting eye. Symmetry on right and left gaze, prompt abolition by moving the eyes a few degrees back toward primary position, and the absence of other neurologic abnormalities generally serve to distinguish end point from pathologic nystagmus. End-point nystagmus is the most common form of nystagmus seen in routine clinical practice and has no clinical significance.

Although OKN is a normal response, its characteristics may be altered in disease. Changes in OKN occur primarily with deep parietal lobe lesions. Vestibular nystagmus occurs normally in response to rotation (e.g., Barany chair) or irrigation of the ear with hot or cold water. Its patterns may be altered by disease.

Nonneuropathologic nystagmus. Types of nystagmus that are not physiologic, but do not result from neurologic disease include drug induced, congenital, and ocular. Drug-induced nystagmus is very common and results from the effects of alcohol, sedative hypnotics, anticonvulsants, and other drugs. It is typically symmetric and gaze evoked horizontally and vertically.

Congenital nystagmus (infantile nystagmus syndrome) is most often horizontal jerk and remains horizontal even in upgaze and downgaze, a pattern unusual in other forms of nystagmus.[11] Congenital nystagmus is frequently asymptomatic. Patients often have a null point of least nystagmus intensity and best vision in slightly eccentric gaze and may adopt a head turn or tilt to maintain gaze in this null zone. The nystagmus typically damps with convergence. The patient with congenital nystagmus characteristically holds reading material extremely close and regards it with a peculiar head tilt, but still has mediocre vision. A virtually pathognomonic feature of congenital nystagmus is "inversion" of OKNs. Moving an OKN tape so as to cause an expected summation with the fast phase of the congenital nystagmus produces instead a diminution or a paradoxical reversal of nystagmus direction. Congenital nystagmus may be familial, inherited as an autosomal recessive, X-linked dominant or recessive.

Latent nystagmus, a form of congenital nystagmus, occurs only when one eye is covered. The slow phase beats toward the covered eye. In manifest latent nystagmus, the nystagmus is present with both eyes open, but only one is fixating. Vision in the other eye is suppressed because of strabismus or amblyopia.

Ocular nystagmus is seen in patients with very poor vision. Visual-loss-induced nystagmus is typically continuous and pendular and usually damps with convergence. When the visual loss is asymmetric, the more prominent nystagmus often occurs in the eye with the least vision (Heimann-Bielschowsky phenomenon).

Neuropathologic nystagmus. Nystagmus is a frequent manifestation of disease of the nervous system. Common types include vestibular, positional, gaze evoked, and gaze paretic nystagmus. Table N.2 summarizes important but less often encountered types of nystagmus.

Vestibular nystagmus. Symmetric, equal activity of the vestibular systems on each side normally maintains the eyes in straight-ahead, primary position. Vestibular imbalance causes the eyes to deviate toward the less active side as the normal side overcomes the weakened tonic activity from the hypoactive side. In an alert patient, the frontal eye fields generate a saccade to bring the eyes back toward primary position, creating the fast phase of vestibular nystagmus. The fast phase beats toward the more active, usually the normal, side. The COWS (cold opposite, warm same) mnemonic refers to the fast phase of the nystagmus after vestibular irrigation. Cold water decreases the tonic activity of the labyrinth and induces nystagmus that beats away from the irrigated side.

Vestibular nystagmus may occur because of central or peripheral disease. Peripheral vestibular nystagmus is due to disorders of the labyrinth or vestibular nerve. It is typically associated with nausea and vomiting. Central vestibular nystagmus is due to disorders of the vestibular nuclei or the vestibular connections in the brainstem or cerebellum. Nausea and vomiting are usually not as prominent, but the patient may have other neurologic symptoms and findings. **Central nystagmus** tends to change directions, has a variable pattern, and is not suppressed by visual fixation; the direction in peripheral nystagmus is usually fixed and is suppressed by visual fixation.[12] Because of the influence of the three different semicircular canals, vestibular nystagmus may beat in more than one direction, the summation of which creates an admixed rotatory component or a mixed horizontal-torsional pattern rarely seen with other conditions. Purely torsional nystagmus usually results from lesions involving the central vestibular pathways; mixed torsional-linear nystagmus is typically due to peripheral vestibular disease.

Positional nystagmus. Degenerative changes in the otoliths frequently produce the syndrome of positional vertigo and nystagmus. On positional testing, nystagmus occurs after a latency of up to 30 seconds, usually beats with the fast phase toward the down ear (**geotropic nystagmus**), quickly fatigues despite holding the position, and adapts with repeated attempts to elicit it (see **Dix-Hallpike maneuver**). Positional nystagmus is a very common condition. While generally peripheral, it may also occur with central disease (tumor, stroke, MS, degenerative disease). The presence of **ageotropic nystagmus** should raise concern about a central lesion. **Minicalorics** are used to evaluate vestibular function by analyzing the responses to irrigation.

Gaze-evoked nystagmus. Any nystagmus not present in primary gaze but appearing with gaze in any direction with the fast phase in the direction of gaze is referred to as gaze-evoked nystagmus (GEN). GEN is the most common form of nystagmus seen in clinical practice and may be physiologic or pathologic (**Video N.1**). The physiologic form is end-point nystagmus. Normal physiologic end-point nystagmus is gaze evoked, but only present horizontally and at extremes of gaze. Abnormal GEN occurs short of extreme gaze and is more sustained than end point.

There are many types of pathologic GEN. When symmetric, the most common cause is medications. Medication-induced GEN is typically symmetric and present on both lateral and upward gaze. Nystagmus with the same appearance in the absence of drug effects is nonspecific but usually indicates disease of the cerebellum or cerebellar connections. GEN is also one of the most sensitive eye signs for CNS or peripheral vestibular pathology. In this case, the GEN is asymmetric, and the amplitude is greater with gaze in the direction of the fast phase.

Gaze paretic nystagmus. Gaze paretic nystagmus is a form of gaze-evoked nystagmus seen in patients with incomplete gaze palsies. Rather than having an absolute inability to gaze in a particular direction, the patient achieves lateral gaze transiently but cannot maintain it. The eyes drift back toward neutral and then spasmodically jerk back in the desired gaze direction.

Acquired pendular nystagmus. With pendular nystagmus, the velocity is equal in each direction. It most often occurs congenitally in association with poor vision. The most common cause of acquired pendular nystagmus is MS (**Video Link N.1**).

Nystagmus with localizing significance. Some forms of nystagmus have localizing significance (see Table N.2).[13] Upbeat nystagmus is spontaneous upbeating nystagmus in primary position (**Video N.2**).[14] Its presence suggests bilateral paramedian lesions of the brainstem, usually at the pontomedullary or pontomesencephalic junction, particularly involving the nucleus intercalatus. Rarely, it occurs in Wernicke's encephalopathy and other conditions. Downbeat nystagmus is spontaneous downbeating nystagmus in primary position (**Video N.3**). It is usually caused by damage to the vestibular nuclei in the floor of the fourth ventricle or bilateral damage to the flocculi and/or the paraflocculi.[15] It occurs with craniocervical junction abnormalities, such as Chiari malformation, cerebellar disorders, Wernicke's encephalopathy, and occasionally from the effects of drugs. Spontaneous vertical nystagmus due to focal central lesions has been attributed to primary dysfunction of the superior vestibular nuclei-ventral tegmental tract pathway, which becomes hypoactive after pontine or caudal medullary lesions, causing upbeat nystagmus, and hyperactive after floccular lesions, causing downbeat nystagmus.[15]

Convergence retraction nystagmus is not true nystagmus but an unusual horizontal eye movement induced by attempted upgaze, consisting of synchronous convergence and retraction of both globes followed by a slow divergence movement.[16] The movements are caused by co-contraction of the extraocular muscles. It occurs as part of the dorsal midbrain (Parinaud's) syndrome; **Video Link N.2**).

Rebound nystagmus occurs when there is gaze-evoked nystagmus in one direction, but the fast phase reverses direction and beats transiently in the opposite direction on return to primary position (see Video N.1). It occurs primarily with cerebellar disease. Periodic alternating nystagmus is horizontal jerk nystagmus that spontaneously changes directions every 30 to 180 seconds (**Video N.4**). The clinical significance is similar to that of downbeat nystagmus. In seesaw nystagmus, one eye rises and intorts as the other eye falls and extorts. The movements are pendular. It occurs with lesions in the region of the mesodiencephalic junction and is particularly associated with lesions of the optic chiasm, such as septo-optic dysplasia (**Video Link N.3**).

Bruns' nystagmus is seen with large CPA lesions. There is coarse gaze paretic nystagmus on looking toward the lesion and fine vestibular nystagmus with gaze in the opposite direction (**Video N.5**). Most patients with CPA tumors only have unilateral vestibular nystagmus on contralateral gaze. In Bruns' nystagmus, there is also gaze-evoked nystagmus on ipsilateral gaze because of damage to the flocculonodular lobe and its brainstem connections, indicative of brainstem distortion or compression. The majority of patients with CPA tumors and Bruns' nystagmus have lesions >3 cm in size, often with fourth ventricular distortion.

Video Links

N.1. Acquired pendular nystagmus. (From Thurtell MJ. Diagnostic approach to abnormal spontaneous eye movements. *Neuro-Ophthalmology.* 2014;20(4):993–1007.) Available at: http://journals.lww .com/continuum/pages/videogallery.aspx?videoId=119&autoPlay=true

N.2. Dorsal midbrain syndrome. Available at: https://www.youtube.com/watch?v=u7D1-zj98l8

N.3. Seesaw nystagmus. (From Thurtell MJ. Diagnostic approach to abnormal spontaneous eye movements. *Neuro-Ophthalmology.* 2014;20(4):993–1007.) Available at: http://journals.lww.com/ continuum/pages/videogallery.aspx?videoId=120&autoPlay=true

References

1. Rubboli G, Tassinari CA. Negative myoclonus. An overview of its clinical features, pathophysiological mechanisms, and management. *Neurophysiol Clin.* 2006;36:337–343.

2. Imamura K, Tajiri Y, Kowa H, et al. Peripheral nerve hypertrophy in chronic inflammatory demyelinating polyradiculoneuropathy detected by ultrasonography. *Intern Med.* 2009;48:581–582.

3. Breit S, Wachter T, Schols L, et al. Effective thalamic deep brain stimulation for neuropathic tremor in a patient with severe demyelinating neuropathy. *J Neurol Neurosurg Psychiatry.* 2009;80:235–236.

4. Jenkyn LR, Walsh DB, Walsh BT, et al. The nuchocephalic reflex. *J Neurol Neurosurg Psychiatry.* 1975;38:561–566.

5. Campbell WW, Jr. The numb cheek syndrome: a sign of infraorbital neuropathy. *Neurology.* 1986; 36:421–423.

6. Brazis PW, Vogler JB, Shaw KE. The "numb cheek-limp lower lid" syndrome. *Neurology.* 1991; 41:327–328.

7. Oravivattanakul S, Coffey M, Teston L, et al. Teaching neuroimages: "numb chin syndrome" in a patient with breast cancer. *Neurology.* 2013;80:e131.

8. Thurtell MJ, Leigh RJ. Nystagmus and saccadic intrusions. *Handb Clin Neurol.* 2011;102:333–378.

9. Rucker JC. An update on acquired nystagmus. *Semin Ophthalmol.* 2008;23:91–97.

10. Stahl JS, Leigh RJ. Nystagmus. *Curr Neurol Neurosci Rep.* 2001;1:471–477.

11. Khanna S, Dell'Osso LF. The diagnosis and treatment of infantile nystagmus syndrome (INS). *ScientificWorldJournal.* 2006;6:1385–1397.

12. Huh YE, Kim JS. Bedside evaluation of dizzy patients. *J Clin Neurol.* 2013;9:203–213.

13. Lee AG, Brazis PW. Localizing forms of nystagmus: symptoms, diagnosis, and treatment. *Curr Neurol Neurosci Rep.* 2006;6:414–420.

14. Adamec I, Gabelic T, Krbot M, et al. Primary position upbeat nystagmus. *J Clin Neurosci.* 2012;19: 161–162.

15. Pierrot-Deseilligny C, Milea D. Vertical nystagmus: clinical facts and hypotheses. *Brain.* 2005;128: 1237–1246.

16. Rambold H, Kompf D, Helmchen C. Convergence retraction nystagmus: a disorder of vergence? *Ann Neurol.* 2001;50:677–681.

Object agnosia: Agnosia for physical objects; see **agnosia.**

Objective tinnitus: Noise audible to both the patient and the examiner, as occurs in carotid stenosis. Most tinnitus is subjective.

O'Connell's test: A root stretch maneuver used in the diagnosis of lumbosacral radiculopathy. SLR is first carried out on the sound limb, then on the affected limb, noting the angles of elevation and location of pain produced. Then both legs are raised together, keeping the knees extended (double straight leg-raising test). The painful leg may be raised higher when both legs are raised together than when either is raised alone. With both legs raised to an angle just short of that which produces pain, the sound limb is lowered; this may result in a marked exacerbation of pain, sometimes associated with paresthesias. The patient may be able to do a sit-up with the knees flexed but not extended (Kraus-Weber test). See **straight leg-raising test.** Milgram's test also involves bilateral straight leg raising but by active contraction, with pain said to indicate disc herniation.

Ocular bobbing: One of several types of unusual spontaneous eye movements that may occur in coma.[1,2] Other types include **ping-pong gaze**, **periodic alternating gaze deviation**, repetitive divergence, nystagmoid jerking, and **ocular dipping**; the particular pattern may have localizing significance.

Classical ocular bobbing consists of intermittent, rapid, conjugate, downward eye movements followed by a slower return to primary position. Most patients with this pattern have large intrinsic lesions of the pons, primarily hemorrhage, but the pattern may also occur with metabolic and toxic encephalopathies. Spontaneous and reflex-induced horizontal eye movements are usually absent.

Several less common variants of ocular bobbing may occur; these are less reliable for localization than is the classical form. In ocular dipping, the eyes move downward slowly with a rapid return to midposition. The "reverse" patterns consist of upward eye movements. Reverse bobbing is characterized by a rapid upward deviation and a slow return to primary position; reverse dipping consists of a slow phase up and a fast phase down (Video Link O.1).

Ocular dipping: See **ocular bobbing.**

Ocular dysmetria: An over- or undershooting of the eyes on rapid refixation of gaze toward either side, or on returning to the primary position, that requires corrective saccades; there may also be overshooting in following movements when the object of regard is suddenly stopped. The lesion is usually in the dorsal vermis and fastigial nuclei of the cerebellum. A slow corrective movement that occurs at the end of a dysmetric movement is referred to as a glissade. Hypometric saccades may occur because of inattention or lack of cooperation; hypermetric saccades are always pathologic.

Ocular flutter: See **saccadic intrusions.**

Ocular myoclonus: A term most often used synonymously with **oculopalatal myoclonus** to describe the eye movements associated with **palatal myoclonus,** but that has also been used to describe **opsoclonus.**

Ocular neuromyotonia: A rare disorder characterized by episodic diplopia, occurring either spontaneously or following sustained eccentric gaze.[3] The condition is similar to **superior oblique myokymia** but may involve any muscle. As with limb **myokymia** and neuromyotonia, many patients have undergone radiotherapy to the sellar and parasellar region, likely affecting the ocular motor nerves.

Ocular tilt reaction: A triad of head tilt, ocular torsion, and **skew deviation**.[4] Skew deviation is a small, vertical misalignment of the eyes. In the ocular tilt reaction (OTR), the head and the upper poles of both eyes tilt toward the hypotropic eye **(Fig. O.1)**. It occurs primarily with peripheral vestibular disease, but can be seen in lateral medullary infarction and in cerebellar lesions. The ocular tilt reaction can simulate fourth nerve palsy since both cause an unusual head tilt. The pathway responsible for the OTR crosses the midline just above the sixth nerve nucleus and ascends in the contralateral MLF, lesions in the lower pons cause an ipsilateral OTR,

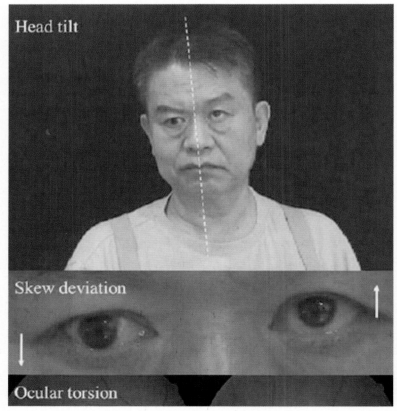

Figure O.1. The ocular tilt reaction refers to the head tilt, ocular torsion, and skew deviation that are ascribed to asymmetry in the otolithic pathway from the utricle. The head tilt and ocular torsion occur toward the hypotropic eye. (From Huh YE, Kim JS. Bedside evaluation of dizzy patients. *J Clin Neurol.* 2013;9:203–213, with permission.)

and more rostral lesions cause a contralateral OTR. Cerebellar lesions may cause either an ipsilateral or contralateral OTR, depending on the structures involved.

Oculocardiac reflex: Bradycardia caused by pressure on the eyeball (Aschner ocular phenomenon).

Oculocephalic response: Turning the head in one direction causes the eyes to turn in the opposite direction (doll's eye response). The oculocephalic response indicates that the pathways connecting the vestibular nuclei in the medulla to the extraocular nuclei in the pons and midbrain are functioning and that the brainstem is intact. It is primarily used in the evaluation of comatose patients. In an alert patient, visuomotor and ocular fixation mechanisms come into play, limiting the drawing of any conclusions about vestibular function. The response is also useful in examining reflex eye movements in patients with supranuclear gaze disorders, such as in PSP.

Oculogyric crisis: Attacks of involuntary conjugate upward deviation of the eyes, which may be transient or last for hours. Classically associated with postencephalitic parkinsonism, these episodes are now seen as a dystonic reaction from phenothiazines and related drugs. Oculogyric crises from neuroleptic drugs may also occur as a tardive syndrome. In absence seizures, there may be brief spasms of upward gaze. See **vestibulo-ocular reflex.**

Oculomasticatory myorhythmia: Rhythmic movements of the eyes and jaw that are pathognomonic of CNS Whipple's disease.[5] Rhythmic jerking of the jaw occurs synchronously with dissociated pendular vergence nystagmus **(Video Link O.2).**[6]

Oculomotor (ocular motor) apraxia (Cogan's syndrome): A congenital inability to make voluntary horizontal saccadic eye movements. Reflex eye movements, including the VOR, are preserved. When attempting to shift gaze horizontally, the patient thrusts the head in the desired direction, using the oculovestibular reflex to acquire the target.

Compensatory blinking or head-thrusting movements develop to shift gaze. Ataxia telangiectasia, Niemann-Pick disease, and Gaucher's disease may cause similar gaze difficulties.

Oculomotor synkinesis: See **aberrant reinnervation of CN III.**

Oculopalatal myoclonus: See **palatal myoclonus.**

Oculopupillary reflex: Constriction of the pupil or dilation followed by constriction in response to painful stimulation of the eye or its adnexa.

Oculosensory reflex: See **oculopupillary reflex.**

Oculosympathetic paresis: See **Horner's syndrome.**

Oculovestibular response: See **vestibulo-ocular reflex.**

OK (pinch, straight thumb) sign: An inability to form the "OK" sign (Fig. O.2). Patients with weakness of the flexor pollicis longus and the flexor digitorum profundus to the index finger are unable to oppose the tips of the thumb and index finger to form a proper circle, but make a triangle instead, touching the finger pads. These muscles are innervated by the anterior interosseous nerve, and the OK sign may be seen in either anterior interosseous or high median neuropathy.

Olecranon reflex: Flexion of the elbow on striking over the olecranon. Wartenberg equated it with the paradoxical triceps jerk (see **inverted reflexes**).[7] Elicitation of the olecranon reflex is actually a technical error that may cause confusion with the paradoxical triceps reflex. In a true paradoxical triceps reflex, the elbow flexes on percussion of the triceps tendon. Elbow flexion can always be produced, even in normals, by percussing too vigorously too far distally over the tip of the olecranon

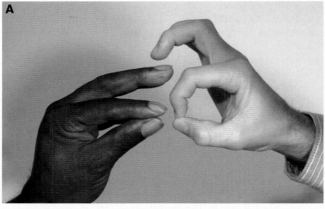

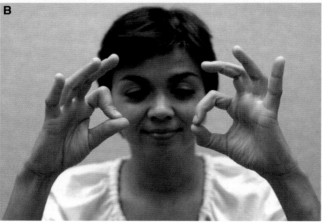

Figure O.2. Anterior interosseous neuropathy; the patient is unable to flex the distal phalanx of the thumb or index finger and is thus unable to make the "OK sign." **A:** Patient on the left, control on the right. **B:** Involved side is the patient's right. (From Campbell WW. *DeJong's the Neurologic Examination.* 7th ed. Philadelphia, PA: Wolters Kluwer Health/Lippincott Williams & Wilkins; 2013, with permission.)

because of the force vectors produced; a biomechanical phenomenon and not a reflex. The trap is that when a paradoxical triceps reflex is present, the finding is so startling when first encountered that the examiner, in trying to reproduce it and convince herself it is real, may stray too far distally and elicit the "olecranon reflex" which then simulates the truly inverted triceps jerk.

Olfaction testing: Examination of the sense of smell. Smell is tested in each nostril separately using nonirritating stimuli, after ensuring that the nasal passages are open. With the patient's eyes closed and one nostril occluded, bring the test substance near the open one. Ask the patient to sniff and indicate whether she smells something and, if so, to identify it. Repeat for the other nostril and compare the two sides. Examine the side that might be abnormal first. Many substances can be used to test smell (e.g., wintergreen, cloves, coffee, cinnamon). At the bedside or in the clinic one can use mouthwash, toothpaste, alcohol, soap, and similar substances. Commercial scratch-and-sniff strips are available. Commercially available quantitative smell and taste tests include the University of Pennsylvania smell identification test (UPSIT) and the Connecticut chemosensory test. The UPSIT requires no trained personnel and may be self-administered. Its forced-choice design helps identify malingering.

The perception of odor is more important than accurate identification. Perceiving the presence of an odor indicates continuity of the olfactory pathways; identification of the odor indicates intact cortical function as well. Since there is bilateral innervation, a lesion central to the decussation of the olfactory pathways never causes loss of smell, and a lesion of the olfactory cortex does not produce **anosmia**. The appreciation of the presence of a smell, even without recognition, excludes anosmia.

Omega sign: See **procerus sign.**

Onionskin (onion peel) sensory loss: See **balaclava helmet sensory loss.**

Ono's hand: See **myelopathy hand.**

Ophthalmoplegia (ophthalmoparesis): Weakness of the eyes. Internal ophthalmoplegia refers to impaired function of the pupil (**iridoplegia**), external ophthalmoplegia to paresis of extraocular muscles. External ophthalmoplegia may be confined to a single muscle, as in a CN VI palsy, or affect all the muscles, as in a mitochondrial myopathy. See **complete ophthalmoplegia.**

Opisthotonos: See **meningeal signs.**

Oppenheim's sign (reflex): (1) Method for eliciting an extensor plantar response; usually done by dragging the knuckles heavily down the anteromedial surface of the tibia from the infrapatellar region to the ankle. An abnormal response is extension of the great toe. The response is slow and often occurs toward the end of stimulation. Oppenheim allegedly did this by raking the handle of his reflex hammer down the shin. Sometimes done in combination with plantar stimulation (see **Babinski's plantar sign**, **pathologic reflexes**). (2) Upper extremity pathological reflex seen with CST disease; rubbing external surface of the forearm causes adduction and flexion of thumb, sometimes with flexion of adjacent digits, more rarely with extension of little finger.

Opsoclonus: See **saccadic intrusions.**

Opsoclonus-myoclonus: See **myoclonus.**

Optic apraxia: See **gaze apraxia.**

Optic (visuomotor) ataxia: Defective hand movements under visual guidance with normal extremity strength and sensation. There is a deficit in the ability to use visual cues to guide extremity movements. Optic ataxia, psychic paralysis of gaze, and **simultagnosia** are characteristic of Balint's syndrome.

Optic atrophy: Loss of substance and demyelination of the optic nerve. In optic atrophy, the disc is paler than normal and more sharply demarcated from the surrounding retina, sometimes having a punched-out appearance (**Fig. O.3**, R.4). The disc margins stand out distinctly; the physiologic cup may be abnormally prominent and extend to the margin of the disc. Loss of myelinated axons and their supporting capillaries with replacement by gliotic scar produce the lack of color, which may vary from a dirty gray to a blue-white color to stark white. Loss of axons causes

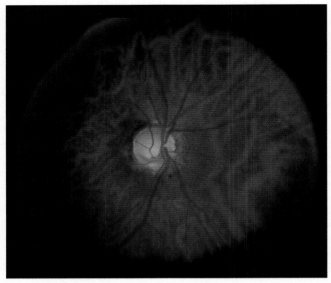

Figure O.3. Primary optic atrophy. (From Campbell WW. *DeJong's the Neurologic Examination.* 7th ed. Philadelphia, PA: Wolters Kluwer Health/Lippincott Williams & Wilkins; 2013, with permission.)

involution of the capillary bed of the disc and allows the sclera to show through, contributing to the pallor. Dark choroidal pigment deposits may be present about the margin of the disc. An atrophic disc may appear perceptibly smaller. **Temporal pallor** may precede definite optic atrophy.

Optic atrophy may follow some other condition, such as optic neuritis or papilledema, and is then referred to as secondary or consecutive optic atrophy. Primary optic atrophy, appearing de novo, occurs as a heredofamilial condition, such as LHON; in some leukodystrophies, lysosomal storage disorders and spinocerebellar degenerations; or after toxic, metabolic, nutritional, compressive, or glaucomatous insult to the nerve. Some causes of optic atrophy are listed in **Table O.1**. In a series of 91 patients with isolated, unexplained optic atrophy, 20% had a compressive lesion on neuroimaging.[8]

Occasionally there is optic atrophy in one eye and papilledema in the other eye: the Foster Kennedy syndrome. The classical cause is an anterior intracranial mass that directly compresses one optic nerve, causing optic atrophy, and then later causes an increase in ICP producing papilledema in the contralateral eye. The atrophic disc cannot swell, resulting in the characteristic ophthalmoscopic findings (Fig. O.4). Intracranial masses now rarely grow to such size undetected, and the finding of optic atrophy in one eye with disc edema contralaterally is more often due to sequential attacks of AION.

Bowtie or **band atrophy** refers to pallor of the disc that may develop in an eye with temporal VF loss following a lesion of the optic chiasm or tract. Cavernous (Schnabel's) optic atrophy is a form of optic atrophy caused by long-standing

Table O.1. Some Causes of Optic Atrophy

Optic neuritis
Glaucoma
Trauma
Chronic papilledema
Ischemic optic neuropathy
Leber's hereditary optic neuropathy
Drugs
Toxins
Optic nerve compression
Deficiency states
Central nervous system syphilis

glaucoma. Pressure-induced and secondary ischemic damage involving the disc result in loss of axons, producing a disc with sharps margins and a characteristically deep optic cup with nasal displacement of the vessels, creating an appearance as if a large divot has been scooped or hollowed out of the nerve head. Pathologically, there is posterior bowing of the lamina cribosa and clear cavernous spaces filled with hyaluronic acid displaced from the vitreous are found in the retrolaminar portion of the nerve.

Optic nerve hypoplasia: A congenitally small, underdeveloped optic nerve. The disc and scleral canal are both small, and there is often a **double ring sign**. The hypoplasia may be unilateral or bilateral and is often associated with other ocular abnormalities, such as astigmatism and **strabismus**. Bilateral optic nerve hypoplasia is a cardinal feature of septo-optic dysplasia (de Morsier's syndrome). It also occurs in fetal alcohol syndrome, fetal anticonvulsant syndrome, and with maternal diabetes.

Optociliary shunt vessels: Abnormal anastomotic channels that sometimes develop in association with compressive optic neuropathy, typically an optic nerve

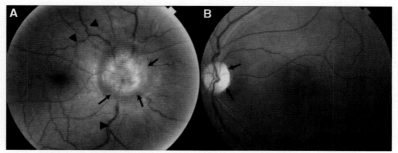

Figure O.4. Foster Kennedy syndrome. Fundoscopy in a 36-year-old man with headaches and loss of vision. **A:** Edema of the optic disk (*arrows*) in the chronic phase ("champagne cork") is visible in the right fundus, with venous tortuosity and dilatation (*arrowheads*). **B:** Left fundoscopy shows a pale optic disk, consistent with axonal death. The lack of color is more marked in the temporal area (*arrows*). (From Pastora-Salvador N, Peralta-Calvo J. Foster Kennedy syndrome: papilledema in one eye with optic atrophy in the other eye. *CMAJ.* 2011;183:2135, with permission. © CMAJ. This work is protected by copyright and the making of this copy was with the permission of Access Copyright. Any alteration of its content or further copying in any form whatsoever is strictly prohibited unless otherwise permitted by law.)

sheath meningioma. Dilated veins joining the central retinal vein and the peripapillary choroid venous system to bypass the obstruction appear at the disc margin (Fig. O.5). The combination of optic atrophy and optociliary shunt vessels has been referred to as the Hoyt-Spencer sign.

Optokinetic nystagmus (OKN, opticokinetic, optomotor): A normal, physiologic type of **nystagmus** sometimes affected by disease.[9] OKN is conjugate nystagmus induced by a succession of moving visual stimuli; it occurs whenever the eyes must follow a series of rapidly passing objects, such as telephone poles zipping by a car or train window. Clinical testing entails moving a striped target, a rotating drum, or a cloth tape bearing stripes or squares in front of the patient and requesting they "count" the stripes or squares. Although OKN is more complex, it can be viewed for clinical purposes as testing pursuit ipsilateral to the direction of target movement, and contralateral saccades. The ipsilateral parieto-temporo-occipital junction mediates pursuit of the acquired stripe via connections that run deep in the parietal lobe. When ready to break off, the PTO junction communicates with the ipsilateral frontal lobe, which then generates a saccadic movement in the opposite direction to acquire the next target. In normal, alert individuals, an OKN stimulus induces brisk nystagmus with the fast phase in the direction opposite tape movement. Responses in one direction are compared with responses in the other direction.

Patients with hemianopias due to occipital lobe disease have a normal OKN response, despite their inability to see into the hemifield from which the tape originates. Because of interruption of the OKN pathways, patients with hemianopias

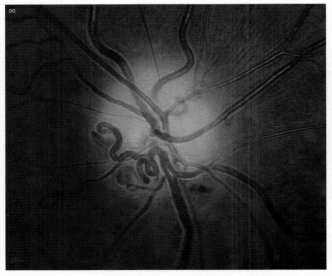

Figure O.5. Pale, elevated optic disc with optociliary shunt vessels in a blind eye; the typical findings of an optic nerve meningioma. (From Savino PJ, Danesh-Meyer HV; Wills Eye Hospital [Philadelphia, PA]. *Neuro-ophthalmology*. 2nd ed. Philadelphia, PA: Wolters Kluwer Health/Lippincott Williams & Wilkins; 2012, with permission.)

due to disease of the optic radiations in the deep parietal lobe have abnormally blunted or absent OKN responses. The patient is unable to pursue normally toward the side of the lesion and is unable to generate contraversive saccades into the blind hemifield. Because tumors are rare in the occipital lobe and much more common in the parietal lobe, a patient with a hemianopia and normal OKN responses is more likely to have an occipital lesion and more likely to have had a stroke. With asymmetric OKNs, the lesion is more likely to be in the parietal lobe and more likely to be nonvascular, i.e., a tumor (Cogan's rule). An asymmetric OKN response has a positive LR of 5.7 for detecting parietal lobe disease.[10]

OKN testing has other uses as well. It may be used to crudely check visual acuity and may provide a clue to the presence of psychogenic visual loss. OKN testing can demonstrate the slowed adducting saccades of a subtle **internuclear ophthalmoplegia** and sometimes accentuate the nystagmus in the abducting eye. OKN-forced upward saccades may induce **convergence retraction nystagmus** in patients with Parinaud's syndrome. OKN abnormalities may be seen early in PSP.

Orbicularis oculi reflex: A reflex contraction of the orbicularis oculi. There are two forms: the nonfocal orbicularis oculi reflex, which causes an eye blink, and a more focal reflex. The nonfocal reflex can be elicited in different ways. Tapping with a finger or percussing with a reflex hammer at many different sites over the forehead and about the eyes may elicit a reflex eye blink. Different names were given to methods of eliciting the reflex by stimulating different areas, all essentially the same response. The most frequently used version currently is the **glabellar tap**.

A more specific orbicularis oculi reflex is the response elicited from one side by a percussion that stretches the muscle (see Video B.4). A fold of the muscle at the temple is pulled taut with the thumb and then percussed to stretch it back toward the ear. Wartenberg thought this reflex useful because it may be decreased in peripheral facial palsy in proportion to the severity of the palsy, but is normal or increased with facial weakness of central origin.

Orbicularis oris reflex: See **snout reflex**.

Organomegaly: Enlargement of an organ, usually meaning liver or spleen or both. In addition to the many general medical conditions causing organomegaly, disorders of particular neurologic interest include alcoholic liver disease, amyloidosis, carnitine deficiency, POEMS, Castleman's disease, Refsum's disease, sarcoidosis, infectious mononucleosis, Wilson's disease, primary biliary cirrhosis, Gaucher's disease, Niemann-Pick disease, hypervitaminosis A, sickle cell disease, Leigh's disease, glycogen storage disorders, and mucopolysaccharidoses.

Orobuccal apraxia: See **buccofacial apraxia**.

Orobuccolingual dyskinesias: See **orofacial dyskinesias**.

Orofacial apraxia: See **buccofacial apraxia**.

Orofacial dyskinesias: Involuntary movements of the mouth, face, jaw, or tongue that may consist of grimacing, pursing of the mouth and lips, "fish-gaping" movements, and writhing movements of the tongue. These often develop as **tardive dyskinesias** after the use of phenothiazines and other psychotropic drugs. Lucey reported orofacial dyskinesias induced by phenytoin (**Video Link O.3**).[11] See **dyskinesias, tardive dyskinesias, rabbit syndrome, bon bon sign**.

Oromandibular dystonia: Abnormal involuntary movements affecting the mouth and jaw. Oromandibular dystonia produces a variety of abnormal movements: jaw opening, jaw closing, lateral movements, bruxism, and combinations of these

(Video Link O.4). Meige's syndrome is oromandibular dystonia and **blepharospasm**. See **dystonia, geste antagoniste**. Video C.3 shows an example of jaw-opening dystonia.

Orthostatic (postural) hypotension: A decrease in BP on standing. In addition to such common causes as volume depletion and medication side effects, there are neurologic conditions in which autonomic dysfunction is a major feature and orthostatic hypotension a common manifestation. Such conditions include MSA, amyloid and other autonomic neuropathies, PD, and porphyria.

At the bedside, BP and pulse are taken with the patient supine and after standing for variable periods, typically the BP is determined at 1, 3, and 5 minutes after standing. Normally, systolic blood pressure (SBP) on standing does not decrease by >20 mmHg, and the diastolic blood pressure (DBP) by not >10 mmHg.[12] There are more stringent diagnostic criteria that permit a 30-point drop in SBP or a 15-point drop in DBP in normals. When routine measurements are unrevealing, orthostatic blood pressure declines can sometimes be detected by having the patient perform 5 to 10 squats and then repeating the measurements. The squat test (1-min standing, 1-min squatting, 1-min standing) provokes large changes in BP and HR.[13] The sustained hand grip, mental stress, and cold pressor tests all look for increases in DBP of at least 15 mmHg or an increase in HR of >10 beats per minute in response to peripheral vasoconstriction induced, respectively, by isometric hand exercise, mental arithmetic, or immersion of the hand in cold water.

The HR should not increase by >30 beats per minute above baseline on standing. In hypovolemia, the most common cause of orthostasis, a reflex tachycardia develops in response to the fall in standing blood pressure. When autonomic cardiovascular reflexes are impaired, the reflex tachycardia may not occur. Patients with the postural orthostatic tachycardia syndrome (POTS) will develop a brisk tachycardia (increased pulse rate more than 30 beats per minute above baseline or more than 120 beats per minute) without orthostatic hypotension.

Orthostatic myoclonus: A condition identified as a cause of gait impairment and unsteadiness in some elderly patients.[14] About half the patients have an associated CNS degenerative disorder, such as MSA, PD, or AD. In most instances, there are complaints of leg jerking, shaking, or trembling, or leg jerking is observed on standing. Symptoms typically lessen with leaning forward onto an object while standing. Gait difficulties often described as **gait apraxia** or **gait ignition failure** is a prominent feature, and NPH or the **orthostatic tremor** syndrome is frequently suspected. Surface EMG studies show nonrhythmic myoclonic bursts with standing, distinct from the findings in orthostatic tremor. In a study of 93 patients, orthostatic myoclonus was slightly more common than orthostatic tremor.[15] Distinguishing between the two conditions may require electrophysiologic studies.

Orthostatic tremor (primary orthostatic tremor, shaky legs syndrome): A type of postural tremor involving the legs that characteristically presents not as tremor but rather as postural unsteadiness and difficulty with standing. The sustained hand grip, mental stress, and cold pressor tests all look for increases in DBP of at least 15 mmHg or an increase in HR of >10 beats per minute in response to peripheral vasoconstriction induced, respectively, by isometric hand exercise, mental arithmetic, or immersion of the hand in cold water.[16] The tremor is high frequency (14–16 Hz) and is maximal when standing, but subsides with walking or sitting. On observation, the legs do not have the appearance of a typical tremor because of the high frequency but just appear tremulous. The tremor may often be appreciated better by palpation of the leg muscles. Orthostatic tremor may be confused with **orthostatic myoclonus**.

Since the legs shake less and the patients are more comfortable when walking, they may prefer to remain in motion. Some patients are not able to tolerate simply standing in one place at all and shuffle around or dart about from spot to spot, pausing only momentarily, a manifestation referred to as the white rabbit sign, after the constantly-on-the-move character in Alice in Wonderland.[17] The tremor can sometimes be brought out by having the patient lie supine and press the feet against a wall.

Oval pupil: See Table P.1
Overflow phenomenon: See **athetosis, dystonia**.
Overpronation: See **pronator drift**.
Oxycephaly: See **craniosynostosis**.

Video Links

O.1. Ocular bobbing and its variants. (From the Robert B. Daroff Collection, Neuro-ophthalmology Virtual Education Library [NOVEL], University of Utah.) Available at: http://stream.utah.edu/m/dp/frame.php?f=adb8a9ee4f938054728

O.2. Oculomasticatory myorhythmia. (From Revilla FJ, de la CR, Khardori N, et al. Teaching neuroimage: oculomasticatory myorhythmia: pathognomonic phenomenology of Whipple disease. *Neurology.* 2008;70:e25.) Available at: http://www.neurology.org/content/suppl/2008/02/03/70.6.e25.DC1/Video.mpg

O.3. Orofacial dyskinesias induced by phenytoin. (From Lucey BP. Teaching video neuroimages: phenytoin-induced orofacial dyskinesias. *Neurology.* 2012; 79:e177.) Available at: http://www.neurology.org/content/suppl/2012/11/01/79.19.e177.DC1/Video_e-1.mpg

O.4. Oromandibular dystonia. Available at: http://www.youtube.com/watch?v=b9roso9B1F0

References

1. Mehler MF. The clinical spectrum of ocular bobbing and ocular dipping. *J Neurol Neurosurg Psychiatry.* 1988;51:725–727.
2. Rosenberg ML. Spontaneous vertical eye movements in coma. *Ann Neurol.* 1986;20:635–637.
3. Frohman EM, Zee DS. Ocular neuromyotonia: clinical features, physiological mechanisms, and response to therapy. *Ann Neurol.* 1995;37:620–626.
4. Huh YE, Kim JS. Bedside evaluation of dizzy patients. *J Clin Neurol.* 2013;9:203–213.
5. Schwartz MA, Selhorst JB, Ochs AL, et al. Oculomasticatory myorhythmia: a unique movement disorder occurring in Whipple's disease. *Ann Neurol.* 1986;20:677–683.
6. Revilla FJ, de la CR, Khardori N, et al. Teaching neuroimage: oculomasticatory myorhythmia: pathognomonic phenomenology of Whipple disease. *Neurology.* 2008;70:e25.
7. Wartenberg R. *The Examination of Reflexes.* Chicago, IL: Year Book Publishers; 1945.
8. Lee AG, Chau FY, Golnik KC, et al. The diagnostic yield of the evaluation for isolated unexplained optic atrophy. *Ophthalmology.* 2005;112:757–759.
9. Buttner U, Kremmyda O. Smooth pursuit eye movements and optokinetic nystagmus. *Dev Ophthalmol.* 2007;40:76–89.
10. McGee S. *Evidence Based Physical Diagnosis.* 3rd ed. Philadelphia, PA: Elsevier/Saunders; 2012.
11. Lucey BP. Teaching video neuroimages: phenytoin-induced orofacial dyskinesias. *Neurology.* 2012;79:e177.
12. Ravits JM. AAEM minimonograph #48: autonomic nervous system testing. *Muscle & Nerve.* 1997;20:919–937.
13. Philips JC, Marchand M, Scheen AJ. Squatting, a posture test for studying cardiovascular autonomic neuropathy in diabetes. *Diabetes Metab.* 2011;37:489–496.
14. Glass GA, Ahlskog JE, Matsumoto JY. Orthostatic myoclonus: a contributor to gait decline in selected elderly. *Neurology.* 2007;68:1826–1830.
15. Gasca-Salas C, Arcocha J, Artieda J, et al. Orthostatic myoclonus: an underrecognized cause of unsteadiness? *Parkinsonism Relat Disord.* 2013;19:1013–1017.
16. Yaltho TC, Ondo WG. Orthostatic tremor: a review of 45 cases. *Parkinsonism Relat Disord.* 2014;20:723–725.
17. Beh SC, Frohman T, Frohman EM. The menagerie of neurology: animal signs and the refinement of clinical acumen. *Neurol Clin Pract.* 2014;4:e1–e9.

Pace test: A maneuver used in the diagnosis of piriformis syndrome; see **piriformis syndrome provocative tests.**

Pachycephaly: See **craniosynostosis.**

Painful arc: See **shoulder examination tests.**

Painful legs and moving toes: Continuous, involuntary movements of the toes associated with pain in the legs. The condition is sometimes a manifestation of peripheral neuropathy, but the responsible cause in many is not clear. Pain occurs first in most cases and is more distressing to patients than the movements.[1] Variants are painful arms and moving fingers, and painless legs and moving toes.

Palatal deviation: See **gag reflex, curtain sign.**

Palatal myoclonus: Involuntary, rhythmic movements of the soft palate and pharynx, sometimes of the larynx, eye muscles, and diaphragm, and occasionally of other muscles.[2] The movements are generally not influenced by drugs or sleep. The palate may bounce up and down, or twitch rhythmically to one side **(Video P.1).** The posterior pharyngeal wall moves laterally, and the larynx moves up and down. Movements involving the diaphragm or larynx may cause a grunting respiratory noise. Opening and closing of the Eustachian tube sometimes causes a clicking sound accompanying the movements, audible to the patient and sometimes to the examiner.

Palatal myoclonus occurs in essential and symptomatic forms. Symptomatic palatal myoclonus occurs with lesions involving the connections between the inferior olivary, dentate, and red nuclei. The Guillain-Mollaret (myoclonic) triangle is a loop: inferior olive → inferior cerebellar peduncle → dentate nucleus → superior cerebellar peduncle → red nucleus → central tegmental tract → inferior olive. A lesion anywhere in this loop, most often brainstem infarction, may cause palatal myoclonus and its variants. Lesions of the central tegmental tract may cause hypertrophy (pseudohypertrophy) of the olive. There is gliosis of the amiculum of the olive, increasing the size of the olive grossly, which may be visualized by MRI.

Palatal myoclonus is also referred to as palatal microtremor. Tremors are due to alternating agonist–antagonist contractions, rhythmic myoclonus to contraction–relaxation cycles of an agonist. In addition, tremors usually disappear in sleep and these palatal movements do not. Whether palatal myoclonus is best characterized as rhythmic myoclonus or a tremor remains unclear.

Patients with ocular involvement are said to have oculopalatal myoclonus. The eye movements have one of two patterns. There is a vertical-torsional form with a greater vertical component in one eye. This "lateral" form is associated with unilateral palatal myoclonus on the same side as the eye with larger vertical nystagmus. In the second "midline" form, there are symmetric, vertical, pendular oscillations with bilateral palatal myoclonus. Patients often have associated signs of brainstem damage.

Paligraphia: Repetitive writing of a word or phrase.

Palilalia: A patient's pathologic repetition of his own spontaneous syllables, words, or phrases.

Palinopsia: Repetitive occurrence of a visual image after the original exciting image has disappeared; most often seen with structural lesions involving the parieto-occipital cortex.[3] Palinopsia is a form of visual perseveration in which the illusory images occur in time. Less common is cerebral polyopia, in which the illusory image occurs in space.[4] Cerebral polyopia may mimic diplopia due to ocular malalignment, but the false image does not disappear with covering one eye.

Pallanesthesia: Loss of vibratory perception.

Palmar reflex: A reflex produced by gentle stroking across the palm of hand, which causes flexion of the fingers or a closing of the hand. The response is minimal or absent in normal individuals beyond the first few months of life. When exaggerated, this response is referred to as a **grasp reflex.**

Palmaris brevis sign: Wrinkling of the skin over the hypothenar eminence with small finger abduction in the face of weakness of the ulnar hand intrinsics; proves the lesion involves the deep palmar branch of the ulnar nerve.[5]

Palmomental (Marinesco-Radovici) reflex: Contraction of the mentalis and orbicularis oris muscles causing wrinkling of the skin of the chin with slight retraction and sometimes elevation of the angle of the mouth in response to scratching or stroking the palm of the ipsilateral hand. The palmomental reflex (PMR), or palm-chin reflex, is best elicited by stroking a blunt point over the thenar eminence, either from wrist toward thumb or vice versa, or by tapping this area. The PMR is classified as a **frontal release sign** or a **primitive reflex.** The PMR is so frequently present in normal persons that significance can only be attached to a marked exaggeration of the response or a conspicuous asymmetry between the two sides. The PMR is weak and fatigable in normals, stronger and more persistent in disease. If the response is marked, the reflexogenic zone may be wide, including the hypothenar area. A trigger area outside the palm probably does not occur in healthy people. In neurological patients, the reflex can sometimes be elicited by stimulation of the forearm, chest, abdomen, or even the sole; changing the name to "mentalis reflex" has been suggested. Spread of the reflex response beyond the chin region may also occur; involvement of the platysma has been termed the palmocervical reflex. The PMR can help in the differential diagnosis of facial palsy—it is absent in peripheral facial palsy and may be exaggerated in central facial paresis. The pollicomental (thumb–chin) reflex is the same response produced by stroking the palmar surface of the thumb.

The localizing value and clinical significance of these reflexes is limited. A unilateral PMR may occur with bilateral, contralateral, or ipsilateral lesions. The pathways involved in the PMR remain uncertain, but it is clear that a unilateral PMR does not have localizing value. The PMR has been reviewed in detail by Owen and Mulley.[6] See pathologic reflexes.

Palpebral reflex: Blinking in response to any of a number of stimuli; usually named by the inciting stimulus. The auditory-palpebral reflex is blinking in response to noise, the visuo-palpebral in response to bright light, the trigemino-palpebral in response to facial sensory stimuli. See **orbicularis oculi reflex**.

Paper test: See **Marie's paper test.**

Papilledema: Swelling of the optic disc due to increased ICP (Fig. P.1). By convention, disc swelling due to increased ICP is referred to as papilledema; under all other circumstances, the noncommittal terms *disc edema* or *disc swelling* are preferred.[7] The ophthalmoscopic appearance of disc edema is similar whatever the etiology,

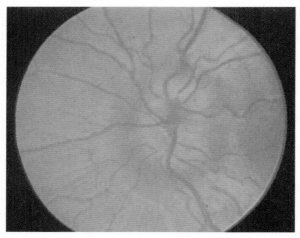

Figure P.1. Severe papilledema. (From Campbell WW. *DeJong's the Neurologic Examination.* 7th ed. Philadelphia, PA: Wolters Kluwer Health/Lippincott, Williams & Wilkins; 2013, with permission.)

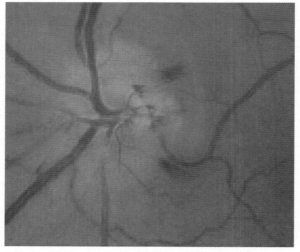

Figure P.2. Swollen, elevated optic disc with blurred margins and peripapillary flame hemorrhages due to ischemic optic neuropathy. (From Nagel MA, Russman AN, Feit H, et al. VZV ischemic optic neuropathy and subclinical temporal artery infection without rash. *Neurology.* 2013;80:220–222, with permission.)

and it is not possible to distinguish papilledema from other causes of disc edema by inspection. Figure P.2 shows a swollen disc due to AION. Visual function provides a critical clue to the nature of disc abnormalities. Patients with acute papilledema and those with disc anomalies (pseudopapilledema) have normal visual acuity, visual fields, and color perception. Impairment of these functions is the rule in patients suffering from optic neuropathies of any other etiology. A critical step in evaluating a questionably abnormal disc is therefore a careful assessment of vision. **Pseudopapilledema** refers to conditions causing an abnormal disc appearance that may be confused with papilledema.

In papilledema, pressure on the optic nerves because of increased ICP impairs axoplasmic flow and produces axonal edema and an increased volume of axoplasm at the disc. The swollen axons impair venous return from the retina, engorging first the capillaries on the disc surface, then the retinal veins, and ultimately causing splinter- and flame-shaped hemorrhages as well as cotton wool exudates in the retinal nerve fiber layer. Further axonal swelling eventually leads to elevation of the disc above the retinal surface.

The four stages of papilledema are early, fully developed, chronic, and atrophic. Fully developed papilledema is obvious, with elevation and expansion of the disc surface, humping of vessels crossing the disc margin, obliteration of disc margins, peripapillary hemorrhages, cotton wool exudates, engorged and tortuous retinal veins, opacification of the nerve fiber layer, and marked disc hyperemia (see Fig. P.1). The recognition of early papilledema is much more problematic (Fig. P.3). Occasionally, the only way to resolve the question of early papilledema is by serial observation. The earliest change is loss of previously observed spontaneous venous pulsations (SVPs). Venous pulsations are best seen where the large veins dive into the disc centrally. The movement is a back-and-forth rhythmic oscillation of the tip of the blood column, which resembles a slowly darting snake's tongue. Side-to-side expansion of a vein is much more difficult to see. The presence of SVPs indicates

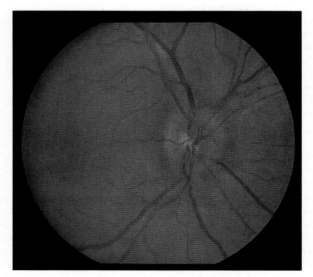

Figure P.3. Early papilledema. (From Campbell WW. *DeJong's the Neurologic Examination.* 7th ed. Philadelphia, PA: Wolters Kluwer Health/Lippincott, Williams & Wilkins; 2013, with permission.)

an intracranial pressure less than approximately 200 mm H_2O. However, since they are absent in 10% to 20% of normals, only the disappearance of previously observed SVPs is clearly pathologic.[8]

As papilledema develops, increased venous back pressure dilates the capillaries on the disc surface, transforming its normal yellowish-pink color to fiery red. Blurring of the superior and inferior margins evolves soon after. However, since these margins are normally the least distinct areas of the disc, blurry margins alone are not enough to diagnose papilledema. There is no alteration of the physiologic cup with early papilledema. With further evolution, the patient with early papilledema will develop diffuse disc edema, cup obscuration, hemorrhages, exudates, and venous engorgement. Frank disc elevation then ensues as the fundus ripens into fully developed papilledema. In chronic papilledema, hemorrhages and exudates resolve and leave a markedly swollen "champagne cork" disc bulging up from the plane of the retina. The disc mushrooms up from the plane of the retina, loses its cup, and often becomes surrounded by exudates. If unrelieved, impaired axoplasmic flow eventually leads to death of axons and visual impairment, which evolves into the stage of atrophic papilledema, or secondary **optic atrophy**. Papilledema ordinarily develops over days to weeks. With acutely increased ICP due to subarachnoid or intracranial hemorrhage, it may develop within hours. Measuring diopters of disc elevation ophthalmoscopically has little utility.

Acute papilledema causes no impairment of visual acuity or color vision. The typical patient has no symptoms related to its presence except for transient visual obscurations. The blind spot may be enlarged, but VF testing is otherwise normal. In patients who develop optic atrophy following papilledema, the visual morbidity can be severe and may include blindness.

With current technology, imaging would usually detect intracranial mass lesions before the development of increased intracranial pressure. As a result, idiopathic intracranial hypertension is the most common cause of papilledema in the developed world. The typical patient is an obese young female with headaches, with no focal findings on neurologic examination, normal imaging except for small ventricles, and normal CSF except for elevated opening pressure. Without adequate treatment, visual loss is a common sequel.

Changes ophthalmoscopically indistinguishable from papilledema occur when conditions primarily affecting the optic nerve papilla cause disc edema. Papilledema is usually bilateral; other causes of disc edema, such as optic neuritis, AION, optic nerve compression or infiltration, central retinal vein occlusion, pappillophebitis, and LHON, are often unilateral. Optic neuropathies generally cause marked visual impairment, including loss of acuity, central or cecocentral scotoma, loss of color perception, and an RAPD. Disease of the optic nerve head is usually due to demyelination, ischemia, inflammation, or compression. Optic neuritis with disc edema is sometimes called papillitis. Papillitis may occur as an isolated abnormality, as a manifestation of MS or as a complication of some systemic illness. Demyelinating optic neuropathies causing papillopathy are common as a feature of MS, but they also can occur as an independent disease process or complicate other disorders such as acute disseminated encephalomyelitis and neuromyelitis optica.

Paracentral scotoma: See **scotoma**.

Paradoxical ankle reflex: See **inverted reflexes, ankle reflex**.

Paradoxical myotonia: **Myotonia** that increases with repetitive movement, rather than decreasing as usual. It occurs primarily in paramyotonia congenita **(Video Link P.1)**. The worsening with exercise may be particularly prominent in the eyelids. See **myotonia**.

Paradoxical pupils: Pupils that constrict in darkness, which may occur in congenital retinal and optic nerve disorders; the mechanism is unknown **(Table P.1)**. Paradoxical pupillary dilation in the eye with an oculosympathetic paresis may occur in some circumstances.

Paradoxical reflexes: See **inverted reflexes.**

Paradoxical triceps reflex: See **inverted reflexes, olecranon reflex.**

Paragrammatism: See **agrammatism.**

Paragraphia: A written **paraphasia,** a common feature in aphasic disorders.

Parakinesia: See **chorea.**

Paralexia: A reading error due to either a paraphasic speech error or a mistake in comprehension, seen in aphasia (see **paraphasia**). Paralexia may also occur in patients with **attentional deficits** when part of a word is not detected.

Paraparesis (paraplegia): Weakness (paralysis) of both legs. Commonly used modifiers include spastic, when there is hyper-reflexia, increased tone, and pathologic reflexes, or flaccid, when there is no change in tone or reflexes; complete or incomplete; and descriptions of severity and acuity. Patients might then have a severe, acute, flaccid paraparesis or a mild, subacute, spastic paraparesis. **Weakness** affecting muscles in the CST distribution (hip flexors, knee flexors, and foot dorsiflexors) more severely than other muscles may provide an early clue that leg weakness is due to myelopathy. Reflex changes and pathologic reflexes are frequently not obvious in an early or mild myelopathy.

    The most common cause is transverse myelopathy from any of a number of conditions causing demyelination, compression, or ischemia.[9] Other conditions that

Table P.1. Some of the Unusual Pupillary Shapes, Reactions, and Behaviors That Occasionally Occur

Pupil	Characteristic
Paradoxical pupils	Constrict in darkness; seen in congenital retinal and optic nerve disorders
Springing pupil	Intermittent, sometimes alternating, dilation of one pupil, lasting minutes to hours seen in young, healthy women, often followed by headache
Tadpole pupil	A benign condition in which a pupil intermittently and briefly becomes comma-shaped because of spasm involving one sector of the pupillodilator
Periodic unilateral mydriasis	May occur in migraine and as an ictal phenomenon
Scalloped pupils	Suggestive of familial amyloidosis
Oval pupils	Usually portend major intracranial pathology; may be a transient phase in evolving injury to the third nerve nuclear complex
Corectopia iridis (ectopia pupillae, Wilson's sign)	Spontaneous, cyclic displacement of the pupil from the center of the iris; it is usually seen in severe midbrain disease

may cause paraparesis include hereditary disorders, such as HSP; metabolic disorders, such as adrenomyeloneuropathy; infection, such as HTLV-1 (tropical spastic paraparesis) or syphilis (Erb's spastic [syphilitic] paraplegia); degenerative disorders, such as primary lateral sclerosis; and the effects of toxins, such as lathyrism and konzo. Rarely, bilateral hemispheric lesions may cause weakness in both legs simulating spinal cord disease. This pattern may occur with a parasagittal mass, classically meningioma, impinging on the medial aspect of the motor cortices bilaterally or from border zone infarction with deep subcortical white matter involvement. Polyneuropathy or polyradiculopathy may sometimes cause weakness of only the legs, as in the paraparetic variant of GBS.[10] In a recent series of 490 GBS patients, 8% had the paraparetic form.[11]

Occasionally, dystonia primarily affecting the legs mimics spastic paraparesis (dystonic paraparesis). This occurs particularly in dopa-responsive dystonia (Segawa's syndrome), causing confusion with such conditions as diplegic cerebral palsy and HSP.[12]

Paraphasia: A speech error in which an aphasic patient substitutes a wrong word or sound for the intended word or sound. In a phonemic (phonologic, literal) paraphasia, there is the addition, deletion, or substitution of a phoneme; however, the word is recognizable and may be clearly pronounced. Substitution of the wrong phoneme would cause the patient to say "blotch" instead of watch, or "thumbness" instead of numbness. Technically, a literal paraphasia is a single-letter substitution. *Phonemic paraphasia* is the preferable term since a single-letter substitution also changes the phoneme, and the brain thinks in phonemes, not letters. In a semantic (verbal) paraphasia, the patient substitutes the wrong word. A semantic paraphasia would cause the patient to say "ring" instead of watch. With phonemic paraphasias, instead of "Hand me the fork," the patient might say, "Land me the pork"; with semantic paraphasias it would be "Foot me the spoon." Paraphasias are similar to the malapropisms, spoonerisms, and sniglets everyone occasionally utters, but aphasic patients make them more often and may not recognize them as wrong. A **neologism** is a novel utterance, a nonword made up on the spot. The patient might call a watch a woshap. Phonemic paraphasias are more typical of anterior and semantic paraphasias more typical of posterior, perisylvian lesions.

Paraplegia in flexion: The posture that results when the primitive **flexion reflex** becomes tonic and permanent, most often in patients with severe myelopathy, usually traumatic. The exaggeration of the **flexion reflex** causes involuntary **flexor spasms** that hold the legs intensely flexed with increasing frequency and for longer and longer periods until they can no longer be actively or even passively extended, terminating eventually in a tonic flexion posture with permanent fixed flexion of the hips and knees and dorsiflexion of the ankles and toes. In the severest cases, the legs and thighs are completely flexed and the knees pressed against the abdomen. The heels may be tucked into the perineum. Lesions at higher levels, such as the cervical spine, are more likely to cause paraplegia in flexion than those at more caudal levels. Paraplegia in extension is more common and more likely to result from incomplete myelopathy. Paraplegia in flexion has become less prevalent with improved care of patients with spinal cord injuries.

Paratonia: An alteration in tone to passive motion that is often a manifestation of diffuse frontal lobe disease. It has been divided into inhibitory paratonia (**gegenhalten,** paratonic rigidity) and facilitory paratonia (mitgehen).[13] Experts defined paratonia as a form of hypertonia with an involuntary variation in tone during passive movement, varying from active assistance to active resistance; the degree of resistance depends on the speed of movement (e.g., slow → low resistance, fast → high resistance) and is proportional to the amount of force applied.[14]

In the limb placement test, the examiner passively lifts the patient's arm, instructs the patient to relax, releases the arm, and notes whether or not it remains elevated. The arm remaining aloft, in the absence of parkinsonism or spasticity, indicates paratonia. In facilitory paratonia, the patient cooperates too much. The patient actively assists the examiner's passive movements, and the limb may continue to move even after the examiner has released it. In demented patients, the severity of paratonia, either inhibitory or facilitory, correlates inversely with the MMSE score.[13]

Paratonic rigidity: See **paratonia, gegenhalten.**

Paresis: See **weakness.**

Parietal drift: A tendency of the arm contralateral to a parietal lobe lesion to drift. In contrast to the much more common **pronator drift**, the involved arm usually rises overhead and moves outward **(Fig. P.4)**. Patients typically have impaired position sense and other parietal findings and the updrift is thought to occur because of deafferentation, referred to as sensory wandering. Associated findings may include **pseudoathetosis** and inco-ordination that may mimic cerebellar ataxia (sensory ataxia, parietal ataxia, pseudocerebellar syndrome).

Parkinsonian tremor (PT): The rest **tremor** that occurs in PD and the various parkinsonian syndromes **(Video P.2)**. Typically, the tremor is slow and coarse, varying in rate from 2 to 6 Hz and averaging 4 to 5 Hz. The movement in the

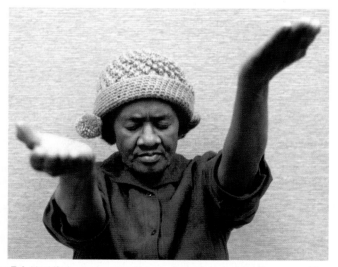

Figure P.4. Updrift due to a parietal lobe lesion with loss of position sense. The patient harbored a mass lesion of the right parietal lobe, a large dermoid that had eroded through the calvarium, hidden beneath the hat. (From Campbell WW. *DeJong's the Neurologic Examination.* 7th ed. Philadelphia, PA: Wolters Kluwer Health/Lippincott, Williams & Wilkins; 2013, with permission.)

hand characteristically involves the flexors, extensors, abductors, and adductors of the fingers and thumb, together with motion of the wrist and arm, including flexion, extension, pronation, and supination. As a result, there is a repetitive movement of the thumb on the first two fingers, together with the motion of the wrist, producing the classical pill-rolling. The tremor is relatively rhythmic, present at rest, and temporarily suppressed by movement. PT may involve the hands, feet, jaw, tongue, lips, and pharynx, but usually not the head. The tremor may be unilateral at onset; it may even begin in a single digit, but in most cases eventually becomes bilateral. The tremor fluctuates, increasing in amplitude but not rate when the patient becomes excited. The tremor is often more apparent when the patient is walking. It disappears during sleep and is aggravated by emotional stimulation, fatigue, and anxiety.

Although the diagnosis of PT is straightforward in most cases, especially when there is pronounced asymmetry or there are accompanying signs of PD or a parkinsonian syndrome, such as **cogwheel rigidity, bradykinesia, masked facies, postural instability, hypophonia,** or a reduced arm swing on one side when walking. If bradykinesia, rigidity, and tremor are all present with asymmetry and no atypical features, there is a positive LR of 4.1 and a negative LR of 0.4 for the diagnosis of PD.[15] In some cases it remains difficult to distinguish PT from **essential tremor,** and in some patients the two diseases may coexist. Tremor features helpful in distinguishing between the two are discussed in the ET section. Also helpful are age of onset, response to alcohol, and family history. Onset in adolescence and young adulthood, or in the senium, favors ET. Large, sloppy handwriting suggests ET; a cramped, small script (**micrographia**) favors PD.

Parkinsonism: The constellation of clinical features seen in PD and related disorders. Parkinsonism is a clinical diagnosis appropriate in the presence of rest **tremor, bradykinesia**, **rigidity**, and impaired **postural reflexes**. PD is but one cause of parkinsonism, and it must be differentiated from other conditions that may have some of its typical features as a component of another disorder.[16] Other disease processes may produce a similar clinical picture, characterized by decreased movement and rigidity; these have been grouped together as the akinetic-rigid syndromes. About 80% of the instances of akinetic-rigid syndrome are due to PD **(Table P.2)**. The terms *parkinson syndrome* or *parkinson plus* are sometimes used to designate such other disorders, and the features that resemble PD are referred to as parkinsonism or parkinsonian. One of the most common causes of parkinsonism is treatment with dopamine-blocking agents (see Table A.2).

Features common in parkinsonism include **masked facies**, resting **tremor, bradykinesia**, cogwheel **rigidity, postural instability, micrographia, hypophonia**, and an abnormal gait and posture (see **gait disorders**). See **parkinsonian tremor**.

Atypical parkinsonism refers to a clinical picture that deviates from that expected for idiopathic PD and often signifies the presence of one of the other parkinsonian syndrome.[17] Such atypical features might include symmetry of findings, as idiopathic PD is typically asymmetric, an extension instead of a flexion posture and a lack of response to levodopa. The presence of other neurological signs, such as eye movement abnormalities, cerebellar signs, early dementia, spasticity, or dysautonomia suggest an alternate diagnosis.

When bradykinesia, rigidity, and tremor are all present with asymmetry and no atypical features, there is a positive LR of 4.1 and a negative LR of 0.4 for the

Table P.2. The Differential Diagnosis of Parkinson's Disease

PD
Parkinsonian syndromes
Progressive supranuclear palsy
Multisystem atrophy (MSA)
MSA-parkinsonian (striatonigral degeneration)
MSA-cerebellar (olivopontocerebellar degeneration, sporadic form)
MSA-autonomic (Shy-Drager syndrome)
Diffuse Lewy body disease
Corticobasal degeneration
Drug-induced parkinsonism
Dopa-responsive dystonia
Other non-Parkinson's akinetic-rigid syndromes
Huntington's disease (rigid or juvenile form)
Wilson's disease
Essential tremor
Depression
Arthritis, polymyalgia, fibromyalgia

From Campbell WW. *DeJong's the Neurologic Examination*. 7th ed. Philadelphia, PA: Wolters Kluwer Health/Lippincott Williams & Wilkins; 2013.

diagnosis of PD.[15] Features suggestive of atypical parkinsonism are an inability to perform 10 tandem steps (negative LR of 5.0 for PD), rapid progression (positive LR 2.5 for MSA), bulbar signs (positive LR of 4.1 for MSA), autonomic dysfunction (positive LR of 4.3 for MSA), cerebellar signs (positive LR of 9.5 for MSA), and pyramidal signs (positive LR of 4.0 for MSA).[15] Features suggestive of arteriosclerotic (vascular) parkinsonism include the presence of pyramidal signs (LR 21.3), findings confined to the legs (LR 6.1), and abrupt onset (LR 21.9).[15]

Parry-Romberg syndrome: See **facial hemiatrophy.**

Past pointing: A deviation of the extremities caused by either cerebellar or vestibular disease **(Video P.3).** These two types of past pointing have different patterns. Testing is usually done with the upper extremities. A quick and effective technique is simply to have the patient close the eyes while doing traditional cerebellar finger-to-nose testing. If past pointing is present, the limb will deviate to the side of the target because of the absence of visual correction. This method will usually bring out past pointing if it is present. The traditional method is to have the patient extend the arm and place his extended index finger on the examiner's index finger; then with eyes closed raise the arm directly overhead; then bring it back down precisely onto the examiner's finger.

With acute vestibular imbalance, the more active (usually the normal) labyrinth will push the limb toward the less active (abnormal) side, and the patient will miss the target. The past pointing will always be to the same side of the target and will occur with either limb. With a cerebellar hemispheric lesion, the ipsilateral limbs have ataxia and incoordination; past pointing occurs only with the involved arm and may be to the side of the lesion or erratically to either side of the target. In vestibulopathy, after a period of compensation the past pointing disappears and may even begin to occur in the opposite direction.

The Quix test is similar. The patient stands with the arms outstretched. Drift of the extremities laterally or body sway consistently to one side suggests the presence of vestibular imbalance.

Patellar reflex: See **knee reflex.**

Pathologic reflexes: Responses not generally found in the normal individual. Some are responses that are minimally present and elicited with difficulty in normals but become prominent and active in disease; others are not seen in normals at all. Some are responses normally seen in infancy that disappear only to reemerge later in the presence of disease. A decrease in threshold or an extension of the reflexogenic zone plays a role in many pathologic reflexes.

Some pathologic reflexes may also be classified as **associated movements**, related to uninhibited spread of motor activity. Some responses that are more in the realm of an associated movement are sometimes referred to clinically as reflexes, such as the Wartenberg thumb adduction sign, an associated movement sometimes called a Wartenberg reflex (see **Wartenberg signs**).

Most pathologic reflexes are related to disease involving the CST and associated pathways. **Frontal release signs**, or **primitive reflexes**, such as the **palmomental, grasp, snout**, and **sucking** reflexes, are responses present in infants and children that disappear with maturation but reappear because of normal aging or neurological disease, particularly frontal lobe disorders. Pathologic reflexes in the lower extremities are more constant, more easily elicited, more reliable, and more clinically relevant than those in the upper limbs. Searching for upper-extremity pathologic reflexes is much less productive and often omitted. The most important pathologic reflex by far is **Babinski's plantar sign**. Other useful lower extremity pathologic reflexes include the **Chaddock** and **Oppenheim**. Many alternate methods have been described to elicit an extensor plantar response (Table M.3).

Some CST responses are characterized by plantar flexion instead of extension. The best known of this group of reflexes is **Rossolimo's sign**. Many similar responses have been described, all variations on the same reflex elicited by striking slightly different parts of the foot. See also **Marie-Foix sign, dorsal foot response, and crossed extensor reflex.**

The upper-extremity pathologic reflexes primarily fall into two categories: **frontal release signs** and exaggerations of or variations on the **finger flexor reflex**. The **Hoffmann** and **Trömner** signs are alternative methods of delivering the stretch stimulus. Certain other reflexes may appear in the upper extremities in the presence of CST pathology. These include the **Klippel-Feil sign, Leri's sign, Mayer's sign**, the **bending reflex**, and the **nociceptive reflex of Riddoch and Buzzard**. These are all of marginal clinical significance.

Patrick's test: See **FABER test.**

Peau d'orange: A rough, textured appearance and feel of the skin likened to an orange peel. It is seen most often in breast cancer, but is also a classic manifestation of eosinophilia-myalgia syndrome and eosinophilic fasciitis.

Pectoralis reflex: One of the occasionally useful DTRs (see Table D.1). Tapping a finger placed on the tendon of the pectoralis major muscle near its insertion on the greater tuberosity of the humerus causes adduction and slight internal rotation of the arm at the shoulder (see Video B.4). The response is feeble normally. In patients with cervical spondylotic myelopathy, a hyperactive pectoralis reflex indicates spinal cord compression at the C2–C3 and/or C3–C4 levels.[18]

Peek (peek-a-boo) sign: One of the eye signs of MG. Because of orbicularis fatigue, the patient is unable to keep the eyes closed tightly.[19] On attempting to maintain lid closure, the lid margins separate, exposing the sclera. The patient thus appears to "peek" at the examiner. The peek sign is very suggestive of MG; it does not occur in control patients or in those with facial weakness due to other disorders.

Peek-a-boo sign: (1) the **peek sign** seen in MG; (2) visibility of the medial aspect of the heel when viewed from the front, indicative of a cavus deformity of the foot (peek-a-boo heel sign).

Pendular nystagmus: See **nystagmus.**

Pendulum test (Wartenberg's pendulum test): A maneuver to compare the tone in the lower extremities.[20,21] The patient sits on the edge of a table, relaxed with legs hanging freely. The examiner either extends both legs to the same horizontal level and then releases them, or gives both legs a brisk, equal backward push. If the patient is completely relaxed and cooperative, there will normally be a swinging of the legs that progressively diminishes in range and usually disappears after six or seven oscillations. The oscillations are smooth and in a straight line. In extrapyramidal rigidity, there is a decrease in swing time and velocity, but usually no qualitative change in the response. In spasticity, there may be little or no decrease in swing time, but the movements are jerky and irregular, the forward movement may be greater and more brisk than the backward, and the movement may assume a zigzag pattern. In hypotonia, the response is increased in range and prolonged beyond the normal. In all of these maneuvers, a unilateral abnormality will be more apparent. A modification was developed to evaluate spasticity at the elbow.[22]

Penguin gait: See **gait disorders.**

Percussion myotonia: See **myotonia.**

Periodic alternating gaze deviation: Unusual spontaneous eye movements seen in patients in coma. The movements are similar to those seen in **ping-pong gaze** but much less frequent, with the gaze deviations changing direction every 2 to 15 minutes, rather than every few seconds. This pattern has been reported primarily in patients with hepatic encephalopathy but occurs with structural lesions as well.[23] See **ocular bobbing.**

Peripheral facial paralysis: See **facial weakness.**

Peripheral nystagmus: See **central nystagmus.**

Peripheral vascular disease signs: Tests for the presence of peripheral vascular disease. These are of interest to the neurologist as markers of vascular pathology in patients with stroke and in the evaluation of exertional leg pain to help separate vascular from neurogenic claudication.

Markers of occlusive peripheral vascular disease include decreased pulses, bruits, changes in the hair and nails, muscle atrophy, splinter hemorrhages, dependent rubor, impaired capillary refill, and distal cyanosis. An involved extremity tends to appear cool and pale. More advanced disease may cause ulcers or gangrene. Arterial ulcers are located distally, involving the feet and toes, and appear as small, dry, often encrusted, punched-out lesions exquisitely tender to touch. Venous ulcers tend to occur at the medial ankle and are moist or weeping. Diabetic foot ulcers tend to involve the forefoot, especially the toes or plantar surface of the metatarsal heads; there is also usually evidence of peripheral neuropathy. Peripheral arterial emboli may cause the "blue toe syndrome." Presence of involved toes on both feet suggests an embolic source proximal to the aortic bifurcation, as might occur with atrial fibrillation or endocarditis.

Either the dorsalis pedis or posterior tibial pulse is sometimes absent in otherwise healthy people, but in only 0% to 2% are both absent. In a symptomatic leg, the signs shown to increase the probability of peripheral vascular disease are absence of both pedal pulses (LR 14.9), a limb bruit (LR 7.3), wounds or sores on the foot (LR 7.0), absence of the femoral pulse (LR 6.1), and asymmetrical coolness of the foot (LR 6.1).[15] Evidence of ischemia with intact pedal pulses suggests small vessel disease, usually due to diabetes.

Buerger's test is performed by raising the recumbent patient's legs as high as possible. With arterial insufficiency, one or both feet become pallid. The patient then sits with the legs over the side of the table. There is a delay in the return of color and venous refill, after which the feet become suffused with a deep, reddish purple color ("sunset foot") that starts with the toes and spreads proximally. In the De-Weese test, the patient runs in place, does toe raises, or flexes and extends the ankle against resistance until leg pain begins. Disappearance of the pedal pulses with the onset of leg pain suggests a vascular origin; pain without a decrease in peripheral pulses suggests neurogenic claudication. The ankle-brachial index is calculated by determining the highest systolic pressure in the posterior tibial or dorsalis pedis artery and dividing by the brachial pressure. Normal values are 1.0 to 1.4; 0.91 to 0.99 is considered borderline, and values of <0.9 are abnormal and suggest peripheral arterial disease. A unilaterally decreased carotid pulse may signify high-grade stenosis or occlusion. A decrease in both the carotid and superficial temporal pulse occurs with occlusion of the common carotid. With internal carotid occlusion, collateral flow through the external carotid may cause an increase in the superficial temporal and other facial pulses.[24] Other causes of inequality between the carotid pulses include aortic aneurysm and coarctation of the aorta. A decrease in both carotid pulses may be seen with Takayasu's arteritis.

Disease involving the aortic arch or subclavian artery, particularly on the left, may produce a decreased radial pulse and lower BP on the involved side. Simultaneous palpation of the radial pulses and taking the BP in both arms are traditional bedside methods used in evaluation of patients with suspected cerebrovascular disease, especially when symptoms suggest subclavian steal syndrome. A systolic BP difference of >20 mm Hg is considered significant. In subclavian steal, 94% of patients have a decrease in BP of 20 mm Hg or more in the affected arm.[15] Most patients also have a decreased, absent, or delayed radial pulse (**radial–radial delay**).

The pulsations of the superficial temporal arteries are palpable just anterior to the tragus. In giant cell arteritis, the superficial temporal pulse may disappear; this finding is reportedly pathognomonic of giant cell arteritis in the appropriate clinical setting. The involved artery may also become nodular, tender, and visually more prominent (Fig. P.5). The presence of necrotic lesions of the scalp or tongue and evidence of AION support the diagnosis. In a meta-analysis of 21 studies, physical findings predictive of the diagnosis are temporal artery beading (positive LR 4.6) prominence (positive LR 4.3), and tenderness (positive LR 2.6). The absence of any temporal artery abnormality was the only clinical factor that modestly reduced the likelihood of disease (negative LR 0.53).[25]

Periungual fibroma (Koenen tumors): One of the characteristic skin lesions of tuberous sclerosis (Fig. P.6).[26] The lesions are skin-colored to reddish nodular deposits that occur mainly around the thumbnails and great toenails and are often mistaken for warts. There are reports of periungual fibromas as the only clinical sign of tuberous sclerosis complex.[27] See **adenoma sebaceum, hypomelanotic macule**, **poliosis, shagreen patch.**

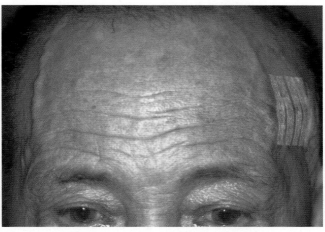

Figure P.5. Biopsy proven giant cell arteritis with an indurated, nonpulsatile tender superficial temporal artery on the right; biopsy site on the left.

Periungual telangiectasias: A sign of DM, see **dermatomyositis skin changes.**

Peroneal (Lust) phenomenon: See **tetany.**

Peroneal (tibialis anterior) reflex: A minor DTR, one of those that may be occasionally useful (see Table D.1, Video B.4). Like the **extensor digitorum brevis reflex,** it is one of the "elusive L5 reflexes" that is normally difficult to elicit and may be depressed in L5 radiculopathy.[28] See **hamstring reflexes.**

Perseveration: The persistence of one reply or one idea in response to various questions (verbal perseveration). Palilalia, echolalia, and perseveration are often manifestations of psychosis, but can occur with organic lesions. In copying tasks involving drawing simple figures with multiple loops, patients with perseveration may insert extra loops. Motor perseveration is the inability to stop performing an action or a movement, the opposite of motor **impersistence.** The patient continues to execute a motor program even after the task is complete or the requirements change.

Pes cavus: A common foot deformity, present to some degree in as many as 20% of the population. The term is used to describe a spectrum of foot deformities that have in common a high arch (Fig. P.7).[29] Pes cavus occurs in several neurologic conditions. Symmetric foot deformities are seen in many of the spinocerebellar degenerations and in CMT disease. Asymmetric pes cavus suggests a spinal dysraphism syndrome such as a tethered cord (Fig. P.8).

A number of terms are used to describe deformed feet, not always with any degree of precision. Clubfoot is often used to describe any type of malformed foot. Talipes is from the Latin for ankle (talus) and foot (pes) and is used as a prefix for particular foot deformities. Equinus is used because horses walk on their toes (digitigrade). Humans normally walk on their soles (plantigrade) but these foot deformities cause the patient to bear weight more on the forefoot. So the common term *talipes equinus* merely translates into a foot deformity associated with a tendency to walk on the toes. Varus deviation is commonly present, so *talipes equinovarus* (or

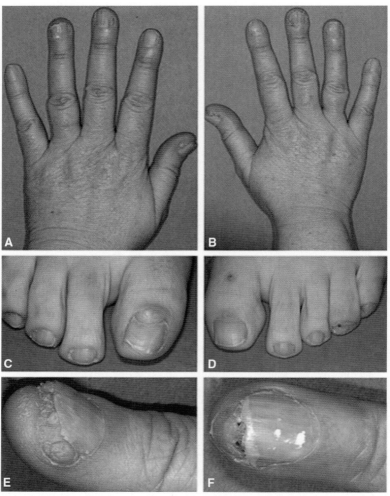

Figure P.6. Isolated Koenen tumors as a sign of tuberous sclerosis complex. Multiple subungual and periungual fibromas. Skin-colored erythematous papules and tumors are seen on the right **(A)** and left **(B)** hand, the right **(C)** and left **(D)** foot, the left thumbnail **(E)**, and the fourth digit of the left hand **(F)**. (From Quist SR, Franke I, Sutter C, et al. Periungual fibroma (Koenen tumors) as isolated sign of tuberous sclerosis complex with tuberous sclerosis complex 1 germline mutation. *J Am Acad Dermatol.* 2010;62:159–161, with permission.)

pes equinovarus) is the medical term for clubfoot. Figure P.7 shows the commonly seen foot deformities. See **hammer toes.**

Orthopedic exactness is not required for neurologic purposes, but the presence of a foot deformity should be recognized as a possibly relevant finding in a patient

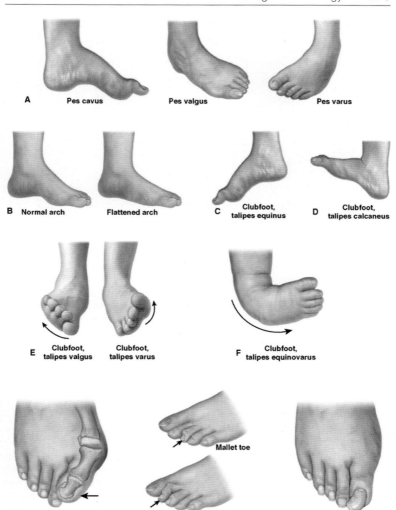

Figure P.7. Disorders of the foot. **A:** Pes Cavus **(Left)**, Pes Valgus **(Middle)**, and Pes Varus **(Right)**. **B:** Normal Arch **(Left)** and Flatfoot **(Right)**. **C:** Clubfoot, Talipes Equinus. **D:** Clubfoot, Talipes Calcaneus. **E:** Clubfoot, Talipes Valgus **(Left)** and Varus **(Right)**. **F:** Clubfoot, Talipes Equinovarus. **G:** Hallux Valgus. **H:** Mallet Toe **(Top)** and Hammer Toe **(Bottom)**. **I:** Oxychogryphosis. (From Pansky B, Gest TR. *Lippincott's Concise Illustrated Anatomy. Vol. 1: Back, Upper Limb & Lower Limb.* Philadelphia, PA: Wolters Kluwer Health/Lippincott Williams & Wilkins; 2012, with permission.)

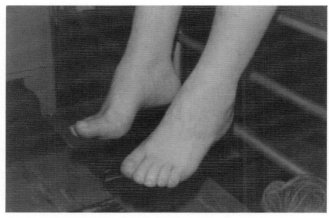

Figure P.8. A unilateral foot deformity in a patient with a tethered cord.

with neurologic complaints. The pes cavus associated with spinocerebellar degenerations such as Friedreich's ataxia is primarily skeletal in origin and is associated with scoliosis and other skeletal deformities. In chronic denervating conditions, such as CMT disease, there is significant atrophy and weakness of the intrinsic foot muscles producing clawing of the toes in addition to the high arch.

Petechiae: See **purpura.**

Petren's gait: See **gait disorders.**

Phalen's test (sign): See **carpal tunnel syndrome provocative tests.**

Phillipson's reflex: See **crossed extensor reflex.**

Phoria: See **strabismus.**

Photostress (light stress) test: A technique used to help distinguish optic nerve disease from macular disease by recording the visual recovery time after exposure to a bright light. The recovery time is prolonged in patients with macular disease, but normal in those with optic nerve disease. To perform the test, the best corrected acuity is recorded in each eye, and then the normal eye is exposed to a bright light directed into the pupil for 10 to 15 seconds with the other eye covered. The time is noted until the patient is able to read one line above the just recorded best acuity. In a young healthy eye, recovery time is usually 15 to 30 seconds, in older individuals 30 to 50 seconds. Then the symptomatic eye is exposed to bright light for the same length of time and the recovery interval noted. Markedly asymmetric recovery times between the two eyes or a recovery time exceeding 60 seconds is abnormal. Photostress recovery time increases with age but is independent of pupil size, ametropia, and visual acuity.[30]

Physiologic tremor: See **tremor** and **enhanced physiologic tremor.**

Piano-playing movements: Choreic movements of the fingers. When asked to hold the hands outstretched, there are constant random movements of individual fingers (see Video C.8).

Pick's sign: **Lid nystagmus** provoked by convergence; seen in cerebellar or medullary lesions.

Pigmentary retinopathy: See **retinitis pigmentosa.**

Pill-rolling tremor: See **parkinsonian tremor.**

Piloerection: Goose flesh (anserina). Piloerection is an involuntary erection of hairs mediated by the sympathetic nervous system. It is one of the cold defense mechanisms, along with vasoconstriction and shivering. Piloerection may also occur as a sign of sympathetic overactivity. Autonomic disturbances, including piloerection, may accompany focal temporal or frontal lobe seizures and as part of the picture of autonomic dysreflexia in spinal cord lesions. In temporal lobe seizures, piloerection, either unilateral or bilateral, may occur in isolation or accompany other signs of sympathetic hyperactivity. When in a unilateral, hemibody distribution, the piloerection is typically ipsilateral to the seizure focus. Loss of piloerection may occur as a manifestation of dysautonomia in peripheral neuropathy, along with changes in skin temperature or color, mottling, alopecia, hypertrichosis, and thickening or fragility of the nails.

Piltz-Westphal reaction: Constriction of the pupils on attempted lid closure; a normal finding.

Pinch sign: See **OK sign.**

Ping-pong gaze: Unusual spontaneous eye movements seen in patients in coma. There are slow, horizontal, conjugate eye movements that alternate every few seconds. These eye movements usually occur with bilateral hemispheric or peduncular infarction. The movements are usually smooth but a saccadic variation has been reported.[31] Some regard ping-pong gaze as a short cycle variant of **periodic alternating gaze deviation.** For a video, see Moccia et al.[32] See **ocular bobbing.**

Pinhole test: A method to exclude refractive error as a cause of impaired vision. The pinhole permits only central light rays to enter the eye and these are less likely to be disrupted by refractive errors such as presbyopia and astigmatism. After obtaining a baseline acuity, the patient should attempt to read further down the acuity card through the pinhole. Improvement of vision by looking through the pinhole suggests impairment related to a refractive error. Visual impairment due to a neurologic process, such as optic neuritis, will not improve with a pinhole. Under some circumstances, such as with a cataract, vision may get worse with the pinhole.

Pinpoint pupils: Bilaterally tiny pupils that still react to light. The pupils are usually about 1 mm in diameter. Bilateral pinpoint pupils occur with acute, severe brainstem lesions, such as pontine hemorrhage or thrombosis of the basilar artery, or with opiate toxicity. The bilateral miosis seen in large pontine lesions is probably due to dysfunction of the descending sympathetic pathways bilaterally. The light reaction is preserved with lesions involving the descending sympathetic system, but may be very difficult to see without magnification when the pupils are extremely small. Focusing on a tiny pupil with the ophthalmoscope, and turning the light off, then back on, may reveal the residual light reactivity. Hypothermia can cause small, unreactive pupils. The most common cause of pinpoint pupils in patients with depressed consciousness is opiate toxicity.

Piriformis syndrome provocative tests: Maneuvers used to provoke pain in patients with suspected piriformis syndrome. Piriformis syndrome is a controversial disorder, and whether these tests have any real clinical utility is conjectural.[33]

The Beatty maneuver seeks to elicit buttock pain on the symptomatic side by having the patient hold the affected leg several inches off the examination table while lying on the unaffected side. In the FAIR test, aka the piriformis test, with the patient lying on the unaffected side, the symptomatic leg is flexed at the hip and knee and forced into adduction and internal rotation by pressing down on the knee. Induction of buttock or sciatic distribution pain with this maneuver supports the diagnosis. Prolongation of the H-reflex in this position has been claimed as an objective sign of the disorder. The Freiburg test seeks to elicit buttock pain with passive, forced internal rotation of the affected leg. The Pace test attempts to elicit buttock pain with resisted abduction of the affected leg. Resisted abduction of the hip in the side-lying position may also provoke pain arising from the SI joint (see sacroiliac joint signs).

Piriformis tests: See **piriformis syndrome provocative tests.**

Pisa syndrome (sign): Tonic, lateral flexion of the trunk with mild backward rotation, causing the patient to lean to one side whenever erect. Originally described by Ekbom as a dystonic reaction due to neuroleptic therapy, other cases without neuroleptic exposure were later described. Pisa syndrome occurs in PD and other parkinsonian syndromes, particularly MSA; Pisa syndrome is one of the features suggestive of atypical parkinsonism.[34] In addition to Pisa syndrome, other postural deformities, such as camptocormia, **anterocollis,** and **scoliosis,** are common and often disabling complications of PD and related disorders.[35]

Pitres' sign: The absence of pain on squeezing the testicles, a classic sign of tabes dorsalis (see also **Abadie's sign** and **Biernacki's sign**).

Plagiocephaly: See **craniosynostosis.**

Plantar grasp reflex: A grasp reflex of the foot, with flexion and adduction of the toes in response to a light pressure on the plantar surface of the foot, especially its distal and medial portions. The plantar grasp is present in the normal newborn but disappears by the end of the first year. It may reappear in adults, along with a grasp reflex of the hand, in disease of the opposite frontal lobe. The plantar grasp may be elicited by drawing the handle of a reflex hammer from the midsole toward the toes, causing the toes to flex and grip the hammer (Fig. P.9). Too far medial stimulation when attempting to elicit **Babinski's plantar sign** may produce a plantar grasp instead.

Plantar muscle reflex: See **Rossolimo's sign.**

Plantar reflex (response): (1) See **Babinski's plantar sign.** (2) Stroking the plantar surface of the foot from the heel forward is normally followed by plantar flexion of the foot and toes. Flexion is the normal response after the first 12 to 18 months of life. In ticklish patients, there may be voluntary withdrawal with flexion of the hip and knee, but in every normal individual there is a certain amount of plantar flexion of the toes on stimulation of the sole of the foot. A tonic plantar reflex with slow, prolonged contraction has been described as a sign of frontal lobe and extrapyramidal disease. The normal plantar response may be difficult to obtain in individuals with plantar callosities. See **plantar grasp reflex.**

Plantar stretch reflex: The reflex elicited by striking the ball (sole) of the foot, or the examiner's hand placed flat against the sole, with the patient supine (see Video B.4). It is considered equivalent to the **ankle reflex** for clinical purposes. For a demonstration, see Stanford Medicine 25, An Initiative to Revive the Culture of Bedside Medicine, Deep Tendon Reflexes (http://stanfordmedicine25.stanford.edu/the25/tendon.html).

Platysma sign: See **Babinski's platysma sign.**

Plegia: See **weakness.**

Plexiform neuroma: One of the characteristic lesions of NF1 (see Table N.1). These are large tumors that develop along the course of a nerve (Fig. P.10). They often occur on the face and can cause severe disfigurement. The lifetime risk of malignant

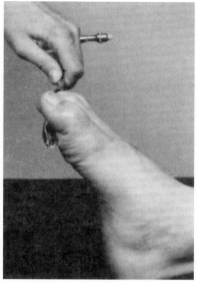

Figure P.9. The plantar grasp reflex with brisk bending of toes to grasp reflex hammer handle. (From Massey EW, Pleet AB, Scherokman BJ. *Diagnostic Tests in Neurology: A Photographic Guide to Bedside Techniques.* Chicago, IL: Year Book Medical Publishers; 1985, with permission.)

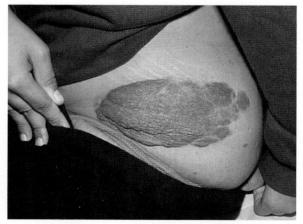

Figure P.10. A plexiform neuroma in a patient with NF1. (From Goodheart HP. *Goodheart's Photoguide of Common Skin Disorders.* 2nd ed. Philadelphia, PA: Wolters Kluwer Health/Lippincott Williams & Wilkins; 2003, with permission.)

degeneration is about 5%. See **café-au-lait spot, neurofibroma, Crowe's sign, Lisch nodule**.

Poliosis (leukotrichia): Localized depigmentation of the hair, usually a patch or streak of white hair, most often a white forelock (Fig. P.11). Some of the neurologically relevant disorders associated with poliosis include Vogt-Koyanagi-Harada disease, tuberous sclerosis, Waardenburg's syndrome, and Apert's syndrome.

Pollicomental reflex: See **palmomental reflex**.

Polydactyly: See **syndactyly**.

Popeye arm: Wasting of the biceps and triceps with sparing of the deltoid and forearm musculature, a characteristic pattern seen in FSH.

Popliteal compression test: See **bowstring sign**.

Porter's tip position: See **waiter's tip position**.

Positional nystagmus: See **nystagmus**.

Posterior column signs: Abnormalities on examination that reflect dysfunction of the posterior columns. Impaired position and vibration sensibility and the presence of a **Romberg sign** are the primary signs. Other abnormalities due to loss of fine, discriminative touch that may be demonstrable include **astereognosis, agraphesthesia,** and loss of **two-point discrimination**.

Posterior fossa stare: See **Collier's sign**.

Posting: See **forearm rolling** and **subtle signs of hemiparesis**.

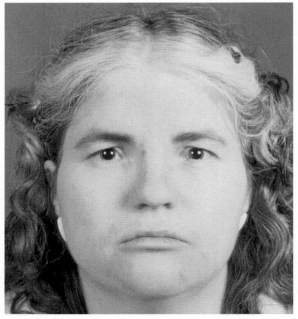

Figure P.11. Poliosis in a patient with Waardenburg's syndrome. (From Gold DH, Weingeist TA. *Color Atlas of the Eye in Systemic Disease.* Baltimore, MD: Wolters Kluwer Health/Lippincott Williams & Wilkins; 2001, with permission.)

Postural instability: Difficulty maintaining balance and an upright posture, usually due to impaired **postural reflexes**, often accompanied by a tendency to fall.[36] Postural instability is a common feature in parkinsonian disorders, especially PD, PSP, and MSA. In PD, impaired postural reflexes lead to a tendency to fall forward (propulsion), which the patient tries to avoid by walking with increasing speed but with very short steps, the **festinating gait.** Falls are common. In PSP, the tendency is to retropulsion and falling backward. Postural stability may be assessed by the pull test.[37] Standing behind the patient, the physician pulls the patient backward by the shoulders or pushes lightly on the sternum, remaining vigilant to prevent a fall (see Video G.4). The push or pull must be hard enough to cause the patient to lose balance and require a rescue response. When postural instability is present, the pull may cause retropulsion or multiple backward steps before the patient is able to regain balance. With severe postural instability, the patient may tend to fall en bloc without taking any steps to regain balance. Postural instability may also occur because of impaired perfusion, such as with orthostatic hypotension, or vestibular dysfunction. When a patient, seated in a chair, is suddenly tilted backward, there is absence of the normal reflex leg extension to counteract the loss of balance (Souques' leg sign).

Postural reflexes: A complex group of reactions that serve to maintain the erect posture and normal position. The reflex mechanisms of standing and righting involve the vestibular system, principally the utricle; proprioceptive impulses from muscles, tendons, and joints; exteroceptive impulses from the body surface; and visual stimuli. Standing may be thought of as a postural reflex, and any interference with the mechanisms mediating postural reflexes may interfere with the act of normal standing. Loss of postural reflexes is an important feature of PD and related disorders, and similar impairment is likely related to the tendency of the elderly to fall (see **postural instability**).

Postural tremor: See **tremor.**

Pourfour du Petit syndrome: See **reverse Horner's syndrome.**

Praxis: The ability to perform complex motor acts. Impaired praxis results in the various forms of **apraxia.**

Prayer sign: An inability to place the palms together in a position of prayer due to flexion contractures of the fingers. The prayer sign is seen in Bethlem myopathy. More common causes are diabetic arthropathy involving the small joints of the hands, an ulnar **claw hand,** Dupuytren's contracture, and scleroderma.

Preacher's hand: See **benediction hand.**

Preretinal hemorrhage: See **Terson's syndrome.**

Presbyopia: Loss of the power of **accommodation** due to advancing age. The **near point of accommodation** lengthens with advancing presbyopia. This may cause significant difficulties in assessing **visual acuity** at the bedside since the best corrected acuity is the relevant function for neurological purposes and patients do not always have correction available. Checking acuity at a distance of 20 feet, as in an eye lane, removes the effects of presbyopia but is frequently not feasible. Acuity cards and electronic devices are available that are designed for testing at 1 m, 2 m, and 6 ft. If one of these is not available, a **pinhole test** may improve the acuity and help resolve whether an impairment is likely ophthalmologic or neurologic in origin.

Pressure provocative test (median nerve compression test): See **carpal tunnel syndrome provocative tests.**

Prévost's (Vulpian's) sign: See **gaze palsy.**

Priapism: Abnormal persistence of penile erection. In neurologic patients, it primarily occurs in patients with chronic SCI and other forms of severe myelopathy. It may occur in isolation or as part of a **mass reflex.** Priapism may also follow acute traumatic SCI, when it tends to occur at the moment of injury. In all myelopathy patients, priapism is associated with complete motor and sensory paraplegia and the presence or absence of priapism may help determine whether or not the lesion is complete.[38] Intermittent, spontaneous priapism provoked by walking occurs in some patients with lumbar spinal stenosis and neurogenic claudication.[39]

Primary deviation: See **strabismus.**

Primary orthostatic tremor: See **orthostatic tremor.**

Primary writing tremor: A 4-to-7-Hz **task-specific tremor** that affects writing in isolation. It may be difficult to distinguish from writer's cramp, a task specific dystonia, as patients with dystonic writer's cramp may have superimposed tremulousness when writing.

Primitive reflexes: Phenomena present in normal infants and children that disappear with maturation but reappear with normal aging or in the face of neurological disease, particularly frontal lobe disorders.[40] Reflexes usually included in this category include the **grasp, palmomental, pollicomental, corneomandibular, sucking, root, snout, glabellar tap,** and **nuchocephalic** reflexes.[41] See **age-related signs, pathologic reflexes,** and **frontal release signs.**

Procerus sign: Facial dystonia causing contraction of the forehead muscles, particularly the procerus and corrugator, with knitting of the brows and widening of the palpebral fissures, producing an expression of surprise, astonishment or worry with knitted eyebrows, lid retraction, and reduced blinking (Fig. P.12).

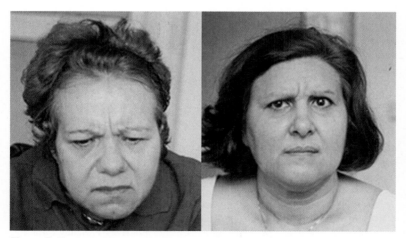

Figure P.12. The expression may be due to a focal dystonia of the procerus muscle plus a combination of reduced blinking and lid retraction. The procerus originates in the nasal bone and inserts in the center of the forehead between the eyebrows; its action forms vertical wrinkles in the glabella region and bridge of the nose. (From Batla A, Nehru R, Vijay T. Vertical wrinkling of the forehead or procerus sign in PSP. *J Neurol Sci.* 2010;298:148–149, with permission.)

The procerus sign is seen most characteristically in PSP and CBD.[42,43] The term *omega sign* has also been used for this facial appearance but in the older literature omega sign also describes the knitted forehead seen in depression, where tonic contraction of the corrugator creates wrinkles in the shape of the Greek letter Ω above the root of the nose.

Prognathism: Abnormal protrusion of the mandible. Prognathism is an integral feature of the facial appearance in acromegaly and pituitary gigantism and may also occur in fragile X syndrome and Apert's syndrome.

Pronation sign of Neri: One of the **associated movement** signs, seen in the paretic limb. The patient lies supine with the upper extremities extended and pronated; when the forearm is flexed and supinated by examiner, the paretic arm returns to pronation; similar to Strümpell's and Babinski's **pronator signs**. The phenomenon could well be due to the higher resting tonus in the pronator muscles that occurs with spasticity (see **pronator catch**, **pronator drift**). It is one of many signs related to the tendency of CST lesions to cause forearm pronation that can be demonstrated in a number of ways **(Table P.3)**.

Pronation-supination test: A test to evaluate for the presence of **dysdiadochokinesia; see rapid alternating movements.**

Pronator catch: A sign of spasticity elicited by manipulation of the forearm. The hypertonicity due to lesions involving the corticospinal pathways differs from that of rigidity because it is not uniform throughout the range of movement and because it varies with the speed of movement. The hypertonia of spasticity varies greatly from muscle to muscle and is often particularly prominent in the forearm pronators. The relationship of the hypertonus to the speed of movement is a key feature distinguishing spasticity from rigidity. In spasticity, if the passive movement is made slowly, there may be little resistance. But if the movement is made quickly, there will be a sudden increase in tone partway through the arc, causing a catch or a block as though the muscle had impacted a stop. In the upper extremity, it is useful to look for spasticity involving the pronator muscles. With the patient's elbow flexed to about 90 degrees and the forearm fully pronated, the examiner slowly supinates the patient's hand. Unless spasticity is severe, there will be little or no resistance to this slow movement. If, after several slow repetitions, the examiner supinates the patient's hand very quickly, a sudden resistance at about the midrange of movement, referred to as a "pronator catch," signals pronator spasticity. The catch will then relax, and the supination movement can be completed. When hypertonus is severe, this maneuver may elicit pronator clonus (see Table P.3).

Table P.3. Signs Related to the Tendency of the Forearm to Pronate Because of CST Lesions, Which Cause Relative Weakness of the Supinators and Increased Resting Tone in the Pronators

Pronator drift (Barré's sign)
Pronation sign of Neri
Pronator catch
Babinski's pronator sign
Wilson's pronator sign
Strümpell's pronator sign

Pronator drift (Barré's sign): One of the **subtle signs of hemiparesis,** one of the types of **drift,** and one of many **pronator signs** (see Table P.3). Pronator drift is seen with mild CST weakness **(Video P.4).** The patient holds the upper extremities outstretched to the front, palms up and eyes closed for 20 to 30 seconds. In normals, the palms will remain flat, the elbows straight, and the limbs horizontal. Any deviation from this position will be similar on the two sides. The patient with a mild CST deficit may demonstrate pronator drift to varying degrees. With mild drift, there is slight pronation of the hand and slight flexion of the elbow on the abnormal side **(Fig. P.13).** With more severe drift, there is more prominent pronation and obvious flexion of the elbow, and there may be downward drift of the entire arm **(Fig. P.14).**

Because of the innervation pattern of the CST, the minimally weak CST-innervated muscles are overcome by the non-CST muscles. With a mild CST lesion, the minimally weak muscles in the upper extremity are the extensors, supinators, and abductors. These are overcome by the uninvolved and therefore stronger muscles: the pronators, biceps, and internal rotators of the shoulder. As these overcome the slightly weakened CST-innervated muscles, the hand pronates, the elbow flexes, and the arm drifts downward. With severe CST weakness, this muscle imbalance produces the posture of spastic hemiparesis **(Fig. P.15).**

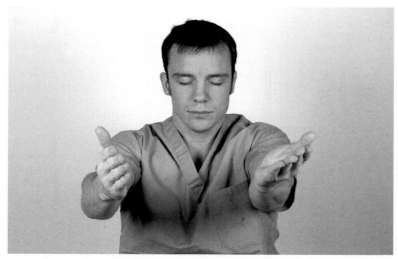

Figure P.13. Technique for testing for pronator drift. In the presence of a corticospinal tract lesion, the selectively weakened muscles are the shoulder abductors and external rotators, the supinators, and the elbow extensors. These muscles are overcome by their antagonists to cause pronation, elbow flexion, and downward drift. This is an illustration of mild pronator drift of the right upper extremity. Patients with mild corticospinal tract lesions may demonstrate a pronator drift or have an abnormal **forearm rolling** or **finger rolling** test in the absence of clinically detectable weakness to formal strength testing. (From Campbell WW. *DeJong's the Neurologic Examination.* 7th ed. Philadelphia, PA: Wolters Kluwer Health/Lippincott Williams & Wilkins; 2013, with permission.)

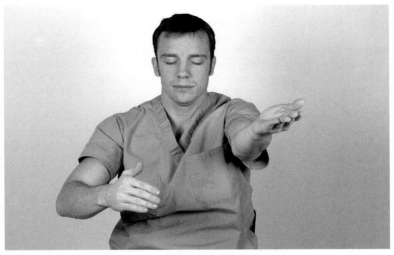

Figure P.14. Moderate drift with further development of the posture. (From Campbell WW. *DeJong's the Neurologic Examination.* 7th ed. Philadelphia, PA: Wolters Kluwer Health/Lippincott Williams & Wilkins; 2013, with permission.)

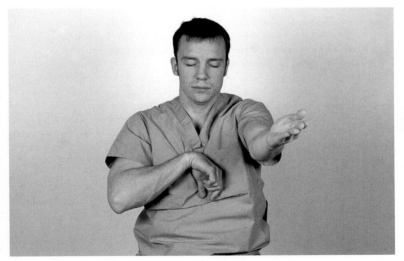

Figure P.15. Further development of pronator drift, with the evolution of "severe" drift to show how marked weakness of the corticospinal innervated muscles produces the posture of spastic hemiparesis. The pathophysiologic basis for pronator drift, for the upper extremity posture of fully developed spastic hemiparesis, and for the upper extremity posture of decorticate rigidity is the same; it is only a matter of degree. A mild corticospinal tract lesion results in mild pronator drift, a severe lesion results in spastic hemiparesis. (From Campbell WW. *DeJong's the Neurologic Examination.* 7th ed. Philadelphia, PA: Wolters Kluwer Health/Lippincott Williams & Wilkins; 2013, with permission.)

Studies of pronator drift have shown a sensitivity of 22% to 91%, a specificity of 93% to 98%, positive LR of 9.6 and negative LR of 0.3 in the detection of contralateral hemispheric disease.[15]

Pronator reflex: One of the occasionally useful DTRs (see Table D.1). With the elbow in semiflexion and the forearm semipronated, tapping over either the volar surface of the distal radius or the dorsal aspect of the styloid process of the ulna may produce brief supination followed by reflex pronation of the forearm (see Video B.4). There may also be flexion of the wrist and fingers. The major muscles participating in this response are the pronator teres and pronator quadratus. This reflex may be exaggerated early when CST lesions develop. Robert Wartenberg thought unilateral exaggeration of the pronator reflex was one of the most sensitive of all pyramidal signs.[44]

Pronator sign: A tendency for the forearms and hands to turn into a position of hyperpronation when the arms are raised overhead in patients with chorea. The term is also used to describe the tendency for pronation to occur because of CST lesions, described in a number of variations, all related to weakness of CST-innervated muscles or increased tone in the pronator muscles, the same phenomenon that underlies **pronator drift** (see Table P.3).

Pronation phenomena have also been described by Babinski and Wilson. In the former, the palmar aspects of the hands are held in approximation with the thumbs up and are then jarred or shaken; the paretic hand falls into a position of pronation. In the latter, there is pronation of the forearm along with internal rotation at the shoulder when the arms are held overhead, palms facing; as a result the affected palm turns outward. Pronation may also occur on the paretic side when the arms are actively abducted with the forearm supinated or when the arms are passively abducted with the forearm supinated and then suddenly released.

Proprioceptive trick: See **geste antagoniste.**

Proptosis: Protrusion of the eye, defined as >2 mm above the normal upper limit (see Fig. C.10). **Exophthalmos** is also used to describe abnormal protrusion of the eye, but generally when the condition is unilateral proptosis is preferred. Thyroid eye disease is the most common cause and is usually, but not always, bilateral. Other causes of proptosis include cavernous sinus thrombosis or carotid-cavernous fistula, cavernous sinus dural AVM, masses within the orbit, orbital pseudotumor, infection within the orbit, Crouzon's syndrome and related disorders, and some systemic diseases, such as amyloidosis. See **chemosis.**

There is a racial difference in normal globe anatomy. Blacks may normally have slightly greater globe projection ($p < 0.025$ for males and $p < 0.01$ for females).[45] Similar differences were seen for measures of interpupillary distance and palpebral fissure width, with greater mean values for black as compared with white adults.

Propulsion: A tendency to lean or fall forward, often a manifestation of impaired **postural reflexes** in PD and related syndromes. Propulsion leads to the **festinating gait.** See **postural instability, retropulsion.**

Prosopagnosia (aprosopagnosia): An inability to recognize familiar faces. In prosopagnosia (face or facial agnosia), the patient may not be able to identify people, even close family members, by looking at their faces, but immediately identify the person by the sound of the voice or other characteristics. The patient may recognize a face as a face but cannot associate it with a particular individual. She learns to identify people using other cues. In extreme examples, the patient is unable to recognize herself in a mirror or a photograph (autoprosopagnosia), which may occur in advanced AD. Patients with prosopagnosia, and other visual agnosias, usually have bilateral lesions of the occipitotemporal area involving the lingual, fusiform, and parahippocampal gyri. Prosopagnosia can occur with unilateral right posterior hemispheric lesions, especially with involvement of the fusiform gyrus. Functional imaging has revealed a focal region in the right fusiform gyrus activated specifically during face perception.[46] Recent literature suggests a hereditary form may affect about 2.5% of the population, and perhaps up to 10% in a very mild form. A common complaint is the inability to keep track of characters in movies. See **agnosia.**

Pseudo-Argyll Robertson pupil: A pupil with **light near dissociation** that occurs in diseases other than neurosyphilis. The pseudo-AR pupil typically lacks the miosis and irregularity characteristic of true AR pupils. Pseudo-AR pupils are seen in conditions such as Wernicke's encephalopathy, sarcoidosis, MS, and **aberrant reinnervation of CN III** (misdirection syndrome). In aberrant reinnervation, the pupillary light reaction is poor to absent, but the pupil constricts on ocular adduction with either convergence or horizontal gaze. The constriction on convergence with an impaired light reaction mimics light near dissociation.

Pseudoathetosis (sensory athetosis): Undulating and writhing movements of the extremities due to loss of position sense as a result of a parietal lobe lesion, or peripheral deafferentation due to such conditions as tabes dorsalis, posterolateral sclerosis, or peripheral nerve disease (Fig. P.16). The movements are more marked when the eyes are closed (Video Link P.2).[47]

Pseudo-Babinski sign: Dorsiflexion of the great toe, usually tonic and sustained, not related to disease of the CST but to basal ganglia disease, producing a **dystonic foot.** The tonically extended toe is also referred to as a **striatal toe.** See **Bajonet posture.**

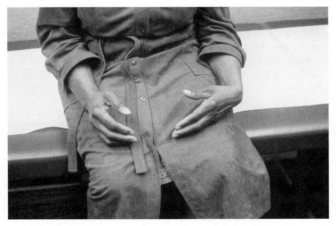

Figure P.16. Pseudoathetosis of the left hand in a patient with a right parietal lobe lesion. The hand exhibited spontaneous writhing and twisting movements. (From Campbell WW. *DeJong's the Neurologic Examination.* 7th ed. Philadelphia, PA: Wolters Kluwer Health/Lippincott Williams & Wilkins; 2013, with permission.)

Pseudo-Graefe sign: See **aberrant reinnervation of CN III.**

Pseudo-Horner's syndrome: See **Horner's syndrome.**

Pseudohypertrophy: Apparent muscle enlargement due to replacement of diseased muscle by fat and fibrous tissue without an actual increase in muscle fiber size or number. **Calf enlargement** in patients with Duchenne muscular dystrophy is a classic example of muscle pseudohypertrophy (see Fig. C.2). When hypertrophy is present, the muscles are firm and hard; in pseudohypertrophy they appear enlarged but may feel doughy or rubbery on palpation. The feel of pseudohypertrophy has been likened to that of a plastic, gelatinous toy such as a slimy, imitation snake. Comparing the circumference of the calf with the knee is often informative. Pseudohypertrophy is common in Duchenne and Becker dystrophy; an alternate term for DMD is *pseudohypertrophic muscular dystrophy.* It occurs in other neuromuscular conditions as well. Pseudohypertrophy may also result from the deposition of abnormal material in muscle, as in amyloidosis.

Pseudomyotonia: A term used to describe delayed muscle relaxation, particularly on elicitation of DTRs, that lacks the characteristics of true myotonia and is not accompanied by myotonic discharges on EMG. There is frequently accompanying muscle stiffness and cramping. Some of the conditions said to cause pseudomyotonia include hypothyroid myopathy, acquired neuromyotonia (Isaac's syndrome), sarcoplasmic reticulum-Ca^{++} ATPase deficiency (Brody's disease), McArdle's disease, and stiff person syndrome. See **hung-up reflex.**

Pseudopapilledema: A condition of the optic disc, usually a congenital anomaly, that can be confused with **papilledema (Table P.4).** A small, cupless disc with **drusen** is the most common cause. Other causes include **tilted discs, myelinated nerve fibers,** a persistent embryonic anterior hyaloid artery causing traction on the disc, a Bergmeister's papilla with epipapillary glial tissue producing anterior traction on the disc or obscuring the disc margins (Figs. P.17 and R.4).

Pseudoptosis: The appearance of **ptosis** in the absence of levator abnormality. Pseudoptosis may occur in a number of situations. **Proptosis** or **eyelid retraction** in one eye may produce the appearance of a droopy lid in the other, healthy eye. A narrow palpebral fissure can occur because of mechanical limitation of levator excursion or **enophthalmos.** In vertical strabismus with the hypertropic eye fixing, the lid of the hypotropic eye may seem to be ptotic, but is not. In Duane's syndrome, the palpebral fissure narrows on ocular adduction because of globe

Table P.4. Characteristics of Papilledema and Pseudopapilledema

Characteristic	Papilledema	Pseudopapilledema
Size of disc	Normal	Small
Optic cup	Initially present	Absent
Optic disc color	Hyperemic	Normal or pale
Disc morphology	Normal	Possibly abnormal
Drusen	Absent	Possibly present
Spontaneous venous pulsations	Absent	Present
Retinal veins	Distended	Normal
Peripapillary hemorrhages	Often present	Absent
Peripapillary nerve fiber layer	Edematous	Normal

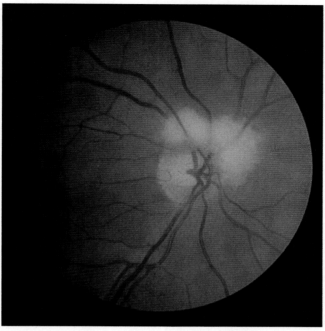

Figure P.17. Myelinated nerve fibers. (From Campbell WW. *DeJong's the Neurologic Examination.* 7th ed. Philadelphia, PA: Wolters Kluwer Health/Lippincott Williams & Wilkins; 2013, with permission.)

retraction, causing dynamic enophthalmos (see Video D.5). Intrinsic abnormalities of the eyelids because of inflammation, trauma or other factors may be mistaken for ptosis. Nonorganic ptosis is rare; it can occur because of voluntary unilateral **blepharospasm**. A telltale clue is that there is contraction of the orbicularis oculi or relaxation of the eyebrow elevators, causing brow ptosis in addition to the appearance of lid ptosis. See **levator dehiscence, dermatochalasis**.

Pseudoradicular syndrome: Sensory loss or sensory symptoms in an apparently radicular distribution but due to a lesion of the contralateral thalamus or sensory cortex. See **thalamic sensory loss**.

Pseudoulnar and pseudopseudoulnar claw hand: See **finger drop, myelopathy hand**.

Psychogenic signs: See **functional signs**.

Psychogenic tremor: Tremor not due to organic neurologic disease. Psychogenic tremor is typically complex and does not fit well into the tremor classification scheme. The patient may have rapidly changing clinical features including variable resting, postural and kinetic components, and disability out of proportion to the tremor. Typical features include abrupt onset with severe involvement and maximal disability immediately, onset in one limb with rapid generalization, spontaneous resolution and recurrence, a decrease in the tremor with distraction, refractoriness to conventional antitremor treatment, and entrainment. Entrainment is a change in the frequency of the tremor to match that of a task performed by another body part. The patient with a psychogenic 10-Hz right-hand tremor asked to pat on the left thigh with the left hand at 3 Hz soon has a 3-Hz right-hand tremor. Normally, tremor amplitude and frequency have an inverse relationship, but a psychogenic tremor may be paradoxically both high amplitude and high frequency, especially when attention is focused on the tremor.

Ptosis (blepharoptosis): Droopiness of the eyelid (see **eyelid position, abnormal**). Ptosis occurs in many neurologic conditions. It may be unilateral or bilateral, partial or complete. Compensatory overcontraction of the frontalis may lead to a worried or surprised appearance; with asymmetric ptosis, covering the eye with the droopy lid may cause the frontalis hypercontraction to disappear. A number of conditions may cause an appearance that simulates ptosis (see Fig. C.17); see **pseudoptosis, levator dehiscence, dermatochalasis**.

Total unilateral ptosis only occurs with complete third nerve palsy (Fig. P.18). Mild to moderate unilateral ptosis occurs as part of **Horner's syndrome**, or with partial third nerve palsy (see Fig. H.14). Rarely, ptosis is the only manifestation of an oculomotor nerve palsy. Mild to moderate bilateral ptosis occurs in some neuromuscular disorders, such as MG, muscular dystrophy, or ocular myopathy. The ptosis in MG is frequently asymmetric and may be unilateral, though it will tend to shift from side to side (Fig. P.19). It characteristically fluctuates from moment to moment and is worsened by prolonged upgaze (fatigable ptosis, Simpson's test). See **Cogan's lid twitch sign, curtain sign, ice pack test**. Ptosis in MG may respond

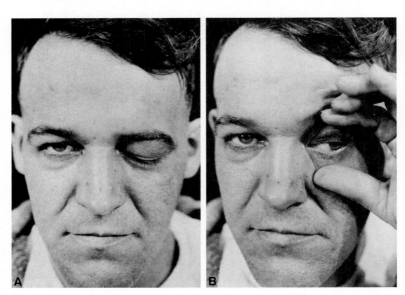

Figure P.18. Paralysis of the left oculomotor nerve in a patient with an aneurysm of the left internal carotid artery. **A:** Only ptosis can be seen. **B:** On elevating the eyelid, the pupil is dilated and the eyeball is deviated laterally. (From Campbell WW. *DeJong's the Neurologic Examination.* 7th ed. Philadelphia, PA: Wolters Kluwer Health/Lippincott Williams & Wilkins; 2013, with permission.)

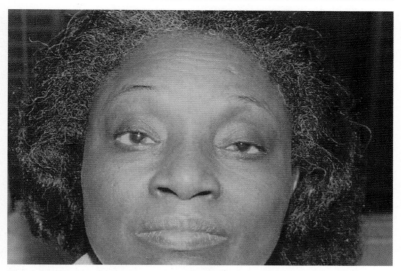

Figure P.19. Typical bilateral, asymmetric ptosis in a patient with myasthenia gravis. There is frontalis hypercontraction as the patient struggles to keep her eyes open.

dramatically to edrophonium **(Fig. P.20)**. Ptosis due to neuromuscular disorders is frequently accompanied by orbicularis oculi involvement, producing weakness of eye closure. The pattern of weakness of both eye opening and eye closure strongly suggests a myopathy or neuromuscular transmission disorder.

Cerebral ptosis is due to supranuclear lesions. Unilateral cerebral ptosis occurs with lesions, usually ischemic, of the opposite hemisphere, and is more common with right hemisphere lesions. Bilateral supranuclear ptosis may occur with unilateral or bilateral hemispheric lesions. Ptosis has been reported in as many as 37.5% of patients with hemispheric strokes. Because of the anatomy of the central caudal nucleus, bilateral ptosis can occur as the only ocular motility abnormality with some midbrain lesions.

Senile or involutional ptosis is very common, but asymmetric lids, **dermatochalasis**, and **levator dehiscence** are more the rule than the exception in the elderly. Congenital ptosis is common; because of levator fibrosis, it may be associated with lid lag in downgaze that is unusual in acquired ptosis. **Jaw winking** often occurs in conjunction. **Blepharospasm** is a focal dystonia causing involuntary eye closure; levator function is normal. In **apraxia of eyelid opening**, the patient has difficulty in voluntarily initiating lid elevation although there is no levator impairment or blepharospasm. Facial weakness never causes ptosis. In fact, the palpebral fissure on the weak side is often wider than normal, and unilateral widening of one palpebral fissure may be an early sign of facial palsy.

Puboadductor reflex: See **symphysis pubis reflex.**

Pull test: See **postural instability.**

Pulsating enopthalmos: A sign of NF1 in which aplasia of the greater wing of the sphenoid and lateral wall of the orbit causes the globe to collapse back into the orbit

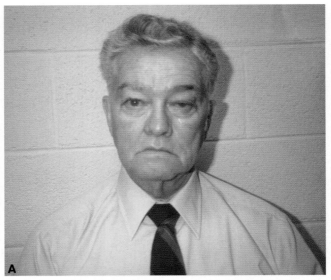

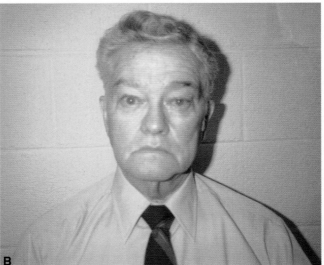

Figure P.20. A: MG causing left ptosis. **B:** Resolution of ptosis after intravenous edrophonium.

and pulsate synchronously with transmitted pulsations from the brain, as shown in the video by Lehn et al.[48] Pulsating exophthalmos can also occur.

Pupil sparing: Lack of involvement of the pupil in a CN III palsy. The pupil is usually involved early and prominently with third nerve compression. Pupillary sparing usually indicates the lesion is ischemic, most often due to diabetes, and not due to compression, but many examples of exceptions to this maxim have been reported.[49] In alert patients with new onset CN III palsy, a normal pupil significantly decreases the probability of an aneurysm or other compressive lesion (LR of 0.2).[15] The apparently reliable "pupil rule" is that complete pupil sparing with otherwise complete and isolated palsy of CN III is never due to an aneurysm. The rule requires careful application in younger patients, when ischemia is less likely. The pupil rule has become less important with the ready availability of advanced noninvasive imaging.

Pupillary dilation lag: See **dilation lag.**

Pupillary escape: See **pupillary light reflex.**

Pupillary light reflex: Constriction of the pupil on exposure to light. The pupillary light reaction is mediated by the macula, optic nerve, chiasm, optic tract, lateral geniculate body, and pretectum. Because of the decussation in the chiasm and the decussation in the posterior commissure, pupillary fibers are extensively commingled and the reflex is bilateral, both direct and consensual.

The light reflex should be tested in each eye individually. The examining light should be shone into the eye obliquely with the patient fixing at distance to avoid eliciting a confounding near response. A common error in pupil examination is to have the patient fixing at near, as by instructing him to look at the examiner's nose. This technique provokes both a light stimulus and a near stimulus simultaneously, and the pupils may well constrict to the near target of the examiner's nose even when the reaction to light is impaired or absent. Using this technique, the examiner might miss **light near dissociation.** Always have the patient fix at distance when checking the pupillary light reaction.

The pupils are normally equal, round, and equally reactive to light and near. A difference of 2 mm in pupil size is a significant degree of **anisocoria.** In some conditions, the pupils become abnormally shaped or exhibit unusual behavior (**Fig. P.21**, Table P.1). The normal pupillary light reflex is brisk constriction followed by slight dilatation back to an intermediate state (pupillary escape). The responses may be noted as prompt, sluggish, or absent, graded from 0 to 4+, or measured and recorded numerically, e.g., 4 mm → 2 mm. The status of the light reflex is judged by comparing the two eyes and by comparing the direct response and the consensual response.

The direct response occurs in the eye stimulated, and the consensual response occurs in the other eye. The eye with a severed optic nerve will show no direct

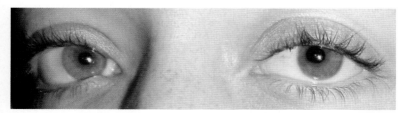

Figure P.21. Tadpole pupil. The left pupil is elongated due to focal dilation of the superonasal sector in a young woman who complained of episodic mydriasis. (From Kawasaki A, Mayer C. Tadpole pupil. *Neurology.* 2012;79:949, with permission.)

Table P.5. Direct and Consensual Light Reaction

| | Complete Lesion CN II OD | | Complete Lesion CN III OD | |
	Response OD	Response OS	Response OD	Response OS
Light stimulus OD	No response	No response	No response	Normal
Light stimulus OS	Normal	Normal	No response	Normal
Near reflex	Normal	Normal	No response	Normal

OD, right eye; OS, left eye.
Comparison of direct and consensual light reflex and pupillary constriction to the near reflex in the presence of a complete lesion of the right optic nerve versus the right oculomotor nerve. In both instances, the right pupil is frozen to direct light stimulation, and the distinction is made by the other reactions.
From Campbell WW. *DeJong's the Neurologic Examination*. 7th ed. Philadelphia, PA: Wolters Kluwer Health/Lippincott Williams & Wilkins; 2013.

response, but a normal consensual response to a light stimulus in the other eye, as well as constriction to attempted convergence **(Table P.5)**. Lesser degrees of optic nerve dysfunction can often be detected by checking for an **afferent pupillary defect**. The pupil frozen because of III nerve palsy will have no near response and no direct or consensual light response, but the other eye will exhibit an intact consensual response on stimulation of the abnormal side.

Pupillary near response (accommodation): Pupillary constriction that occurs as part of the near response, along with convergence and rounding up of the lens for efficient near vision. Normally, the light and near responses are of the same magnitude. **Light near dissociation** is present when the responses are not comparable.

Pure word mutism: An unusual aphasic syndrome in which the patient is totally unable to speak but auditory comprehension, reading, and writing are normal. It is probably a severe form of **apraxia of speech**, usually due to a small lesion of the posterior inferior frontal area.

Purpura: Skin lesions due to the extravasation of blood into the skin or mucous membranes **(Fig. P.22)**. Purpura is divided into palpable and nonpalpable (macular) forms. Nonpalpable purpura is usually noninflammatory in origin, while palpable purpura typically indicates vasculitis. Nonpalpable purpura is divided into petechiae (<3 mm) and ecchymosis (>5 mm). A lack of blanching on pressure is characteristic of all of these lesions. A hemorrhagic rash refers to a rash that has one or more of these features.

Neurologically relevant conditions that produce purpura include bacterial endocarditis, Rocky Mountain spotted fever, meningococcemia (Waterhouse-Friderichsen syndrome), thrombotic thrombocytopenic purpura, disseminated intravascular coagulation, leptospirosis, West Nile fever, fat embolism, and toxic shock syndrome. Any condition that causes a coagulopathy, such as idiopathic thrombocytopenic purpura, can also produce a hemorrhagic rash.

Palpable purpura occurs in bacterial endocarditis, Rickettsial diseases, cryoglobulinemia, and in various forms of vasculitis.

Puusepp's sign: See **little toe reflex of Puusepp**.

Pyramidal syndrome: See **long tract signs**.

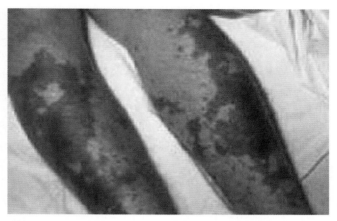

Figure P.22. Meningococcemia. Purpuric lesions showing large ecchymoses and small satellite petechiae. (From Betts RF, Chapman SW, Penn RL. *Reese and Betts' a Practical Approach to Infectious Diseases*. 5th ed. Philadelphia, PA: Wolters Kluwer Health/Lippincott Williams & Wilkins; 2003, with permission.)

Video Links

P.1. Paradoxical myotonia in paramyotonia congenita. (From Statland JM, Barohn RJ. Muscle channelopathies: the nondystrophic myotonias and periodic paralyses. *Musc Dis.* 2013;19(6):1598–1614.) Available at: http://journals.lww.com/continuum/pages/videogallery.aspx?videoId=108&autoPlay=true

P.2. Pseudoathetosis. (From Lo YL, See S. Images in clinical medicine. Pseudoathetosis. *N Engl J Med.* 2010;363:e29.) Available at: http://www.nejm.org/doi/full/10.1056/NEJMicm0907786

References

1. Hassan A, Mateen FJ, Coon EA, et al. Painful legs and moving toes syndrome: a 76-patient case series. *Arch Neurol.* 2012;69:1032–1038.
2. Pearce JM. Palatal Myoclonus (syn. Palatal Tremor). *Eur Neurol.* 2008;60:312–315.
3. Gersztenkorn D, Lee AG. Palinopsia revamped: a systematic review of the literature. *Surv Ophthalmol.* 2015;60:1–35.
4. Blythe IM, Bromley JM, Ruddock KH, et al. A study of systematic visual perseveration involving central mechanisms. *Brain.* 1986;109:661–675.
5. Pleet AB, Massey EW. Palmaris brevis sign in neuropathy of the deep palmar branch of the ulnar nerve. *Ann Neurol.* 1978;3:468–469.
6. Owen G, Mulley GP. The palmomental reflex: a useful clinical sign? *J Neurol Neurosurg Psychiatry.* 2002;73:113–115.
7. Van Stavern GP. Optic disc edema. *Semin Neurol.* 2007;27:233–243.
8. Jacks AS, Miller NR. Spontaneous retinal venous pulsation: aetiology and significance. *J Neurol Neurosurg Psychiatry.* 2003;74:7–9.
9. Jeffery DR, Mandler RN, Davis LE. Transverse myelitis. Retrospective analysis of 33 cases, with differentiation of cases associated with multiple sclerosis and parainfectious events. *Arch Neurol.* 1993;50:532–535.
10. Ropper AH. Unusual clinical variants and signs in Guillain-Barre syndrome. *Arch Neurol.* 1986;43:1150–1152.
11. van den Berg B, Fokke C, Drenthen J, et al. Paraparetic Guillain-Barre syndrome. *Neurology.* 2014;82:1984–1989.
12. Jan MM. Misdiagnoses in children with dopa-responsive dystonia. *Pediatr Neurol.* 2004;31:298–303.
13. Beversdorf DQ, Heilman KM. Facilitory paratonia and frontal lobe functioning. *Neurology.* 1998;51:968–971.
14. Hobbelen JS, Koopmans RT, Verhey FR, et al. Paratonia: a Delphi procedure for consensus definition. *J Geriatr Phys Ther.* 2006;29:50–56.

15. McGee S. *Evidence Based Physical Diagnosis.* 3rd ed. Philadelphia, PA: Elsevier/Saunders; 2012.
16. Aerts MB, Esselink RA, Post B, et al. Improving the diagnostic accuracy in parkinsonism: a three-pronged approach. *Pract Neurol.* 2012;12:77–87.
17. Stamelou M, Hoeglinger GU. Atypical parkinsonism: an update. *Curr Opin Neurol.* 2013;26:401–405.
18. Watson JC, Broaddus WC, Smith MM, et al. Hyperactive pectoralis reflex as an indicator of upper cervical spinal cord compression. Report of 15 cases. *J Neurosurg.* 1997;86:159–161.
19. Osher RH, Griggs RC. Orbicularis fatigue: the "peek" sign of myasthenia gravis. *Arch Ophthalmol.* 1979;97:677–679.
20. Brown RA, Lawson DA, Leslie GC, et al. Does the Wartenberg pendulum test differentiate quantitatively between spasticity and rigidity? A study in elderly stroke and Parkinsonian patients. *J Neurol Neurosurg Psychiatry.* 1988;51:1178–1186.
21. Brown RA, Lawson DA, Leslie GC, et al. Observations on the applicability of the Wartenberg pendulum test to healthy, elderly subjects. *J Neurol Neurosurg Psychiatry.* 1988;51:1171–1177.
22. Lin CC, Ju MS, Lin CW. The pendulum test for evaluating spasticity of the elbow joint. *Arch Phys Med Rehabil.* 2003;84:69–74.
23. Averbuch-Heller L, Meiner Z. Reversible periodic alternating gaze deviation in hepatic encephalopathy. *Neurology.* 1995;45:191–192.
24. Fisher CM. Facial pulses in internal carotid artery occlusion. *Neurology.* 1970;20:476–478.
25. Smetana GW, Shmerling RH. Does this patient have temporal arteritis? *JAMA.* 2002;287:92–101.
26. Ghosh SK, Bandyopadhyay D, Chatterjee G, et al. Mucocutaneous changes in tuberous sclerosis complex: a clinical profile of 27 Indian patients. *Indian J Dermatol.* 2009;54:255–257.
27. Quist SR, Franke I, Sutter C, et al. Periungual fibroma (Koenen tumors) as isolated sign of tuberous sclerosis complex with tuberous sclerosis complex 1 germline mutation. *J Am Acad Dermatol.* 2010;62:159–161.
28. Berlin L. A peroneal muscle stretch reflex. *Neurology.* 1971;21:1177–1178.
29. Aminian A, Sangeorzan BJ. The anatomy of cavus foot deformity. *Foot Ankle Clin.* 2008;13:191–198, v.
30. Margrain TH, Thomson D. Sources of variability in the clinical photostress test. *Ophthalmic Physiol Opt.* 2002;22:61–67.
31. Sieben A, Crevits L, Santens P. Saccadic ping pong gaze in coma. *Neurologist.* 2007;13:161–163.
32. Moccia M, Allocca R, Erro R, et al. Ping-pong gaze: Sherrington would not have done it better. *JAMA Neurol.* 2014;71:1450.
33. Campbell WW, Landau ME. Controversial entrapment neuropathies. *Neurosurg Clin N Am.* 2008;19:597.
34. Hozumi I, Piao YS, Inuzuka T, et al. Marked asymmetry of putaminal pathology in an MSA-P patient with Pisa syndrome. *Mov Disord.* 2004;19:470–472.
35. Doherty KM, van de Warrenburg BP, Peralta MC, et al. Postural deformities in Parkinson's disease. *Lancet Neurol.* 2011;10:538–549.
36. Visser M, Marinus J, Bloem BR, et al. Clinical tests for the evaluation of postural instability in patients with Parkinson's disease. *Arch Phys Med Rehabil.* 2003;84:1669–1674.
37. Munhoz RP, Li JY, Kurtinecz M, et al. Evaluation of the pull test technique in assessing postural instability in Parkinson's disease. *Neurology.* 2004;62:125–127.
38. Todd NV. Priapism in acute spinal cord injury. *Spinal Cord.* 2011;49:1033–1035.
39. Baba H, Maezawa Y, Furusawa N, et al. Lumbar spinal stenosis causing intermittent priapism. *Paraplegia.* 1995;33:338–345.
40. van Boxtel MP, Bosma H, Jolles J, et al. Prevalence of primitive reflexes and the relationship with cognitive change in healthy adults: a report from the Maastricht Aging Study. *J Neurol.* 2006;253:935–941.
41. Schott JM, Rossor MN. The grasp and other primitive reflexes. *J Neurol Neurosurg Psychiatry.* 2003;74:558–560.
42. Morimatsu M. Procerus sign in progressive supranuclear palsy and corticobasal degeneration. *Intern Med.* 2002;41:1101–1102.
43. Batla A, Nehru R, Vijay T. Vertical wrinkling of the forehead or Procerus sign in Progressive Supranuclear Palsy. *J Neurol Sci.* 2010;298:148–149.
44. Wartenberg, R. *The Examination of Reflexes.* Chicago, IL: Year Book Publishers; 1945.
45. Barretto RL, Mathog RH. Orbital measurement in black and white populations. *Laryngoscope.* 1999;109:1051–1054.
46. Barton JJ, Press DZ, Keenan JP, et al. Lesions of the fusiform face area impair perception of facial configuration in prosopagnosia. *Neurology.* 2002;58:71–78.
47. Lo YL, See S. Images in clinical medicine. Pseudoathetosis. *N Engl J Med.* 2010;363:e29.
48. Lehn A, Airey C, Boyle R. Pulsating enophthalmos in neurofibromatosis 1. *JAMA Neurol.* 2013;70:644–645.
49. Jacobson DM. Relative pupil-sparing third nerve palsy: etiology and clinical variables predictive of a mass. *Neurology.* 2001;56:797–798.

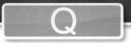

Quadrantopia: See **visual field defects.**
Quadriceps reflex: See **knee reflex.**
Quadriparesis (quadriplegia): Weakness (paralysis) involving all four extremities. The same considerations discussed under paraparesis apply for the most part. The most common cause is transverse myelopathy due to demyelination, compression, or ischemia. See **weakness.**
Quix test: See **past pointing.**

Rabbit syndrome (tremor): A rhythmic perioral tremor, generally associated with the use of psychotropics but sometimes associated with PD or occurring spontaneously. Compared with the movements of tardive dyskinesias, these are more rapid and regular and do not involve the tongue.[1,2] See **orofacial dyskinesias, tardive dyskinesias, bon bon sign.**

Raccoon (Panda) eyes: Bilateral periorbital ecchymoses characteristically seen in basilar skull fracture; may also be seen in other conditions, such as amyloidosis, multiple myeloma, migraine, sarcoidosis, and after continuous positive airway pressure use.[3]

Radial deviation: The tendency of the wrist to deviate radially on extension in posterior interosseous neuropathy; see **finger drop.**

Radial–radial delay: A difference in the arrival times of the radial pulses at the wrists, a potential indicator of significant brachiocephalic atherosclerosis with subclavian stenosis on the side of the delayed pulse, as might occur in patients with subclavian steal syndrome. The pulse asymmetry is usually accompanied by a difference in blood pressure in the two arms. See **peripheral vascular disease signs.**

Radial periosteal (radioperiosteal) reflex: See **brachioradialis reflex.**

Radialis sign (of Strümpell): An abnormal **associated movement** seen in **hemiparesis**; attempts to close the fingers or make a fist on the paretic side are accompanied by dorsiflexion of the wrist.

Radovici sign: See **palmomental reflex.**

Raimiste's arm sign: Elbow is placed on a table, with hand and forearm held upright by the examiner; when the sound hand is released it remains upright, and when the paretic hand is released, it flexes to an angle of about 130 degree; a sign of flaccidity rather than spasticity; may be present immediately after the onset of an organic **hemiparesis.**

Raimiste's leg sign: A pathologic **associated movement** of a paretic limb, which may be seen even when the patient is unable to voluntarily move the affected extremity. When the sound leg is forcefully abducted or adducted against the examiner's resistance, the paretic leg will carry out a movement identical with that attempted on the normal side. With the patient supine and the lower extremities abducted, an attempt to adduct the sound leg against resistance causes the paretic leg to also adduct, drawing the legs together. With attempted abduction of the sound leg, the paretic leg also abducts. See **abductor sign, Hoover's sign.**

Rapid alternating movements: Movements that require precise coordination of the contractions of the agonist and antagonist. The reciprocal relationship is particularly impaired in cerebellar disease, but rapid alternating movements (RAM) may also be disturbed by disorders of the CST or by extrapyramidal conditions. Abnormal RAMs are referred to as **dysdiadochokinesia.**

Rebound nystagmus: See **nystagmus.**

Rebound phenomenon: Contraction of the antagonist after a load is unexpectedly removed during strong contraction of the agonist, leading to a slight movement in the opposite direction. Rebound is the jerk back in the opposite direction, the recoil, on release of the restraint and is present normally, exaggerated in spastic limbs, and decreased or lost in cerebellar disease. Cerebellar disease causes disruption of the reciprocal relationship between agonist and antagonist, and it is the absence of rebound (usually accompanied by impairment of the **checking reflex**) in limbs affected by cerebellar disease that is abnormal. Many sources, including neurology textbooks, are confused on this point and imply that the presence of rebound is abnormal in cerebellar disease; in fact, the reverse is the case. Human and animal studies of the abnormalities associated with cerebellar dysfunction have shown the cerebellum contributes to the timing of the individual components of a movement, controls the amount of muscular activity, and coordinates the sequence of activation of agonists and antagonists.[4]

Loss of rebound may be detected with the Holmes rebound test (see **checking reflex**). The rebound test may also be carried out in other ways. Elbow extension against resistance may be tested instead of flexion. With both arms outstretched in front of the patient, the examiner may press either down or up on them as the patient resists and then suddenly lets go. This technique allows comparison of the rebound phenomenon on the two sides.

Recurring utterance: See **monophasia.**

Red desaturation: See **color desaturation.**

Red lens (red glass) test: See **diplopia rules.**

Red reflex: A quick screening method for evaluating vision, most often used in children. Shining a direct ophthalmoscope into both eyes from a distance of approximately 2 feet produces a red reflex that fills the pupil and a small white **corneal light reflex** symmetrically centered on both sides. Opacities in the media or major retinal pathology are sometimes apparent with a simple assessment of the red reflex. A cataract may cause black dots against the red background or block the red reflex, causing it to appear dark or dull; occasionally a white color is seen (leukocoria). Vitreous hemorrhage may block the red reflex. Strabismus causes a brighter red reflex in the deviated eye and decentralization of the corneal light reflex. Major differences in refractive error between the two eyes may cause asymmetry of the red reflex.

Reemergent tremor: See **essential tremor.**

Refined Romberg test: See **Romberg sign.**

Reflex grasping: See **grasp reflex.**

Reflex reinforcement: Methods to enhance **deep tendon reflex** activity. In some patients, DTRs are markedly diminished, or even apparently absent, although there is no other evidence of nervous system disease. Reinforcement may increase the amplitude of a sluggish reflex or bring out a latent reflex not otherwise obtainable. Reflexes that are normal on reinforcement, even though not present without reinforcement, may be considered normal. In elderly patients with absent ankle jerks, the reflexes appeared with reinforcement 70% of the time.[5]

A reflex can be reinforced or brought out using several methods (see Video B.4). In the Jendrassik manoeuver, the patient attempts to pull the hands apart with the fingers flexed and hooked together, palms facing, as the tendon is percussed (Fig. R.1). The effect is very brief, lasting only 1 to 6 seconds, and is maximal for only 300 milliseconds. The Jendrassik maneuver is obviously useful only for lower-extremity reflexes. Other techniques include having the patient clench one

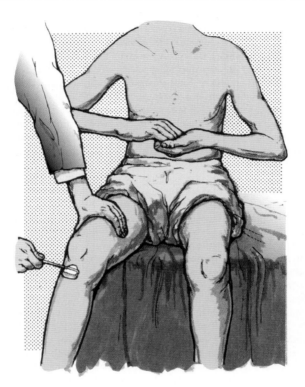

Figure R.1. The Jendrassik maneuver to reinforce the knee reflex. (From Campbell WW. *DeJong's the Neurologic Examination.* 7th ed. Philadelphia, PA: Wolters Kluwer Health/Lippincott Williams & Wilkins; 2013, with permission.)

or both fists, firmly grasp the arm of the chair, side of the bed, or the arm of the examiner. Reinforcement may also be carried out by having the patient look at the ceiling, grit the teeth, cough, squeeze the knees together, take a deep breath, count, read aloud, or repeat verses at the time the reflex is being tested. A sudden loud noise, a painful stimulus elsewhere on the body—such as the pulling of a hair or a bright light flashed in the eyes—may also be a means of reinforcement. The physiologic explanation for the Jendrassik potentiation remains a matter of debate, but it is certainly more complex than simply distracting the patient.[6]

Another method to reinforce the reflex response is to have the patient tense the muscle being tested. A simple and effective method to reinforce a knee or ankle jerk is to have the patient maintain a slight, steady contraction of the muscle whose tendon is being tested (e.g., slight plantar flexion by pushing the ball of the foot against the floor or the examiner's hand to reinforce the ankle jerk). The patient may tense the quadriceps by extending the knee slightly against resistance as the knee jerk is being elicited. Slight muscle contraction due to inability to relax may be one reason for the slightly hyperactive reflexes often seen in patients who are tense or anxious. See **Babinski's reinforcement sign.**

Relative afferent pupillary defect: See **afferent pupillary defect.**

Reptilian stare: An appearance of the face in PD and related disorders. The decreased rate of blinking (5–10 per minute rather than the normal 12–20), **masked facies** and slight **eyelid retraction** causes patients with parkinsonism to have a fixed, staring expression. A reduced spontaneous blink rate accompanied by exaggerated blinking on **glabellar tap** (Myerson's sign) is characteristic of PD. See **Stellwag's sign, eyelid retraction, Collier's sign.**

Respiratory failure, signs of: Neurological disorders are a common and important cause of respiratory failure **(Table R.1)**. Restrictive lung diseases affect the chest wall, lung, or respiratory muscles and reduce respiratory function without affecting airway flow. Restrictive defects produce proportional decreases in FEV_1 and FVC; the FEV_1/FVC ratio remains normal or slightly elevated. Obstructive pulmonary diseases involve the airways and cause a reduction in airflow. Spirometry shows a reduced FEV_1 and FEV_1/FVC ratio due to airflow impairment with a relatively normal FVC. Neurologic and neuromuscular diseases typically produce restrictive disease; some, such as myotonic dystrophy, also cause defects in central ventilatory drive. Acutely ill neurological patients may also develop respiratory failure due to atelectasis, aspiration pneumonitis, pulmonary edema, or pulmonary embolism.

Once respiratory muscles are affected by neuromuscular disease, respiratory failure may ensue abruptly because of intercurrent illness, particularly infection, or develop slowly over months or years resulting in chronic hypercapnic respiratory failure. In most neuromuscular disorders, respiratory muscle weakness develops insidiously along with weakness of other muscle groups. Occasionally, respiratory failure may be the presenting manifestation of a neuromuscular disorder. This is particularly likely to occur with ALS, MG, adult-onset acid maltase deficiency, and mitochondrial myopathy. Respiratory failure occurs commonly in GBS.

Table R.1. Neurologic and Neuromuscular Causes of Respiratory Failure

Level	Common Etiologies
Upper motor neuron	
Hemisphere or brainstem	Stroke
Spinal cord	Trauma
Lower motor neuron	
Anterior horn cell	ALS
	Poliomyelitis
Peripheral nerve	Phrenic nerve palsy
	GBS/CIDP
	Critical illness polyneuropathy
Neuromuscular junction	MG
	Botulism
Muscle	Muscular dystrophy
	Acid maltase deficiency
	Critical illness myopathy

Tachypnea (>20/min) at rest is common as respiratory muscle weakness worsens. This is followed by evidence of a high respiratory workload, including nasal flaring, sweating, tachycardia, and intercostal and subcostal retraction. If there is diaphragmatic or intercostal weakness, the accessory muscles that act in deep inspiration are brought into play, and breathing recruits the scaleni, sternocleidomastoids, serrati, and pectorals. Arterial blood gas abnormalities usually do not develop until late and cannot be used as a parameter to judge the need for ventilatory support. Spirometry generally shows a restrictive pattern. Serial measurement of FVC is vital to follow the progression of respiratory muscle weakness and in determining when ventilatory support is necessary. With rapidly progressive respiratory failure, as may occur in GBS and MG, a decrease of FVC to <15 to 20 mL/kg or <1 L usually indicates the need for intubation and ventilatory support. Normal FVC is approximately 40 to 70 mL/kg. Static pressures are also very useful. Decrease in the peak expiratory pressure (PEP) and peak inspiratory pressure (PIP) to <50 cm H_2O or <-50 cm H_2O, respectively, generally indicate the need to consider intubation. One recommendation for critical values are a VC <20 mL/kg, a PIP of <30 cm H_2O, and a PEP of <40 cm H_2O: the 20/30/40 rule **(Table R.2)**.[7]

The inability to count out loud to 20 at 1 number per second is another useful marker for impending respiratory failure. Quick, forceful diaphragmatic contractions are impaired; one manifestation of this may be the inability to sniff. Manifestations of developing hypoxia include restlessness, impaired arousal, tachypnea, tachycardia, and occasionally hypertension.

Neuromuscular disorders may cause weakness of the intercostals or the diaphragm, or both. Normally, both the abdomen and thorax expand synchronously during inspiration as the diaphragm descends, pushing the abdomen outward and pulling air into the lungs. Weakness of the intercostal muscles causes abdominal respiration, with alternate bulging and retraction of the epigastrium as exaggerated diaphragmatic contraction compensates for the intercostal weakness. The intercostal spaces may retract during inspiration, and the ribs do not rise and separate.

The manifestations of diaphragmatic weakness vary depending on the etiology and whether the weakness is unilateral or bilateral. Unilateral diaphragmatic weakness is difficult to detect clinically. Normally, the chest and abdomen both expand on inspiration because of descent of the diaphragm. Disturbance of the normal pattern of chest wall and abdominal movements is referred to as paradoxical respiration. Abnormal paradoxical motion of the thorax and abdomen may indicate impending respiratory failure or diaphragm weakness. When bilateral paralysis of the diaphragm is present, the excursion of the costal margins is increased and the epigastrium does not bulge during inspiration. With severe diaphragmatic weakness, the abdomen may move inward with inspiration, a phenomenon known as

Table R.2. Indications for Assisted Ventilation

Progressively declining respiratory reserve
Vital capacity <20 mL/kg
Peak inspiratory pressure <30 cm H_2O
Peak expiratory pressure <40 cm H_2O
paO_2 <60 mm Hg
$paCO_2$ >50 mm Hg
Inadequate protection of airway

paradoxical abdominal movements. When the accessory muscles attempt to compensate for diaphragm weakness, they produce greater negative intrathoracic pressure on inspiration, sucking the chest inward with inspiration (Video Link R.1).

In patients with neuromuscular disease, paradoxical abdominal movements detect diaphragm weakness with a sensitivity of 95% and specificity of 70%, with a positive LR of 3.2.[8] Paradoxical inward abdominal movements on inspiration that worsen when supine strongly suggest severe diaphragm weakness. When supine, the diaphragm alone is responsible for the majority of the inspiratory effort. With bilateral diaphragmatic weakness, the vital capacity may decrease dramatically when supine (>30%), compared with the usual minimal drop.

Response, automatic: See **Stroop test.**

Rest test: See **ice pack test.**

Rest tremor: See **tremor, parkinsonian tremor, essential tremor.**

Retinal artery occlusion: Occlusion of a retinal artery, either the central retinal artery (CRAO) or a branch artery (BRAO). Examination in the early stages shows blockage of the involved artery; opaque, grayish white, edematous retina in its distribution; minor retinal hemorrhages; cotton wool spots, and obscuration of the features of the pigment epithelium and choroid. CRAO may produce a **cherry red spot**. The most common cause is atherosclerotic vascular disease, especially retinal emboli from disease of the carotid bifurcation. A **Hollenhorst plaque** or other type of embolic material may be visible. Other causes of retinal artery occlusion, especially BRAO, include vasculitis, such as giant cell arteritis; a hypercoagulable state; sickle cell disease; Susac's syndrome; antiphospholipid syndrome; fat emboli; and Behcet's disease.

Retinal lesions: The various lesions that may be apparent on fundoscopic examination and useful in the diagnosis of neurologic disorders. There are of course many types of retinal lesions, the ones most relevant in a neurologic context include the following. Retinal hamartomas are common in tuberous sclerosis, sometimes as the first objective sign of the disorder, and occur occasionally in NF1. Ophthalmoscopically, the appearance varies from relatively flat, smooth, semitranslucent lesions to large, elevated, nodular lesions resembling mulberries (Fig. R.2).

Hemangiomas and hemangioblastomas of the retina are a feature of von Hippel-Lindau disease (Fig. R.3). Retinal AVMs occur in Wyburn-Mason syndrome and many patients harbor cerebral AVMs in addition. Facial hemangiomas in the trigeminal distribution may also occur, ranging from subtle discoloration to large port wine nevi similar to those seen in Sturge-Weber disease.

Retinal vascular sheathing: An appearance of the retinal blood vessels, primarily the veins, with white or yellowish streaks running in parallel on either side of the vessel (Fig. R.4). Sheathing occurs in 5% to 10% of MS patients, possibly more. See **Table R.3** for other conditions associated with vascular sheathing or retinal vasculitis.[9] In some instances, the appearance of sheathing may be due to unusual light reflexes related to draping of the nerve fiber layer over otherwise normal retinal veins.

Although retinal periphlebitis clearly occurs in a substantial percentage of patients with MS, it is not clear that sheathing correlates with disease activity or severity. However, some studies suggest that the incidence of sheathing is higher than the 5% to 10% usually cited.[10] When these changes are observed in a patient with otherwise isolated optic neuritis, they may indicate that clinically evident demyelinating diseases is likely to develop within the next several years.

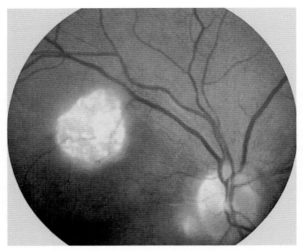

Figure R.2. Multiple retinal astrocytomas (astrocytic hamartomas) in a patient with tuberous sclerosis. Larger lesion is located just above center of macula, and small lesion is located just temporal to optic disc. (From Tasman W, Jaeger E. *The Wills Eye Hospital Atlas of Clinical Ophthalmology*. 2nd ed. Philadelphia, PA: Wolters Kluwer Health/Lippincott Williams & Wilkins; 2001, with permission.)

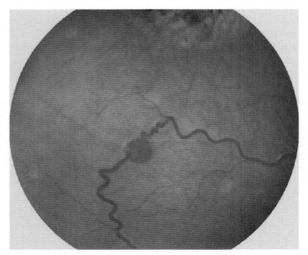

Figure R.3. Capillary hemangioma of retina (von Hippel tumor). Fundus photograph shows small red intraretinal tumor fed and drained by prominent dilated tortuous retinal blood vessels. Superior to the lesion is an area of chorioretinal atrophy subsequent to prior cryotherapy of another retinal capillary hemangioma. (From Tasman W, Jaeger E. *The Wills Eye Hospital Atlas of Clinical Ophthalmology*. 2nd ed. Philadelphia, PA: Wolters Kluwer Health/Lippincott Williams & Wilkins; 2001, with permission.)

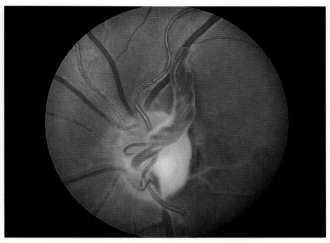

Figure R.4. Prepapillary arterial loop surrounded by a fibroglial sheath that is probably a remnant of Bergmeister's papilla. The optic disc is pale, and the cilioretinal artery is sheathed secondary to the effects of toxemia of pregnancy 15 years earlier. (From Tasman W, Jaeger E. *The Wills Eye Hospital Atlas of Clinical Ophthalmology*. 2nd ed. Philadelphia, PA: Wolters Kluwer Health/Lippincott Williams & Wilkins; 2001, with permission.)

Table R.3. Conditions Associated with Retinal Vascular Sheathing

Multiple sclerosis
Sarcoidosis
Behcet's disease
Amyloidosis
Diabetes
Sickle cell disease
Retinitis (e.g., toxoplasmosis, Lyme disease, HIV)
Hypertensive retinopathy
Retinitis pigmentosa
Unusual light reflexes in normals

Retinal vein pulsations: See **papilledema.**

Retinitis pigmentosa (pigmentary retinopathy): Retinal degeneration associated with abnormalities of the retinal pigment epithelium. RP occurs in several hereditary disorders associated with a primary abnormality of the photoreceptor–retinal pigment epithelium complex. The classic triad of retinitis pigmentosa is "bone-spicule" retinal pigmentation, arteriolar attenuation, and waxy pallor of the optic disc (Fig. R.5). Patients typically have prominent night blindness and impaired peripheral vision but well-preserved central visual acuity until late in the course. A ring **scotoma** is often present on VF examination. Some of the conditions associated with retinitis pigmentosa include Refsum's disease; abetalipoproteinemia (Bassen-Kornzweig syndrome); Friedreich's ataxia; neuronal ceroid lipofuscinosis; Kearns-Sayre syndrome; syphilis; NARP (neuropathy, ataxia, retinitis pigmentosa);

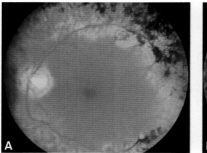 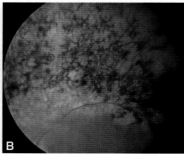

Figure R.5. A: Retinitis pigmentosa fundus photo demonstrating optic nerve waxy pallor, vascular attenuation, and midperipheral "bone spicule" pigmentary retinopathy. **B:** Higher magnification photograph of midperipheral "bone spicule" retinopathy. (From Nelson LB. *Pediatric Ophthalmology*. Philadelphia, PA: Wolters Kluwer Health/ Lippincott Williams & Wilkins; 2012, with permission.)

some lysosomal storage disorders, mitochondopathies, and spinocerebellar degenerations; and Usher's syndrome.

Retraction–convergence nystagmus: See **convergence retraction nystagmus.**

Retrocollis: See **cervical dystonia.**

Retropulsion: A tendency to lean or fall backward, often a manifestation of impaired **postural reflexes** in **parkinsonism**, especially in PSP. See **postural instability.** The **pull test** is one method to test for a tendency for retropulsion (see Video G.4).

Reverse Chaddock: See **Chaddock's sign.** The reverse Chaddock is the same in all respects except the stimulus moves from the small toe toward the heel.

Reverse Horner's syndrome: See **Horner's syndrome.**

Reverse jaw winking: See **inverse jaw winking.**

Reverse Marcus Gunn phenomenon: See **inverse jaw winking.**

Reverse ocular bobbing/dipping: See **ocular bobbing.**

Reverse straight leg raising test: See **femoral nerve stretch test, Ely's test.**

Revilliod's sign: Acquired inability to wink the eye, reportedly an early sign of corticobulbar tract dysfunction.

Rey-Osterreith test: A very complicated figure with multiple elements used in the **mental status examination** (Fig. R.6). The Rey-Osterreith complex figure (ROCF) is used to assess visuospatial abilities, visual perception, and visual organization, functions that largely depend on the right hemisphere. Executive functioning, particularly planning and organization, and nonverbal memory are also important in ROCF performance. One of the key features is the assessment of visual memory. The ROCF is used frequently in the evaluation of suspected dementia.[11] In patients with various types of dementia, ability to reproduce the ROCF correlates significantly with tests of working memory. Both the immediate copy and the delayed recall abilities are related to age.[12]

The Rey-Osterrieth figure is very complex and can bring out subtle constructional apraxia. Constructional tasks are particularly useful for differentiating psychiatric from neurologic disease. Impaired constructional ability is a sensitive indicator of lesions involving various parts of the brain, but in patients with psychiatric disease constructional ability is preserved.

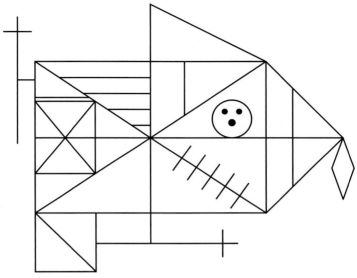

Figure R.6. The Rey-Osterrieth complex figure. (From Campbell WW. *DeJong's the Neurologic Examination.* 7th ed. Philadelphia, PA: Wolters Kluwer Health/Lippincott Williams & Wilkins; 2013, with permission.)

Rhinolalia: See **nasal speech.**
Rhinorrhea: See **cerebrospinal fluid rhinorrhea.**
Riddoch mass reflex: See **nociceptive reflex of Riddoch and Buzzard.**
Riddoch's phenomenon: See **akinetotopsia.**
Rigidity: A type of **hypertonia** creating an involuntary resistance to passive movement, seen primarily in extrapyramidal disorders. The relationship of the hypertonia to the speed of movement is a key feature distinguishing **spasticity** from rigidity. Rigidity is present to more or less the same degree regardless of the speed of the movement and throughout the range of motion of a limb. Spasticity is more apparent with fast than slow movements and is most marked near the middle of the range of motion.

Two forms occur commonly: cogwheel rigidity and lead pipe rigidity. In lead pipe (plastic) rigidity, there is smooth resistance throughout the range of movement with no variability related to the speed or direction of movement. Lead pipe rigidity occurs in **paratonia, gegenhalten, and decerebrate** and **decorticate rigidity**. Lead pipe rigidity, less so cogwheel rigidity, also occurs as a prominent feature of NMS and serotonin syndrome.

In cogwheel rigidity (**Negro's sign**), there is a ratchety, jerky, tremulous variation in the hypertonicity. As the part is manipulated, it seems to give way in a series of small steps as if the limb were attached to a heavy cogwheel or ratchet. The jerky quality of the resistance may be due to **tremor** superimposed on lead-pipe rigidity. The frequency of the jerkiness corresponds to the frequency of the postural tremor. Cogwheel rigidity possibly results from alterations in extrapyramidal regulation of supraspinal motor neurons, causing changes in the response of lower motor neurons to activation. Cogwheel rigidity is most commonly encountered in PD and other parkinsonian syndromes. It appears first in proximal muscles and then spreads distally. It may affect any muscle, but there is predominant involvement of neck and trunk muscles and the flexor muscles of the extremities. The rigidity on one side may be exaggerated by active movements of the contralateral limbs (**Froment's sign**). Poor relaxation in patients with other forms of tremor may also produce cogwheeling.

Ring scotoma: See **scotoma, retinitis pigmentosa.**

Rinne test: A bedside tuning fork test of hearing that compares air conduction (AC) and bone conduction (BC). The fork should be heard twice as long by AC as by BC. The Rinne test is normal or positive when AC is better than BC. In **conductive hearing loss**, BC is better than AC, and the Rinne is said to be negative. Sound is not conducted normally through the canal or from the tympanic membrane through the ossicular chain to the cochlea, but the sensorineural mechanisms are intact; AC is impaired but BC is preserved. In **sensorineural hearing loss**, both AC and BC are impaired while retaining their normal relationship of AC better than BC; the Rinne is positive or normal. Because of inconsistent use of the terms positive and negative, it is preferable to state that AC is better than BC or that the Rinne is normal (see Table C.5).

Risus sardonicus: The peculiar "smile" characteristic of Wilson's disease. The face has a fixed, forced grinning expression with the mouth open and the upper lip drawn back due to facial dystonia (Fig. R.7). In a series of 119 patients with Wilson's disease, risus sardonicus was present in 72%.[13] The term has also been used to describe the facial expression in cephalic tetanus and reported to occur in MSA.[14]

Rocket sign: The tendency of patients with PSP to launch themselves up from a chair, then fall backward into it because of **postural instability** due to impaired **postural reflexes**.[15]

Roger's sign: See **numb chin syndrome.**

Romberg (Brauch-Romberg) sign: A comparison of balance with eyes open and eyes closed, exploring for imbalance due to proprioceptive sensory loss.[16] When proprioception is disturbed, the patient may be able to stand with eyes open, but sways or falls with eyes closed (Video R.1). The Romberg is a sensitive **posterior column sign.** The patient stands with the feet as close together as will allow the maintenance of eyes open balance. A normal individual can stand feet together and eyes open without difficulty, although some allowance is necessary in the elderly. Normally, closing the eyes causes at most a transient and minor loss of balance. In patients with impaired proprioception, eye closure produces increased swaying or frank loss of balance with the necessity to take a step to regain it, and rarely a near fall.

The Romberg sign is often misunderstood and misinterpreted. The essential finding is a difference between standing balance with eyes open and closed. In order to test this function, the patient must have a stable stance eyes open and then demonstrate a decrease in balance with eyes closed, when visual input is eliminated and the patient must rely on proprioception to maintain balance. Romberg described this sign in patients with tabes dorsalis and thought it was pathognomonic. Romberg did not actually state that the feet should be placed together; that was a later addition. Nor did he comment on arm positioning. It is common practice to

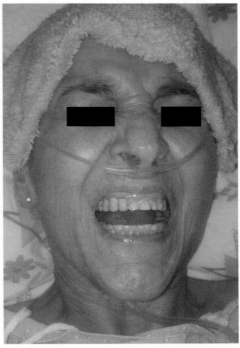

Figure R.7. Facial dystonia causing a fixed grimace in a patient with tetanus. (From Cohen R. Risus sardonicus. *Int J Infect Dis.* 2014;20:79, with permission.)

have the patient hold the arms outstretched in front, but this is in order to check simultaneously for **pronator drift** or to perform finger-to-nose testing; it is not what Romberg described. Some authorities recommend holding the arms at the sides, others crossing the arms on the chest. Whether arm position makes any difference in test sensitivity is unknown. Turning the head side to side eliminates vestibular clues and increases the reliance on proprioception (Ropper's[17] refined Romberg test). The critical observation is eyes-open versus eyes-closed stability. Inability to maintain balance with eyes open and feet together is not a positive Romberg.

There is some variability, even among expert examiners, in how the Romberg test is performed and interpreted. Many patients sway slightly with eyes closed, and minimal amounts of sway, especially in elderly patients, are seldom significant. Minor, normal swaying may stop if the patient is simply asked to stand perfectly still. Most clinicians discount sway at the hips and insist on seeing sway at the ankles before calling the test positive; some require the patient take a corrective step to the side; and some that the patient nearly fall. Some require the patient be barefoot. One definition of a positive Romberg is the inability to stand with feet together and eyes closed for 60 seconds. In one study, all the healthy controls and over half of those with cerebellar ataxia could stand for 60 seconds, but half the sensory ataxia patients could only stand for 10 seconds.[8]

The "sharpened" or tandem Romberg (von Stein test) is done by having the patient stand in tandem position with eyes open and closed; the limits of normality for this variation are conjectural. In relatively young patients with a low likelihood of neurological disease, a quick and effective substitute for the Romberg is simply to have the patient close the eyes while walking tandem. This is a difficult maneuver and has high value as a screening test. In one study, this "walking Romberg" was more sensitive than the standard Romberg.[18]

The Romberg sign is used as a test of proprioceptive, not cerebellar, function. The pioneering 19th-century clinicians thought it was particularly useful in separating tabes dorsalis from cerebellar disease. In fact, patients with cerebellar disease, particularly disorders of the vestibulocerebellum or spinocerebellum, may have some increase in instability with eyes closed, but not usually to the degree seen with impaired proprioception. Patients with cerebellar disease, or those with severe weakness, may not have a stable base eyes open. It may help to have the patient widen stance to the point of stability eyes open, then close the eyes, and check for any difference. Only a marked worsening of balance with eyes closed qualifies as a positive Romberg sign. Some histrionic patients will sway with eyes closed in the absence of any organic neurological impairment (**false Rombergism**).

The Romberg is also useful in the evaluation of vestibular disease. In unilateral vestibulopathy, if balance is lost with eyes closed the patient will tend to fall toward the side of the less active labyrinth, usually the side of the lesion, as the normal contralateral vestibular system pushes him over. If the patient has spontaneous nystagmus due to a vestibular lesion, the fall will be in the direction of the slow phase. In peripheral vestibular disease, the direction of the fall can be affected by changing head position; the patient will fall toward the abnormal ear. With a right vestibulopathy and facing straight ahead, eye closure will cause the patient to fall to the right; looking over his right shoulder, he will fall backward; and looking over his left shoulder, he will fall forward.

Roos test: See **Elevated Arm Stress Test.**

Rooting (root, searching) reflex: A **primitive reflex** or **frontal release sign.** The lips, mouth, and even head deviate toward a tactile stimulus delivered beside in the mouth or on the cheek. A grossly exaggerated response may include automatic opening of the mouth, smacking, chewing, and even swallowing movements, even when the object fails to touch the lips but is only brought near them.

Rosenbach's sign: A fine tremor of the eyelids; may occur in hyperthyroidism.

Rossolimo's sign: An abnormal plantar muscle reflex seen in CST disease, consisting of contraction of the toe flexors elicited by tapping the ball of the foot, or the plantar surfaces of the toes. The response is quick plantar flexion of the toes, especially the smaller ones; in normals, there is no movement or slight dorsiflexion of toes. Many variations have been described elicited by striking slightly different parts of the foot. See **pathologic reflexes.**

Rotatory nystagmus: The pattern characteristic of **vestibular nystagmus.** The nystagmus vectors occur in multiple directions simultaneously because of the influence of the three different semicircular canals, producing a torsional or rotational component not often seen with other types of nystagmus.

Rubral (Holmes, cerebellar outflow, midbrain) tremor: A severe, large-amplitude, relatively slow (2–5 Hz) tremor, involving both proximal and distal muscles, present at rest but made worse with action. The clinical picture resembles a combination of **parkinsonian tremor** and **cerebellar tremor**. It may be unilateral and is usually due to stroke or trauma. Formerly thought to result from an abnormality of the red nucleus, it is now believed to be due to a lesion involving cerebellar efferent and nigrostriatal fibers coursing through the midbrain.

Rust's sign: A sign most typically seen with cervical spine injuries in which the patient holds his head in his hands to provide support and stability. Patients with neck extensor weakness, such as from MG or ALS may also hold their head in their hands; see **dropped head**.

Video Link

R.1. Paradoxical respiration in a patient with ALS. Available at: https://www.youtube.com/watch?v=fdaB6VWNi6A

References

1. Lees AJ. Odd and unusual movement disorders. *J Neurol Neurosurg Psychiatry.* 2002;72(suppl 1): I17–I21.
2. Catena M, Fagiolini A, Consoli G, et al. The rabbit syndrome: state of the art. *Curr Clin Pharmacol.* 2007;2:212–216.
3. Beh SC, Frohman T, Frohman EM. The menagerie of neurology: animal signs and the refinement of clinical acumen. *Neurol Clin Pract.* 2014;4:e1–e9.
4. Diener HC, Dichgans J. Pathophysiology of cerebellar ataxia. *Mov Disord.* 1992;7:95–109.
5. Impallomeni M, Kenny RA, Flynn MD, et al. The elderly and their ankle jerks. *Lancet.* 1984;1:670–672.
6. Gregory JE, Wood SA, Proske U. An investigation into mechanisms of reflex reinforcement by the Jendrassik manoeuvre. *Exp Brain Res.* 2001;138:366–374.
7. Hilton-Jones D, Turner MR. *Oxford Textbook of Neuromuscular Disorders.* Oxford, UK: Oxford University Press; 2014.
8. McGee S. *Evidence Based Physical Diagnosis.* 3rd ed. Philadelphia, PA: Elsevier/Saunders; 2012.
9. Vine AK. Retinal vasculitis. *Semin Neurol.* 1994;14:354–360.
10. Birch MK, Barbosa S, Blumhardt LD, et al. Retinal venous sheathing and the blood-retinal barrier in multiple sclerosis. *Arch Ophthalmol.* 1996;114:34–39.
11. Cherrier MM, Mendez MF, Dave M, et al. Performance on the Rey-Osterrieth Complex Figure Test in Alzheimer disease and vascular dementia. *Neuropsychiatry Neuropsychol Behav Neurol.* 1999;12:95–101.
12. Luzzi S, Pesallaccia M, Fabi K, et al. Non-verbal memory measured by Rey-Osterrieth Complex Figure B: normative data. *Neurol Sci.* 2011;32:1081–1089.
13. Machado A, Chien HF, Deguti MM, et al. Neurological manifestations in Wilson's disease: report of 119 cases. *Mov Disord.* 2006;21:2192–2196.
14. Wenning GK, Geser F, Poewe W. The "risus sardonicus" of multiple system atrophy. *Mov Disord.* 2003;18:1211.
15. Rehman HU. Progressive supranuclear palsy. *Postgrad Med J.* 2000;76:333–336.
16. Lanska DJ, Goetz CG. Romberg's sign: development, adoption, and adaptation in the 19th century. *Neurology.* 2000;55:1201–1206.
17. Ropper AH. Refined Romberg test. *Can J Neurol Sci.* 1985;12:282.
18. Findlay GF, Balain B, Trivedi JM, et al. Does walking change the Romberg sign? *Eur Spine J.* 2009;18:1528–1531.

Saccadic dysmetria: See **ocular dysmetria.**

Saccadic intrusions (fixation instability): Brief, involuntary, spontaneous, conjugate interruptions of steady fixation that move the eyes away from a fixation target, followed by a quick return.[1,2] Some intrusions may be more apparent when viewing the fundus. While saccadic intrusions can occur in normals, especially the elderly, they are usually a sign of brainstem or cerebellar disease. The pathology often involves the fastigial nuclei. Movements included as saccadic intrusions are square-wave jerks, macro square-wave jerks, macrosaccadic oscillations, ocular flutter, and opsoclonus. Distinguishing saccadic intrusions from nystagmus is difficult clinically; eye movement recordings are often required to make the distinction and the movements are named for their appearance on such recordings. In saccadic intrusions, the initial movement away from primary position is at saccadic velocity, in contrast to nystagmus, where the initial movement is slow. Both are then followed by a quick corrective saccade back to fixation.

Saccadic intrusions may occur normally but are increased in certain disease states. Square-wave jerks occur normally, producing saccadic movements of <2 degrees followed by a return to fixation after an interval of 200 to 400 ms, occurring at a rate of <10 per minute. Square-wave jerks are not visible to the naked eye. They can be a feature of some spinocerebellar ataxias, and also occur in extrapyramidal disorders, especially PSP. Macro square-wave jerks have the same general characteristics as square-wave jerks, but the amplitude is greater, usually >5 degrees. These have been reported in MS and MSA. Macrosaccadic oscillations are repetitive hypermetric saccades with overshoot of the target in each direction, which may cause continuous to-and-fro movements about the target. Macrosaccadic oscillations occur in diseases affecting the cerebellar fastigial nuclei or their outputs.

Ocular flutter and opsoclonus differ from the other types of saccadic intrusions because there is no pause between movements, creating back-to-back saccades with no intersaccadic interval. Flutter and opsoclonus cause rapid, usually high amplitude, to and fro oscillations that are clinically striking. In ocular flutter, the movements are horizontal. In opsoclonus, the movements occur at all directions: horizontal, vertical, and torsional **(Video Links S.1 and S.2)**.[3,4]

Ocular flutter and opsoclonus are a continuum. Flutter causes intermittent, rapid, back-to-back horizontal saccades producing a quivering or shimmering movement. The pathology involves the cerebellum or brainstem cerebellar connections, particularly the dentate nucleus. In opsoclonus, there are continuous, involuntary, random, chaotic saccades in any direction (saccadomania, dancing eyes, lightning eye movements). The etiology in children is often occult neuroblastoma (dancing eyes–dancing feet; opsoclonus–myoclonus syndrome, Kinsbourne syndrome). The etiology in adults may be paraneoplastic, usually occult lung or breast carcinoma with anti-Ri antibodies; encephalitis, typically parainfectious; or cerebellar disease. Both flutter and opsoclonus may occur due to systemic illness, such as hyperosmolar coma or viral hepatitis, or as an effect of drugs or toxins.

Saccadic lateropulsion: A disorder of saccadic movement seen primarily in Wallenberg's lateral medullary syndrome. The movements are analogous to those seen with past pointing of the limbs due to vestibulopathy. Involvement of the vestibular nuclei on the side of the infarction produces vestibular imbalance, so that the intact vestibular apparatus on the opposite side causes the eyes to deviate toward the side of the lesion.[5] This is responsible for the nystagmus that is usually present, which beats with the fast component away from the side of the lesion. The effects of the vestibular imbalance are also seen when the patient makes horizontal and vertical saccades. Because of the added vestibular input horizontal saccades ipsilateral to the lesion are hypermetric and those contralateral to the lesion are hypometric. Vertical saccades are also affected, so that attempted vertical eye movements veer ipsilaterally and the movements are oblique rather than vertical.

In Wallenberg's syndrome, there is ipsipulsion toward the side of the lesion. Saccadic contrapulsion away from the side of the lesion has been reported in disorders of the rostral cerebellum, such as infarction in the distribution of the superior cerebellar artery.[6]

Saccadic pursuit (cogwheel eye movements): A condition in which pursuit eye movements, normally smooth, are disrupted by superimposed saccades, creating ratchety or jerky movements. The finding is nonspecific and can occur bilaterally with fatigue, inattention, decreased consciousness, basal ganglia disorders, diffuse hemispheric disease, drug effects, or if the target velocity is too fast **(Video Link S.3)**.[7]

Saccadomania: See **opsoclonus.**

Sacral sparing: Preservation of sensation in a saddle distribution in the face of sensory loss otherwise present below a certain spinal level. The lateral spinothalamic tract is somatotopically organized. Lowermost, sacral and lumbar, fibers entering first are displaced progressively more laterally by subsequently entering fibers. As the tract ascends the sacral fibers come to lie most lateral and superficial, nearer to the surface of the cord, with cervical fibers most medial. Since the sacral fibers lie most laterally, an intramedullary spinal cord lesion, such as a neoplasm, may produce sacral sparing. A spinal cord level with "sacral sparing" suggests intraparenchymal spinal cord pathology rather than a myelopathy due to external pressure.

Sacroiliac joint signs: Maneuvers that reproduce sacroiliac joint pain, primarily by extending the hip. SI joint pain has been defined as pain localized in the region of the SI joint, reproducible by stress and provocation tests and relieved by anesthetic injection. SI joint disease can cause pain in the lower back, buttock and posterior thigh that may mimic radicular pain. By some estimates, the prevalence of SI joint pain among patients with axial low back pain may be as high as 30%.[8] Many different methods have been described for evaluation of the SI joints by bedside examination.[9,10] In Gaenslen's test, the patient clutches one knee to the chest to stabilize the pelvis, then extends the leg to be tested. The test may be done with the patient lying on one side and the examiner forcefully pulling the test leg backward. Alternatively the patient may lie supine with the buttock on the side to be tested partially off the table, allowing the leg to drop toward the floor **(Fig. S.1)**. Reproduction of pain suggests SI joint disease. Another variation is to perform the test with the patient standing on one leg and leaning backwards, which additionally stresses the facet joints and pars interarticularis. Pain with this maneuver may also indicate spondylolysis or spondylolisthesis. Another variant is Yeoman's sign,

S

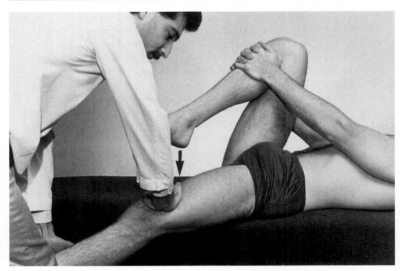

Figure S.1. Gaenslen's test. Flexion of one thigh stabilizes the pelvis, dropping the other leg off the examination table stresses the sacroiliac joint and reproduces the pain in SI joint disease. (From Cipriano JJ. *Photographic Manual of Regional Orthopaedic and Neurological Tests.* 4th ed. Philadelphia, PA: Wolters Kluwer Health/Lippincott Williams & Wilkins; 2003, with permission.)

passive extension of the hip with the patient prone and the knee flexed. This movement is similar to the **femoral nerve stretch test** and **Ely's sign**. All of these involve hip extension and may provoke pain of SI joint origin.

Pain from the SI joint may also occur with simultaneous downward pressure in the region of the anterior superior iliac spines with the patient supine. The pressure may be directed medially (squish test) or laterally with crossed-arms (sacroiliac stretch or gapping test). With the patient side-lying, downward pressure on the iliac crest may cause pain (approximation or compression test). For the sacroiliac rocking test, the patient lies supine and the examiner flexes the knee and hip, forces the knee toward the opposite shoulder and moves back and forth. For the sacral thrust test, with the patient prone the examiner presses downward over the sacrum. Another provocative maneuver is resisted abduction of the hip in the side lying position. This is essentially the same as the **Pace test** and other maneuvers used to diagnose piriformis syndrome, and the pain that might be produced is in the same general location. Pain arising from the SI joint may also increase with the **FABER test**. With all of these, only reproduction of the patient's pain is significant, as nonspecific discomfort can occur. In the Fortin finger test, the patient points to the exact site of pain. Pointing to the posterior superior iliac spine or within 2 cm of it, correlates well with relief of pain by SI joint anesthetic injection and with other evidence of SI joint disease.[11,12]

Saddle anesthesia: The reverse of **sacral sparing**, saddle anesthesia is sensory loss restricted to the buttocks, perineum and inner thighs; the area deliberately anesthetized in an obstetric "saddle block." Saddle anesthesia occurs most commonly with lesions involving the cauda equina or conus medullaris.

Saddle nose: Depression of the bridge of the nose. Saddle nose is a classical sign of congenital neurosyphilis (Fig. S.2). The deformity may also result from trauma, e.g., boxing, Wegener's granulomatosis, relapsing polychondritis, and cocaine abuse.

Scalloped pupils: See Table P.1.

Scalp rugae: An increase in the folds and ridging of the scalp. May occur as a feature of hereditary brachial plexopathy (see Fig. H.24).

Scanning speech: See **dysarthria.**

Scaphocephaly: See **craniosynostosis.**

Scapular winging: Elevation of the scapula away from the chest wall during movement of the arm. Normally, the medial border of the scapula remains close to the chest wall when the arms are raised. However, with weakness of either the serratus anterior or the trapezius, the vertebral border or the entire scapula protrudes posteriorly, away from the thoracic wall. This causes the deformity known as "winging" (Fig. S.3).

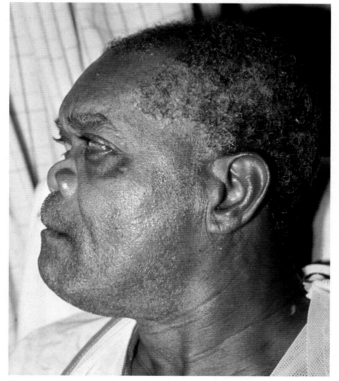

Figure S.2. Saddle nose deformity in a patient with congenital syphilis.

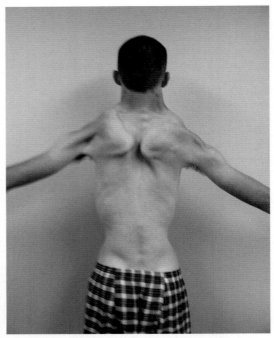

Figure S.3. A patient with facioscapulohumeral muscular dystrophy, showing atrophy of the muscles of the shoulders and upper arms and pronounced scapular winging. (From Campbell WW. *DeJong's the Neurologic Examination.* 7th ed. Philadelphia, PA: Wolters Kluwer Health/Lippincott Williams & Wilkins; 2013, with permission.)

The serratus anterior is primarily a protractor of the scapula and functions during forward arm elevation. When the serratus is weak, the inferior angle is shifted medially and the entire vertebral border rides up from the chest wall **(Video Link S.4)**. Serratus anterior weakness causes winging that is more obvious when trying to elevate the arm in front, in the sagittal plane of the body; it is less obvious when the arms are abducted to the sides. This difference aids in differentiating serratus anterior winging (as from a long thoracic nerve palsy) from the flaring of the scapula that occurs with trapezius weakness (as from a spinal accessory nerve palsy). The trapezius is a rotator and retractor of the scapula and functions primarily during abduction of the arm to the side in the coronal plane of the body. When the trapezius is weak, scapular winging is more apparent on attempted abduction of the arm than on forward elevation. Trapezius winging may be made more conspicuous by having the patient bend forward at the waist so the upper body is parallel to the ground, then raise the arms to the sides, as if beginning a swan dive. This requires strong action by the trapezius to retract the scapula and accentuates the posterior displacement of the shoulder girdle. With winging due to trapezius weakness, the jutting of the inferior angle lessens when the arm is raised anteriorly; in winging due to serratus anterior weakness, it worsens.

Serratus winging may be accentuated by having the patient protract the scapula by pushing forward against resistance. The traditional provocative test is pushing against a wall. Another method to bring out mild serratus winging is to have the patient slowly lower the outstretched arms. This downward movement may exacerbate the winging, and at a certain point as the arms descend the scapula will suddenly snap backward. In the muscular dystrophies, particularly facioscapulohumeral (FSH) dystrophy, there is often weakness of all the shoulder girdle muscles, with prominent scapular winging, typically bilateral.

Schaefer's sign: (1) A **minor extensor toe sign** (see Table M.3); (2) an upper extremity **pathological reflex** in which pinching the flexor tendons at wrist causes adduction and flexion of thumb, sometimes with flexion of adjacent digits, more rarely with extension of little finger, the same response as the **Marie-Foix sign** and very similar to Wartenberg's thumb adduction sign (see **Wartenberg's signs**).

Schirmer's test: A quantitative test of tear production used in the evaluation of **xerophthalmia**. Commercially available filter strips are placed in the inferior conjunctival sac and left in place for 5 minutes. The advancing edge of moisture down the strip is proportional to the moisture in the eye; the results are expressed in millimeters. This test is simple and does not require referral to an ophthalmologist. Normal wetting is 10 to 25 mm, 5 to 10 mm is borderline and <5 mm is abnormal. A modification uses the wetting in 1 minute × 3 to approximate the wetting in 5 minutes. Ophthalmologists can evaluate tear production by the lacrimal glands in a number of ways.

Schnabel's cavernous optic atrophy: See **optic atrophy.**

Schwabach test: A method of assessing hearing in which the examiner with good hearing compares the patient's hearing with his or her own. A tuning fork is placed over the patient's mastoid and when the tone disappears the examiner places the fork on his own mastoid. If the examiner has normal hearing there is no difference. With sensorineural hearing loss, the examiner continues to hear the fork after the patient can no longer hear it. With conductive loss, the patient may hear the fork longer than the examiner can. Because of its limitations the test is seldom used.

Sciatic scoliosis (sciatic list): The tendency of patients with acute lumbosacral radiculopathy to lean toward one side. Most often the patient leans away from the symptomatic side to gain some pain relief. In the past, it was believed that patients might lean toward or away from the side of the lesion depending upon whether the disc herniation was medial or lateral to the nerve root, but these rules have not proven useful. Bending forward may make sciatic scoliosis more obvious while recumbency lessens it. Worsening of the curve with flexion and disappearance with recumbency differentiate sciatic from fixed structural scoliosis.

The patient with acute sciatica tends to adopt a slightly flexed posture when standing, and has a flat lumbar lordosis. The hip and knee on the symptomatic side are often held in slight flexion to take tension off the nerve root. Sometimes the patient will stand on tiptoe because putting the heel down exacerbates the pain (see **Bragard's sign, Minor's sign**).

Scissoring: See **gait disorders.**

Scleral show: Persistent visibility of sclera with the eye in full abduction or adduction. Patients can normally "bury the limbus" with both eyes in full lateral gaze in each direction, somewhat better on adduction than abduction. In full lateral gaze, the temporal limbus abuts the lateral canthus; in full medial gaze, about the inner third of the nasal limbus is buried. A small rim of sclera showing on extreme abduction is not abnormal. Normally, the amount of scleral show on abduction is symmetric in the two eyes. Greater scleral show on full abduction in one eye than the other is a subtle sign of abduction impairment.

Scoliosis: Lateral curvature of the spine (Fig. S.4). Idiopathic thoracic scoliosis is present in up to 5% of school-aged children and adolescents. Scoliosis is a feature of or is associated with a number of conditions of neurological relevance, including: Chiari malformation, Klippel-Feil deformity, syringomyelia, muscular dystrophy, congenital myopathy, spinal muscular atrophy, spinocerebellar degeneration

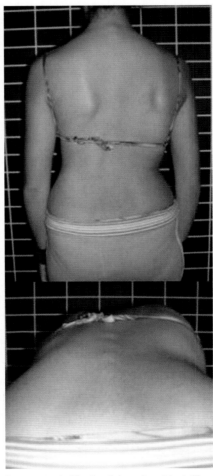

Figure S.4. Scoliosis accentuated by the Adams bend test. (From Rigo M, Negrini S, Weiss HR, et al. SOSORT consensus paper on brace action: TLSO biomechanics of correction (investigating the rationale for force vector selection). *Scoliosis* 2006;1:11.)

(especially Friedreich's ataxia), hereditary neuropathy, osteogenesis imperfecta, and spinal cord tumor.

Subtle scoliosis is often difficult to appreciate with the patient erect, but bending forward may disclose an asymmetry in the contour of the chest and make spinal curvature more obvious. The Adams bend test is carried out by having the patient bend forward with the examiner observing from behind. Other signs of scoliosis include elevation of one shoulder or scapula, prominence of one scapula, an asymmetrical waist or a greater gap between the arm and the thorax on one side. Many patients also have **kyphosis**. Severe scoliosis may cause a slowly progressive thoracic myelopathy. Functional scoliosis of the lumbosacral spine may occur in patients with lumbosacral radiculopathy, see **sciatic scoliosis**. Functional scoliosis disappears with recumbency but fixed scoliosis does not.

Scotoma: An area of impaired vision in the visual field, with normal surrounding vision. There are many types of scotomas. With an absolute scotoma, there is no visual function; with a relative scotoma, visual function is depressed but not absent. A positive scotoma causes blackness or a sense of blockage of vision, as though an object were interposed; it suggests disease of the retina, especially the macula or choroid. A negative scotoma is an absence of vision, a blank spot as if part of the field had been erased; it suggests optic nerve disease but can occur with lesions more posteriorly.

Scotomas are described by their location or their shape. A central scotoma involves the fixation point and is seen in macular or optic nerve disease, such as optic neuritis **(Fig. S.5A)**. A paracentral scotoma involves the areas adjacent to the fixation point. A cecocentral scotoma extends from the blind spot to fixation, and strongly suggests optic nerve disease **(Fig. S.5B)**. Any scotoma involving the blind spot implies optic neuropathy.

An arcuate scotoma is a crescent defect arching out of the blind spot, usually due to glaucoma, less often due to optic neuropathy, with the brunt of damage falling on the fibers forming the superior and inferior nerve fiber layer arcades **(Fig. S.6)**. A junctional scotoma (syndrome of Traquair) is caused by a lesion (usually a mass) located at the junction of one optic nerve with the optic chiasm. The junctional scotoma is an optic nerve defect in one eye (central, paracentral, or cecocentral scotoma) and a superior temporal defect in the opposite eye **(Fig. S.5C)**. A ring scotoma is visual field attenuation in the midportion of the visual field with relative preservation centrally and peripherally; it is the characteristic field defect in **retinitis pigmentosa** (Fig. S.7).

Although scotomas most often result from disease of the retina or optic nerve, they may also be caused by cerebral lesions. Other types of scotomas occur from primary ocular disease, such as retinitis, chorioretinitis, and glaucoma, which are not related directly to disease of the nervous system. Subjective scotomas cannot be delineated in the visual field examination. Subjective scotomas include the scintillating scotomas of migraine, and the annoying but harmless vitreous floaters that many normal individuals experience.

Scratch collapse test: A maneuver touted as useful in the diagnosis of CTS and UNE. To perform the test, the examiner stands facing the patient, who stands with the elbows at the sides and flexed 90 degrees with the wrists neutral. The examiner compares the power of external rotation at the shoulder simultaneously in both arms by pressing inwardly on the wrists. The examiner then scratches or rubs over

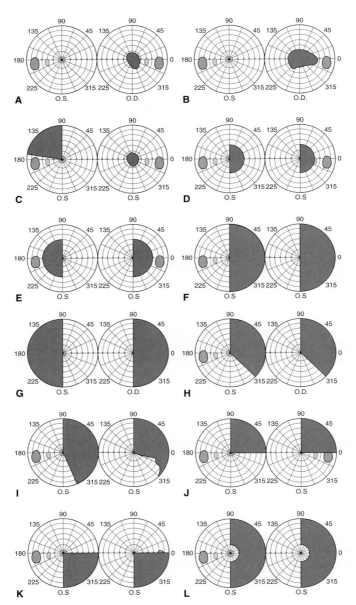

Figure S.5. Types of visual field defects. **A:** Central scotoma. **B:** Cecocentral scotoma. **C:** Junctional scotoma. **D:** Homonymous scotomas. **E:** Heteronymous scotomas. **F:** Right homonymous hemianopia. **G:** Bitemporal hemianopia. **H:** Congruous right homonymous hemianopia. **I:** Incongruous right homonymous hemianopia. **J:** Right superior quadrantopia ("pie in the sky"). **K:** Right inferior quadrantopia. **L:** Macular-sparing right homonymous hemianopia. (From Campbell WW. *DeJong's the Neurologic Examination.* 7th ed. Philadelphia, PA: Wolters Kluwer Health/Lippincott Williams & Wilkins; 2013, with permission.)

Central 24-2 Threshold Test

Fixation Monitor: Gaze/Blind Spot	Stimulus: III, White	Pupil Diameter: 5.1 mm	Date: 03-08-2011
Fixation Target: Central	Background: 31.5 ASB	Visual Acuity:	Time: 12:48 PM
Fixation Losses: 2/17	Strategy: SITA-Standard	RX: + 1.75 DS DC X	Age: 70

False POS Errors: 5%
False NEG Errors: 2%
Test Duration: 07:01

Fovea: OFF

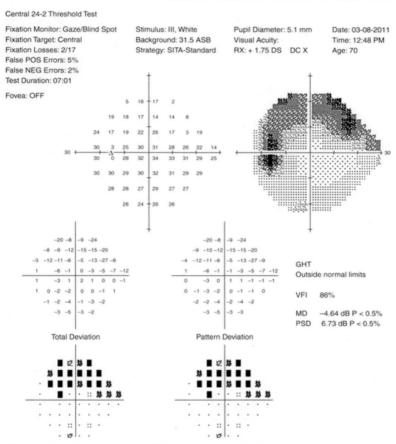

GHT
Outside normal limits

VFI   86%

MD   −4.64 dB P < 0.5%
PSD   6.73 dB P < 0.5%

Total Deviation

Pattern Deviation

Figure S.6. Humphrey visual field examination showing a supero-nasal arcuate scotoma. (From Gerstenblith AT, Rabinowitz MP. *The Wills Eye Manual: Office and Emergency Room Diagnosis and Treatment of Eye Disease.* 6th ed. Philadelphia, PA: Wolters Kluwer Health/Lippincott Williams & Wilkins; 2012, with permission.)

the median nerves at the wrist bilaterally, then again immediately attempts to force the shoulders into internal rotation by pressing on the wrists as the patient resists. If the arm collapses inwardly on one side, this is said to indicate that the patient has CTS on that side. Proponents claim this abrupt loss of external rotation power may also follow scratching of the ulnar nerve at the elbow in patients with ulnar neuropathy.

The rationale behind this test is not apparent. When studied in a blinded fashion for the diagnosis of CTS, the scratch collapse test had a sensitivity of about 30%, less than random chance, and significantly worse than the other **carpal tunnel syndrome provocative tests**, which have also been shown to be of little use.[13,14]

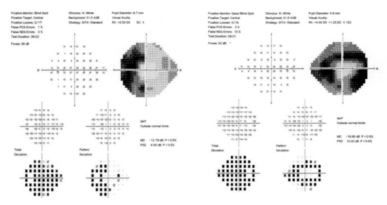

Figure S.7. Humphrey 24-2 visual field test showing generalized depression as well as a full ring scotoma in the right eye and a partial ring scotoma in the left eye. (From Garg SJ. *Uveitis*. Philadelphia, PA: Wolters Kluwer Health/Lippincott Williams & Wilkins; 2012, with permission.)

Scrotal (fissured) tongue: A relatively common condition in which prominent fissures or grooves are present on the dorsal surface of the tongue, creating an appearance resembling the rugae of the scrotum (Fig. S.8). The condition is asymptomatic, but it may occur in association with certain diseases. A scrotal or **geographic tongue** is a feature of Melkersson-Rosenthal syndrome, a cause of recurrent facial paralysis. Scrotal tongue may also occur in Down's syndrome.

Scrotal reflex: A slow, writhing, vermicular contraction of the scrotal skin on stroking the perineum or thigh or applying a cold object to the scrotum. Not to be

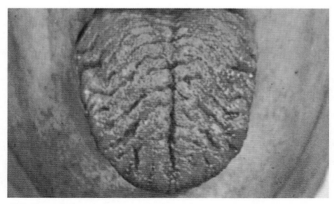

Figure S.8. Scrotal tongue. Furrows or grooves in the tongue create rugae resembling those of the scrotum. A fissured tongue usually has little significance but may be associated with certain diseases. (From Robinson HBG, Miller AS. *Colby, Kerr, and Robinson's Color Atlas of Oral Pathology*. Philadelphia, PA: JB Lippincott; 1990, with permission.)

confused with the **cremasteric reflex,** which is a quick retraction movement of the testicle.

Secondary deviation: See **strabismus.**

Seesaw nystagmus: See **nystagmus.**

Segmental dystonia: See **dystonia.**

Self-grasping: Seen in patients who have active grasp responses, one hand grasps the contralateral forearm. When this sign is present unilaterally it suggests a contralateral frontal or parietal lobe lesion. When it occurs bilaterally, there is no localizing value.

Semantic fluency: See **category fluency.**

Semantic memory: See **memory.**

Semantic paraphasia: See **paraphasia.**

Semimembranosus/semitendinosus reflex: See **hamstring reflexes.**

Senile gait: See **gait disorders.**

Senile ptosis: See **ptosis.**

Senile tremor: See **essential tremor.**

Sensorineural hearing loss (SNHL): Impaired hearing due to disease of the cochlea (e.g., Ménière's disease, Susac's syndrome, syphilis) or eighth cranial nerve (e.g., acoustic neuroma). As a generality, **conductive hearing loss** (CHL) affects low frequencies and SNHL affects high frequencies. Ménière's disease is a notable exception, causing predominantly low-frequency hearing loss, at least early in the course. Despite its disability for the patient, high-frequency SNHL of the type associated with presbycusis and acoustic trauma is not generally of neurologic significance; the use of high-pitched sounds, such as a ticking watch, seldom provides useful information for neurological examination purposes. Only a few conditions of neurologic importance cause bilaterally symmetric hearing loss (e.g., mitochondropathies, adrenoleukodystrophy, Refsum's disease and a few other, primarily hereditary, disorders), and an examination designed to detect auditory asymmetry usually suffices. Useful sounds for bedside testing include whispered voice, finger rub, and pure tones created by a tuning fork. For detecting significant hearing loss, the whispered voice test has a positive LR of 6.0 and the inability to hear a faint finger rub a positive LR of 3.9.[15] How useful tuning fork tests are for general screening has been questioned. But the primary usefulness of the **Weber** and **Rinne tests** is not as a screening tool but to make an initial differentiation between SNHL and CHL in a patient complaining of unilateral symptoms of hearing loss or tinnitus (see Table C.5).

Sensory ataxia: See **ataxia, cortical sensory loss, finger-to-nose test, parietal drift.**

Sensory trick: See **geste antagoniste.**

Sensory wandering: See **parietal drift.**

Serpentine tongue: A dyskinesia producing incessant writhing movements.

Setting sun sign: Sustained downgaze with retracted eyelids; usually seen in children with obstructive **hydrocephalus** ballooning the posterior third ventricle and rostral aqueduct, creating mass effect on the upper dorsal midbrain. The downward **gaze deviation** is a corollary of an **upgaze palsy** related to Parinaud's syndrome (see Fig. H.16). The upgaze paresis is so severe that the eyes are forced into sustained downgaze with **eyelid retraction.** See **Collier's sign.**

Shagreen patch: One of cutaneous manifestations of tuberous sclerosis (Fig. S.9).[16] Shagreen patches are relatively uncommon. The lesions occur most often over the

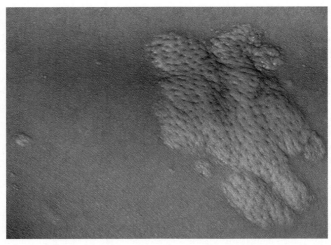

Figure S.9. Tuberous sclerosis with peau d'orange-appearing plaque (shagreen patch). (From Burkhart CN, Morrell D. *VisualDx: Essential Pediatric Dermatology.* Philadelphia, PA: Wolters Kluwer Health/Lippincott Williams & Wilkins; 2010, with permission.)

lumbosacral region and are skin-colored, soft plaques with prominent folliculi creating a **peau d' orange** appearance that may be solitary or multiple and of variable size up to several inches. The name is a French term derived from the resemblance to a type of rough, pock-marked leather. See **adenoma sebaceum, hypomelanotic macule, periungual fibroma, poliosis.**

Shaky legs syndrome: See **orthostatic tremor.**

Shawl sign: See **dermatomyositis skin changes.**

Sheathing: See **retinal vascular sheathing.**

Short neck: An abnormally short neck, often accompanied by a low hairline. A short neck is seen in a number of conditions, such as platybasia, basilar invagination, Klippel-Feil syndrome, Chiari malformation, Turner's syndrome and C1–C2 anomalies, such as congenital atlantoaxial dislocation.

Short stature: A feature of many congenital dysmorphic syndromes. Some of the conditions in which short stature occurs in association with prominent involvement of the nervous system include several of the mitochondrial orders, especially MERRF, MELAS, and Kearns-Sayre syndrome; Schwartz-Jampel syndrome; Refsum's disease; Andersen-Tawil syndrome; Marinesco-Sjögren syndrome; Niemann-Pick disease; CADASIL; hereditary neuralgic amyotrophy and Prader-Willi syndrome.

Short-term memory: See **memory.**

Shoulder abduction sign: See **Bakody's sign.**

Shoulder enlargement, painless: Neuropathic shoulder joint, evidence of syringomyelia.[17]

Shoulder examination tests: Maneuvers useful in the examination of patients with neck, shoulder and arm pain. Patients with shoulder disease occasionally present to the neurologist because the symptoms are confused with those of cervical radic-ulopathy. Common shoulder conditions include subacromial bursitis, biceps ten-donitis, rotator cuff disease, impingement syndrome, adhesive capsulitis, calcific tendinitis, glenohumeral arthritis, and tears of the glenoid labrum are all common causes of shoulder pain. At least a rudimentary shoulder examination should be part of the skill set of the neurologist in order to avoid diagnostic errors and un-necessary testing.

The Apley scratch test is a convenient way to assess active ROM of the shoulder, a useful screen for shoulder pathology (Video S.1). The patient makes three moves as if to scratch: (a) reaching to the opposite shoulder to touch it from the front, (b) from behind the neck as if to touch the upper vertebral border of the opposite scapula, and (c) from behind the lower back as if to touch the lower tip of the opposite scapula (Fig. S.10; Videos S.1 and S.2). The latter two can be combined by having the patient try to touch the fingertips together in the interscapular space, one hand from above and the other from below. Conditions that may cause a positive test include rotator cuff disease, subdeltoid bursitis and acromioclavicular or glenohumeral joint abnormalities. The Apley scratch maneu-ver is a good test of global shoulder joint function, but is more a general range of motion screen than a specific test for any particular condition.[18]

The tendons of four muscles, the supraspinatus, infraspinatus, subscapularis, and teres minor, converge to form a common tendon that covers the top, front, and back of the humeral head. The actions of these rotator cuff muscles abduct the hu-merus and rotate it internally and externally. The rotator cuff tendons are prone to develop degenerative changes. The changes range from inflammation and edema to frank tendon rupture and the symptoms range from mild discomfort to severe pain and weakness. While the biceps tendon is not part of the rotator cuff, degenerative changes in its tendon often accompany rotator cuff tendinopathy. In addition, a slip of the subscapularis extends superiorly and helps to anchor the tendon of the

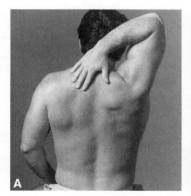 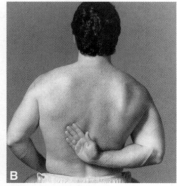

Figure S.10. The Apley scratch test. Exacerbation of the patient's pain indicates de-generative tendinopathy of one of the rotator cuff tendons, usually the supraspinatus. (From Cipriano JJ. *Photographic Manual of Regional Orthopaedic and Neurological Tests*. 4th ed. Philadelphia, PA: Wolters Kluwer Health/Lippincott Williams & Wilkins; 2003, with permission.)

long head of the biceps in the bicipital groove. Disease of the subscapularis may allow the biceps tendon to sublux on contraction, and recurrent microtrauma due to the increased mobility of the biceps tendon leads to the development of biceps tendonitis.

The tests usually performed for biceps tendonitis include Lippman's test, Speed's test and Yergason's test. In Lippman's test, palpation of the biceps tendon over the bicipital groove and moving the tendon from side to side reproduces the pain (Fig. S.11, Video S.1). Vigorous palpation can cause some discomfort even in the absence of pathology, so it is useful to compare the pain produced on the symptomatic and asymptomatic sides. In Speed's test, the elbow is held extended and supinated and the patient flexes the shoulder (not the elbow) against resistance (Fig. S.12, Video S.1) This movement causes the biceps tendon to slide in the bicipital groove and causes anterior shoulder pain in patients with bicipital tendonitis. Speed's test may also be positive due to rotator cuff disease involving the subscapularis. Many patients with biceps tendinopathy also have rotator cuff disease and Speed's test is now often used in the diagnosis of subacromial impingement syndromes in general. A positive Speed test increases the probability of rotator cuff disease with an LR of 1.9.[15] Because the biceps tendon originates from the glenoid

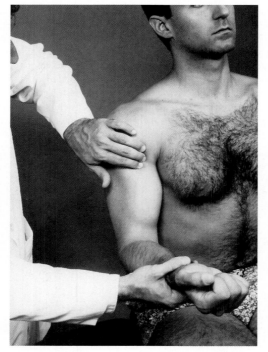

Figure S.11. Lippman's test; moving the biceps tendon back and forth in the bicipital groove reproduces the pain in biceps tendonitis. (From Cipriano JJ. *Photographic Manual of Regional Orthopaedic and Neurological Tests.* 4th ed. Philadelphia, PA: Wolters Kluwer Health/Lippincott Williams & Wilkins; 2003, with permission)

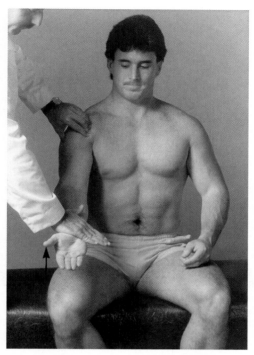

Figure S.12. Speed's test: Elicitation of pain from the anterior shoulder in bicipital tendonitis by flexion of the shoulder against resistance. (From Cipriano JJ. *Photographic Manual of Regional Orthopaedic and Neurological Tests*. 4th ed. Philadelphia, PA: Wolters Kluwer Health/Lippincott Williams & Wilkins; 2003, with permission.)

labrum, the movement may also cause pain with a SLAP lesion (Superior Labral tear from Anterior to Posterior).

Yergason's test (sign) is a test primarily for bicipital tendonitis. With the elbow flexed to 90 degrees and the forearm pronated, the patient attempts to simultaneously flex the elbow and supinate the hand against the examiner's resistance (Fig. S.13, Video S.1). The biceps is an elbow flexor and supinator, and this test uses both motions to cause the biceps to contract and its tendon to move in the bicipital groove, reproducing pain in the anterior shoulder in bicipital tendonitis. The test may also be positive due to inflammation or a tear of the subscapularis tendon in rotator cuff disease and in SLAP lesions. Yergason's test is relatively poor at detecting biceps tendinopathy, with a sensitivity of 41%, a specificity of 79%, a positive LR of 1.86, a negative LR of 0.74, PPV of 0.48, and NPV of 0.74.[18] A positive Yergason test increases the probability of rotator cuff disease with an LR of 2.8.[15]

The impingement sign is evidence of rotator cuff disease of the shoulder, or occasionally of subacromial bursitis. Of the many impingement signs described, two are in common use; both produce pain by trapping the rotator cuff tendons between the humeral head and the acromion or coracoacromial ligament during

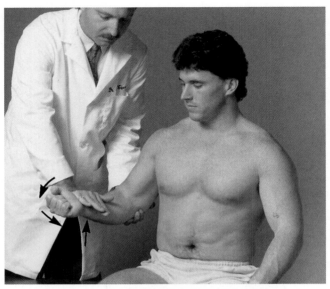

Figure S.13. Yergason's sign: Elicitation of pain from the anterior shoulder in bicipital tendonitis by flexing and supinating the elbow against resistance, which stresses the biceps tendon in its groove. (From Cipriano JJ. *Photographic Manual of Regional Orthopaedic and Neurological Tests.* 4th ed. Philadelphia, PA: Wolters Kluwer Health/ Lippincott Williams & Wilkins; 2003, with permission.)

passive movement of the shoulder (see Video S.1). In the Neer impingement test, the arm is internally rotated, then raised directly overhead with the palm facing outward **(Fig. S.14)**.[19,20] In the Hawkins (Hawkins-Kennedy) impingement test, the arm is held in abduction and external rotation, then forcefully rotated internally, driving the supraspinatus tendon through the subacromial space **(Fig. S.15)**. In another method, the elbow is flexed and the shoulder internally rotated as if to lay the forearm across the abdomen; the arm is then raised so that the forearm passes in an arc in front of the face and overhead.

Internal rotation is a key part of the maneuver in the impingement tests, as it rotates the greater tuberosity anteriorly and narrows the space beneath the acromion. Inflamed and tender tendons are then trapped between the greater tuberosity and the acromion, causing pain during the maneuver. After injection of a small amount of local anesthetic into the subacromial space, these movements may be made painlessly, confirming the diagnosis of impingement syndrome. The pain may also lessen when the patient bends forward and lets the arm hang limp, distracting the inflamed tendons from the point of impingement, or if the examiner supports the flexed forearm at the elbow and pulls gently downward.

Available studies for the different impingement signs indicate a sensitivity of 80% to 90%, a specificity of 25% to 50% and a negative LR of 0.3.[18] For the Neer and Hawkins signs, the positive LR is relatively low (1.6), largely because shoulder pain of all types increases with these maneuvers, causing a low specificity and many false positives.[15]

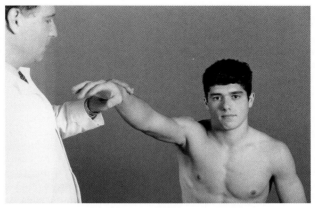

Figure S.14. Elicitation of Neer's impingement sign. With the arm pronated, elevation entraps the supraspinatus tendon under the coracoacromial arch. (From Cipriano JJ. *Photographic Manual of Regional Orthopaedic and Neurological Tests*. 4th ed. Philadelphia, PA: Wolters Kluwer Health/Lippincott Williams & Wilkins; 2003, with permission.)

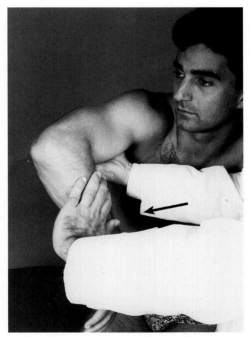

Figure S.15. Elicitation of the Hawkins impingement sign. Rotation forces the rotator cuff tendons beneath the coracoacromial arch. (From Cipriano JJ. *Photographic Manual of Regional Orthopaedic and Neurological Tests*. 4th ed. Philadelphia, PA: Wolters Kluwer Health/Lippincott Williams & Wilkins; 2003, with permission.)

A combination of positive impingement signs, supraspinatus weakness, and infraspinatus weakness increases the LR to 48. A combination of a positive Hawkins sign, a painful arc (see below) and infraspinatus weakness increases the LR to 15.9.[15]

The empty can (Jobe) test is a maneuver designed to examine the supraspinatus muscle and tendon, used primarily in assessing suspected rotator cuff disease. Both the deltoid and supraspinatus participate in simple shoulder abduction, and both are active throughout the range of motion. The common teaching that the supraspinatus effects the first 15 degrees of abduction and can be tested in isolation in that range has been disproven. To perform the empty can test, the patient abducts the arm to shoulder level, moves it forward about 30 degrees, and then hyperpronates the hand so that the thumb points to the floor and the small finger to the ceiling, simulating the action of pouring the contents from a can. This position isolates the supraspinatus insofar as is possible. The examiner then presses down on the extremity. Weakness or pain suggests the presence of supraspinatus muscle weakness or tendinopathy. Because the supraspinatus tendon is often involved early and prominently in rotator cuff disease this test is particularly useful in detecting degenerative changes in its tendon. Studies have shown sensitivities in the range of 65% to 85% and specificities of 50% to 55% with a positive LR of 2.0 for pain indicating a rotator cuff tear, and sensitivities in the range of 40% to 80% and specificities of 60% to 70% for weakness indicating a rotator cuff tear.[15] The so-called full-can test is simply testing infraspinatus strength by having the patient externally rotate the shoulder against resistance with the forearm semi-pronated and thumb up.

The lift-off test is a maneuver in which the patient places the hand against the lower back and attempts to push backward against resistance. Sources on peripheral nerve disease list this as a test of rhomboid strength because it requires rhomboid contraction to stabilize the scapula. Sources on shoulder disease list it as a test of subscapularis strength. The subscapularis is one of the rotator cuff muscles. Its action is to internally rotate the shoulder and lifting the hand from the small of the back is a contorted version of internal rotation.

A painful arc is a finding often present in rotator cuff disease and impingement syndrome. In impingement syndrome, the diseased tendons pass beneath the acromion in the arc between 60 and 120 degrees of abduction. Abduction out to 60 degrees may be painless, but the arc between 60 and 120 degrees is very uncomfortable; and beyond 120 degrees, after the swollen and tender supraspinatus tendon has cleared the narrow confines of the subacromial space, motion is again painless (see Video S.1). The "painful arc sign" is elicited either by having the examiner elevate the patient's arm passively to 180 degrees, then having the patient lower the arm actively, or having the patient actively abduct from 0 degrees to 180 degrees. The sign is positive with pain in the 60 degrees to 120 degrees range and not at the extremes. The painful arc sign has high sensitivity as a single finding, making it helpful in ruling out rotator cuff tendinopathy when absent. For rotator cuff disease the LR is 2.8.[15] The **drop (dropped) arm** sign is another sign of rotator cuff disease.[21] It is related to the painful arc, but rather than complaining of pain the arm simply collapses.

In the presence of a ruptured supraspinatus tendon, the abducted arm may collapse suddenly with the application of minimal resistance or during active range of motion. The examiner places the arm overhead, and then asks the patient to slowly lower it. The patient may not be able to lower the arm slowly because of pain or weakness, causing it to drop abruptly at about 100 degrees of abduction. Studies have shown a sensitivity of only 10% but a specificity of 98% with a positive LR of >10.[18]

The crossed body adduction (scarf) test is a maneuver to detect acromioclavicular joint pathology. The patient crosses the symptomatic arm horizontally as far as possible, as if reaching past the opposite shoulder. This compresses the acromioclavicular joint and aggravates the pain.

Shoulder shaking test: A test to evaluate muscle tone. The examiner places her hands on the patient's shoulders and shakes them briskly back and forth, observing the reciprocal motion of the arms. With extrapyramidal disease, there is a decreased range of arm swing on the affected side. With **hypotonia**, especially that associated with cerebellar disease, the excursions of the arm swing are greater than normal.

Shuffling gait: See **gait disorders.**

Sialorrhea: Increased salivary flow that often leads to drooling. Hypersalivation may occur because of excessive salivation, or the inability to swallow normal secretions. It is a common manifestation of PD and may occur in other **parkinsonism** syndromes. Drooling because of impaired swallowing occurs with bulbar involvement in motor neuron disease and MG. Drooling due to an inability to secure the corner of the mouth is common in peripheral facial palsy (see **facial weakness**). Sialorrhea may occur as a pharmacologic effect, as a side effect of cholinergic drugs or because of anticholinesterase toxicity, as in organophosphate poisoning.

Sicard's sign: An enhancement of the **straight leg raising test**; passively dorsiflexing the patient's great toe just at the elevation angle at which the increased root tension begins to produce pain causes a further increase in pain (see Video B.5). The term Spurling sign is also used for the same maneuver. See **Bragard's sign bowstring sign, popliteal compression test.**

Signe de l'éventail: The fanning of the toes on eliciting **Babinski's plantar sign**.

Simian (ape) hand: The hand posture seen in severe median neuropathy, when atrophy and paralysis of abduction cause the thumb to lie in an adducted and rotated position with the thumbnail parallel rather than perpendicular to the fingernails, falling into the plane of the palm (aka "monkey paw").

Simian posture (stance): A posture of generalized flexion most characteristically associated with **parkinsonism**, especially idiopathic PD (see Video G.4). The patient stands with the trunk and hips flexed, shoulders hunched forward and head down; see **bent spine syndrome**. The simian stance also been reported as a feature of spinal stenosis.[22] Flexion opens the spinal canal and patients are generally less symptomatic when the lumbosacral spine is flexed. When patients with neurogenic claudication are acutely symptomatic they will often seek a posture of flexion by bending or leaning forward, as over a grocery cart.

Simpson's test: See **ptosis.**

Simultagnosia: The inability to perceive more than one object at a time, or specific details but not a picture in its entirety. The patient may see parts but not the whole of a pattern. Simultagnosia is a type of **apperceptive visual agnosia** that causes an inability to see the panoramic view. It occurs as a part of **Balint's syndrome**. The term is also used to refer to the inability to perceive more than one tactile stimulus at a time, see **extinction.**

Skew deviation: A small, vertical misalignment of the eyes that typically results from a prenuclear lesion involving the brainstem or cerebellum (Fig. S.16).

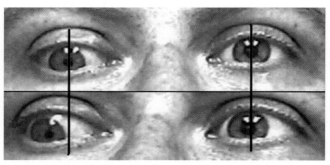

Figure S.16. Skew deviation in a patient with multiple sclerosis and a lesion involving the left dorsal midbrain syndrome with a left hyperdeviation and a left internuclear ophthalmoparesis (on attempted right gaze as seen in the lower figure). (From Brodsky MC, Donahue SP, Vaphiades M, et al. Skew deviation revisited. *Surv Ophthalmol.* 2006;51:105–128, with permission.)

The deviation is usually comitant, remaining about the same in all directions of gaze, and the lesion is most often on the side of the hypotropic eye.[23] Skew deviation is seen most commonly in association with vascular lesions of the pons or lateral medulla. The **ocular tilt reaction** consists of skew deviation with torsion of the eyes and a head tilt. Skew deviation is sometimes associated with an INO, with the lesion on the side of the hypertropic eye. In alternating skew deviation, the hypertropia changes sides spontaneously or with the direction of gaze. The lesion is typically in the midbrain and involves the interstitial nucleus of Cajal.

Skin roll test: See **Waddell signs.**

Skin tag: See **hairy patch and gluteal skyline test.**

Skin wrinkling test: A test used in the evaluation of peripheral nerve injury. The hands are immersed in warm water until wrinkling occurs. Denervated skin does not wrinkle and the lack of wrinkling may outline the distribution of the nerve injury.

Slapping gait: See **gait disorders.**

Slipping clutch gait: See **gait disorders.**

Slump test: See **straight leg raising test.**

Sneeze reflex: See **nasal reflex.**

Snout (orbicularis oris) reflex: Puckering and protrusion of the lips, primarily the lower, often with depression of the lateral angles of the mouth, in response to pressing firmly backward on the philtrum of the upper lip, a minimal tap to the lips, or sweeping a tongue blade briskly across the lips. When exaggerated, the response may include not only puckering and protrusion of the lips, but also sucking and even tasting, chewing, and swallowing movements. Reflex movement of the perioral muscles may persist despite lack of voluntary movement in UMN **facial weakness.** The snout reflex is considered a **frontal release sign** or **primitive reflex.** See **pathologic reflexes.**

Souques' leg sign: See **postural instability.**

Spasm (spasticity) of conjugate gaze: Lateral conjugate deviation of the eyes with forced eyelid closure. In a normal **Bell's phenomenon,** the eyes deviate up or up and out. In some patients with unilateral cerebral lesions, the eyes deviate laterally or obliquely. There is **gaze deviation** with the eyes closed not present with the eyes open. The deviation is contralateral to the side of the lesion in 80% of patients, and ipsilateral in 20%.[24] Patients usually have other CNS signs, such as hemiparesis, hemianopia, or aphasia but no abnormalities of gaze. The lesion is usually parieto-temporal, less frequently occipital; the phenomenon has not been reported with frontal lobe lesions. The mechanism is unclear.

Spasm of the near reflex (convergence spasm): An overactivity of the vergence subcomponent of the supranuclear ocular motor control system resulting in excessive convergence for the distance of the object and an inability to focus at distance. Convergence spasm causes esotropia on lateral gaze that can mimic a CN VI palsy. The disorder is usually functional and caused by voluntary convergence interrupting normal lateral gaze. As the patient looks laterally, the sudden convergence halts the abducting eye in midflight and simulates weakness of the lateral rectus. The mechanism is betrayed by pupillary constriction accompanying the eye movement that indicates the patient is converging. The miosis disappears when one eye is occluded. Convergence spasm has been reported as an isolated finding in a patient with midbrain compression.[25]

Spasmodic dysphonia: A condition that produces **dysphonia** by causing spasm of the vocal cords. If the spasm draws the cord toward the midline to approximate with the opposite cord, the voice is high-pitched, strained, and squeaky (adductor spasmodic dysphonia). If the spasm forces the involved cord away from the midline (abductor spasmodic dysphonia), the voice sounds hoarse and breathless.

Spastic diplegia: See **diplegia.**

Spastic gait: See **gait disorders.**

Spastic kick: See **spasticity.**

Spastic paretic facial contracture: A type of facial contracture causing a fixed expression with wrinkling of the forehead, narrowing of the palpebral fissure, drawing up or twisting of the angle of the mouth, and increased depth of the nasolabial fold. Facial contracture may follow a facial paralysis, or occur de novo. Careful testing may reveal that the affected muscles are still paretic, even though in a state of contracture. This type of spastic paretic facial contracture may occur with a progressive lesion of the pons and is suspicious for neoplasm. When **facial myokymia** and spastic paretic contracture occur together, the likelihood of pontine neoplasm is very high. The contracture may give the faulty impression of weakness on the opposite side.

Spasticity: Hypertonia that is velocity dependent, most evident with rapid movements, and that tends to decrease abruptly near the end of the range of movement. Spasticity results from lesions of the CST and is usually accompanied by hyperactive **deep tendon reflexes, clonus,** absence of **superficial reflexes,** extensor plantar responses and other **pathologic reflexes** (see **long tract signs**). The spasticity results in part because of segmental hyperexcitability of the alpha motoneuron pool.[26] The increase in tone is most marked in the flexor and pronator muscles of the upper limb and the extensors of the lower, and more apparent with an attempt to extend or supinate the muscles of the upper extremity or flex those of the lower. The relationship of the hypertonus to the speed of movement is a key feature distinguishing spasticity from **rigidity.** Passive motion may be carried out with little difficulty if done through a small range of movement, but resistance increases if an attempt is made to move the extremities through a greater range. Slow, passive movement may be carried out with relative ease, but on rapid movement there is a "blocking" or "catching," often with a waxing followed by a sudden waning of tone at the extremes of the range of motion (**clasp-knife response**). Patients with spasticity are at particular risk for **contractures**, especially of the calf muscles.

Testing for a **pronator catch** may bring out upper extremity spasticity. A similar slow then rapid motion technique can be used to detect lower-extremity spasticity. With hands behind the knee, the examiner slowly flexes and extends the knee of the supine and relaxed patient. With adequate relaxation the foot remains on the bed. After several slow repetitions, from the position of full extension, the examiner abruptly and forcefully pulls the knee upward. When tone is normal, the foot will scoot back, remaining in contact with the bed. When there is spasticity, the foot flies upward in a kicking motion (spastic kick). In the heel- or foot-dropping test, the examiner holds the patient's leg flexed at the knee and hip, one hand behind the knee, the other supporting the foot. The foot is suddenly released. Normally its descent is smooth, but when there is spasticity in the quadriceps muscle the foot may hang up and drop in a succession of choppy movements. Similar erratic descent may occur on the **arm dropping test**.

No devices for quantitating spasticity exist, and clinical evaluation remains the most useful tool. The Ashworth scale is commonly used to quantitate spasticity on a scale from 1 (no increase in muscle tone) to 5 (affected part rigid in flexion or extension). Its validity and reliability have been questioned.[27]

Spasticity is often accompanied by sustained contraction of specific groups of muscles. With hemiparesis or hemiplegia, spasticity is most marked in the flexor and pronator muscles of the upper and the extensor muscles of the lower extremity; this causes a posture of flexion of the arm and extension of the leg, the posture of spastic hemiplegia (see Video P.4). The arm is adducted, flexed at the elbow, and the wrist and fingers are flexed. The lower extremity is extended at the hip, knee, and ankle, with inversion and plantar flexion of the foot; there may be marked spasm of the hip adductors. With bilateral lesions the increased tone of the hip adductors causes a **scissoring** of the gait (see Video G.3). Severe spasticity in the lower extremities due to myelopathy may result in **paraplegia in flexion**.

Spatial neglect: See **attentional deficits**.

Speed's test: A test primarily for bicipital tendonitis. See **shoulder examination tests**.

Spinal Injuries Center (SIC) test: A maneuver used to detect nonorganic leg weakness. Patients unable to raise their knees spontaneously have a positive test, indicating nonorganic weakness, when their knees remain up after being lifted by the examiner (**Video Link S.5**).[28,29] The SIC test, or knee lift test, has a sensitivity of 97%, a specificity of 86%, a positive LR of 30.7, and a negative LR of 0.04.[15] See **abductor sign, Hoover's sign, Raimiste's leg sign**.

Spontaneous venous pulsations: See **papilledema**.

Speech apraxia: See **apraxia of speech**.

Spinal myoclonus: See **myoclonus**.

Spinal percussion test: Elicitation of tenderness to percussion over the spinous processes, using either the fist or a reflex hammer. Pain with percussion can occur with localized processes such as spinal epidural hematoma or abscess, or a vertebral fracture.

Split hand: A curious but characteristic presentation of ALS.[30] Although still without explanation, the split hand pattern appears relatively specific for ALS and is rarely seen in any other condition. There is weakness and wasting of the muscles of the lateral aspect of the hand, the thenar muscles and the FDI, with relative sparing of the hypothenar muscles. The FDI is often even more involved than the APB.

Spoon test: See **anhidrosis.**

Spooning: A characteristic hand posture seen in hypotonicity, especially that associated with cerebellar disease or Sydenham's chorea. With the arms and hands outstretched, there is flexion of the wrists and hyperextension of the fingers.

Spread (irradiation) of reflexes: Contraction of muscles not directly stretched during elicitation of a **deep tendon reflex.** Common examples are finger flexion with the **brachioradialis reflex** and the **crossed adductor reflex.** Some spread may occur normally when the DTRs are very active, but pronounced spread suggests an element of **spasticity.** Stronger stimuli are more likely to produce spread. An **inverted reflex** occurs when there is no or little contraction of the muscle directly stretched and the primary response is the spread to other muscles. Sherrington was interested in these "compound" or "combined" reflexes in experimental animals and may have coined the term irradiation. Uncertainty remains regarding the relative importance of central versus peripheral mechanisms.

Springing pupil: See Table P.1.

Spurling's sign (foraminal compression test): A maneuver used to provoke pain in cervical radiculopathy. See **cervical radiculopathy signs.**

Square-wave jerks: See **saccadic intrusions.**

Squint: See **strabismus.**

S-shaped lid: An eyelid deformity sometimes seen in patients with NF1 due to a diffuse neurofibroma distorting the lid margin **(Fig. S.17).**

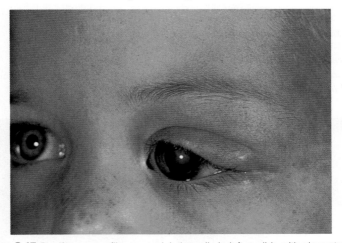

Figure S.17. Plexiform neurofibroma mainly laterally in left eyelids with characteristic S-shaped contour of left upper lid, cafe-au-lait spots in left temple, and buphthalmic left globe displaying an enlarged cornea, dilated pupil and cataract. (From Gold DH, Weingeist TA. *Color Atlas of the Eye in Systemic Disease.* Baltimore, MD: Wolters Kluwer Health/Lippincott Williams & Wilkins; 2001, with permission.)

S

St. Anthony's (St. Guy's, St. Vitus's) dance: See **chorea**.

Stamping gait: See **gait disorders**.

Stapedial reflex (acoustic reflex): A measure of the function of the stapedius muscle in response to loud sounds. The reflex arc is via CN VIII, brainstem interneurons, and CN VII. An impaired reflex may cause hyperacusis in patients with Bell's palsy and can be tested at the bedside with the stethoscope loudness imbalance test. With the patient wearing the stethoscope a slightly vibrating tuning fork is applied to the diaphragm and the patient asked to compare the intensity. With an impaired stapedial reflex the sound may be louder on the side of the facial weakness.

Starfish hand: Severe hand dystonia with spreading of the fingers in a "starfish" pattern **(Fig. S.18)**.[31]

Star walking (compass gait): A test for vestibular imbalance. The patient, eyes closed, takes several steps forward then several steps backward, over and over. A normal individual will begin and end oriented approximately along the same line. A patient with acute vestibulopathy will drift toward the involved side walking forward, and continue to drift during the backward phase (see Video P.3). The resulting path traces out a multipointed star pattern. See **Unterberger-Fukuda stepping test, head impulse test**.

Start-hesitation: See **freezing**.

Startle disease (response): See **hyperekplexia**.

Statokinetic dissociation: See **akinetotopsia**.

Steely hair: See **kinky hair**.

Stellwag's sign: An eye sign primarily associated with hyperthyroidism but that can occur in **parkinsonism**. Definitions vary with some sources stating Stellwag's sign is **eyelid retraction**, others that it is infrequent blinking, and others both. The term is frequently used in the description of the **reptilian stare** seen in parkinsonism. According to some, Stellwag's sign refers to unilateral eyelid retraction, as opposed to Dalrymple's sign where retraction is bilateral.

Steppage gait: See **gait disorders**.

Stepping test: See **Unterberger-Fukuda stepping test**.

Stereoanesthesia: See **astereognosis**.

Stereopsis: Depth perception. Stereopsis requires the development of normal binocular vision. Failure to acquire stereopsis occurs in the face of congenital or other

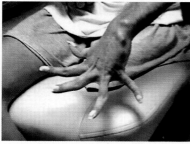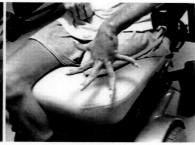

Figure S.18. "Starfish" hand dystonia following a right middle cerebral artery stroke involving the caudate. (From Ho BK, Morgan JC, Sethi KD. "Starfish" hand. *Neurology.* 2007;69:115, with permission.)

long-standing visual disturbances that interfere with ocular alignment and prevent normal binocular vision. Testing for stereopsis is useful in the evaluation of unexplained nystagmus, diplopia or ocular malalignment because lack of stereopsis suggests a long-standing problem, such as a decompensated squint, rather than a recently acquired abnormality.

Stereotypy: A repetitive, purposeless but often seemingly purposeful, involuntary, patterned motor activity. Common foot shaking and other mannerisms are examples of simple stereotypies. More complex stereotypies may involve ritualistic behavior, such as the compulsions of obsessive-compulsive disorder. Stereotypies most commonly occur in psychiatric disorders: Anxiety, obsessive-compulsive disorder, schizophrenia, autism, and mental retardation. They may also be a part of neurologic disorders, such as **tardive dyskinesia** and Tourette's syndrome. The hand wringing in Rett's syndrome is a stereotypy. Stereotypies may resemble motor **tics**, but do not share the suppressability, variability, or mounting-tension compulsion to make the movement.

Sterling's sign: A pathologic **associated movement**. Adduction of the normal shoulder against resistance causes shoulder adduction on hemiparetic side.

Sternal splitting: See **midline splitting.**

Sternutatory reflex: See **nasal reflex.**

Stethoscope loudness imbalance test: See **stapedial reflex.**

Stimulus-bound behavior: Behavior governed by environmental stimuli. Stimulus-bound behavior is a manifestation of **defective response inhibition** and **environmental dependency**, which is particularly likely to occur with frontal lobe disease. The patient is unable to suppress the compunction to respond to environmental stimuli. The patient may repeat the words (see **echolalia**) or gestures (see **echopraxia, imitation behavior**) of another person. **Utilization behavior** is the tendency to reach out and use whatever tool or implement is in the immediate vicinity. See **antisaccade task, applause sign, automatic responses, Stroop test,** and **Go/No-Go test.**

Strabismic amblyopia: See **amblyopia ex anopsia.**

Strabismus: A nonconcordance of the visual axes. Strabismus may be paralytic or nonparalytic. Ordinary strabismus, or congenital squint, occurs when the cerebral cortical mechanisms designed to maintain binocular vision fail for some reason, but the eyes are otherwise normal. Nonparalytic, congenital strabismus is very common in children. In acquired strabismus one or more eye muscles fails to function normally. Acquired strabismus is often paralytic (e.g., from CN III palsy). There is an ocular malalignment, which is worse in the field of action of the affected muscle or muscles.

Comitance describes the consistency of the deviation in various fields of gaze. A **phoria** or **tropia** may be comitant or noncomitant. A comitant strabismus shows the same degree of deviation in all directions of gaze. Congenital, nonparalytic strabismus is typically comitant. Paralytic strabismus is characterized by noncomitance: The ocular malalignment varies with the direction of gaze and is greatest in the direction of action of the paretic muscle. In neurologic patients, strabismus is typically paralytic and noncomitant. In comitant strabismus, as occurs congenitally, **ductions** are normal; in noncomitant strabismus, ductions reveal a limitation of ocular movement.

A patient with right lateral rectus weakness will have no abnormality while looking to the left, because the right lateral rectus has no role to play in left gaze. In primary

S

gaze, the affected eye might drift into esophoria. In right lateral gaze, the right lateral rectus insufficiency would become very obvious. The eye deviation varies with the direction of gaze: none in left gaze, mild in primary gaze, and moderate in right gaze. This variability is noncomitance and is the hallmark of paralytic strabismus.

Primary and secondary deviations are related to which eye is abnormal and which eye is fixing. In paralytic strabismus, the secondary deviation is greater than the primary deviation. The primary deviation is the deviation of the affected eye with the nonaffected eye fixing; the secondary deviation is the deviation of the good, nonaffected, eye with the bad eye fixing. In paralytic strabismus, the affected eye deviates away from the field of action of the involved muscle. With a right CN VI palsy, in primary gaze the right eye will be slightly adducted. With equal vision in the two eyes, the noninvolved left eye will fixate so that in primary gaze the left eye is fixing and the right eye is deviated toward the nose. This deviation of the right eye is the primary deviation. If a target is moved into the field of action of the paretic muscle, to the right, and the left eye is covered so that the right eye is forced to fixate, the left medial rectus (the yoke muscle of the right lateral rectus) will receive equal and simultaneous innervation per Hering's law. On the **cover test**, because the right lateral rectus is contracting in an attempt to fixate, the left medial rectus is simultaneously contracting under cover and the left eye is markedly adducting into right lateral gaze. Removal of the cover reveals deviation of the left eye, termed the secondary deviation.

Not all noncomitant strabismus is paralytic. Some conditions, such as **spasm of the near reflex**, cause dramatic ocular malalignment on testing **versions**, but **ductions** are normal. Some causes of noncomitant esotropia include CN VI palsy, Duane's syndrome, Möebius syndrome, **spasm of the near reflex**, **thalamic esotropia**, MG, muscle entrapment, and thyroid eye disease.

Some causes of noncomitant exotropia include CN III palsy, **internuclear ophthalmoplegia**, especially the WEBINO syndrome, paralytic pontine exotropia, MG, muscle entrapment, and thyroid eye disease.

Perfect eyes are orthophoric (Gr. orthos "straight") in all fields of gaze; the visual axes are precisely parallel during all versional eye movements, even without a stimulus to fusion. Any deviation from perfection is termed heterophoria or heterotropia, usually shortened to phoria and tropia, respectively. In heterotropia, the malalignment is evident at rest. Esotropia is a manifest medial deviation (convergent or internal strabismus; "cross eye," Figs. S.19 and E.2); Exotropia is a manifest lateral deviation (divergent or external strabismus; "wall eye"). Hypertropia is elevation and hypotropia is depression. Heterophoria is a latent tendency for deviation, which only becomes apparent when the stimulus to fusion fails under certain circumstances, such as fatigue or when binocular fusion is deliberately broken, as by covering one eye. Congenital exophoria is very common. Exophoria may occur with myopia, esophoria with hyperopia. When an eye with exophoria is not fixing, it tends to drift back to its anatomical position of slight abduction. Strabismus is evaluated using the **cover tests (Video Links S.6 and S.7)**.

Soto-Hall test: Some sources list this test as a method to reproduce pain in cervical or lumbosacral radiculopathy (see **straight leg raising test);** others describe it as a variant of **Lhermitte's sign** with the addition of downward pressure on the sternum.

Straight leg raising test (Lasègue sign): The primary root stretch sign used in the evaluation of lumbosacral radiculopathy (LSR). As with the physical diagnosis in

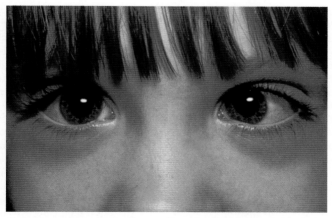

Figure S.19. Esotropia due to strabismus. (From Gold DH, Weingeist TA. *Color Atlas of the Eye in Systemic Disease.* Baltimore, MD: Wolters Kluwer Health/Lippincott Williams & Wilkins; 2001, with permission.)

cervical radiculopathy, most signs have high specificity with low or moderate sensitivity.[32,33] SLR is performed supine by slowly raising the symptomatic leg with the knee extended (see Video B.5). The L5 nerve root normally stretches as much as 2.5 cm during the full range of SLR. Tension is transmitted to the nerve roots between about 30 degrees and 70 degrees and pain increases. Pain at <30 degrees raises the question of nonorganicity, and some discomfort and tightness beyond 70 degrees is routine and insignificant. Caveats are required. Some very symptomatic patients may well have a positive SLR at <30 degrees. Back pain at low levels of elevation may occur with SI joint disease and pain at higher levels may indicate facet arthropathy.

There are various degrees or levels of positivity of the SLR. Ipsilateral leg pain is the lowest level, pain in the back more significant and radiating pain down the leg highly significant. When raising the good leg produces pain in the symptomatic leg (crossed straight-leg-raising sign, Fajersztajn's sign, well-leg raising), the likelihood of a root lesion is very high. Rarely, SLR may even cause numbness and paresthesias in the distribution of the affected nerve root. The **buckling sign** is knee flexion during SLR to avoid sciatic nerve tension. Raising the pelvis may also reduce root stretch and has the same significance. Neri's bowing sign refers to buckling occurring while standing and bending forward (see **Minor's sign**). **Kernig's sign** is an alternate way of stretching the root.

SLR is less useful in older that in younger patients. In younger patients, the discs are more turgid and herniation creates more mass effect and stretch on the root. Aging causes desiccation of the disc and the development of osteophytes (hard disc) and radiculopathy may occur with less mass effect and root tension.

Various SLR modifications may provide additional information, such as by performing the SLR with the thigh and leg adducted and internally rotated (**Bonnet's sign**), or by passively dorsiflexing the patient's foot (see **Bragard's sign**) or great toe (see **Sicard's sign**) if routine SLR does not elicit pain. The **bowstring sign** employs a quick stretch to the sciatic nerve in the popliteal fossa. In severe cases, pain may

S

be elicited merely by dorsiflexion of the foot or great toe as the patient lies supine with legs extended. A similar modification may be carried out by flexing the thigh to an angle just short of that necessary to cause pain, and then flexing the neck; this may produce the same exacerbation of pain that would be brought about by further flexion of the hip (Lindner's, Soto-Hall or Hyndman's sign). Occasionally, the pain may be brought on merely by passive flexion of the neck when the patient is recumbent with legs extended (also Lindner's sign). All these are essentially supine variants of the slump test (see below). See **Brudzinski's sign**.

The pain with SLR should be about the same with the patient supine or seated (see Video B.2). The SLR in fact is often even more positive in the seated position because sitting vastly increases intradiscal pressure and there is often more pressure and tension on the root seated than standing. The symptoms of LSR are characteristically worse when sitting, to the point that very symptomatic patients may take their meals standing up. Failure of a patient with a positive supine SLR to complain or lean backward (positive "flip sign") when the knee is extended while seated (e.g., under the guise of doing the planter response) suggests complicating psychosocial issues (see **Waddell signs**). In **Bechterew's test**, the seated patient may be able to extend each leg alone, but extending both together causes radicular pain; the term is also used to refer simply to the one-sided seated SLR. The **O'Connell test** also employs raising both legs, but with the patient supine, and noting the angles of elevation and location of pain produced. The slump test is essentially a seated SLR with the addition of the examiner forcing the patient's head and trunk forward into a slumped position. If this kind of extreme maneuver is required to reproduce pain, it is unlikely of neurologic significance.

The Valsalva test seeks to elicit radicular symptoms by distending the epidural veins and CSF reservoirs. Maneuvers exploiting this mechanism of eliciting root signs seem more useful in cervical than lumbosacral radiculopathy (see **Naffziger's sign**).

Patients with hip or SI joint disease may have pain on raising the leg whether the knee is bent or straight, those with root stretch signs only have pain when the knee is extended. Pain from hip disease is maximal when the hip is flexed, abducted and externally rotated (see **FABER test**). There are other procedures for checking the SI joints (see **sacroiliac joint signs**). The **femoral nerve stretch test** (reverse straight leg raising test) is a way of eliciting root stretch in the evaluation of high lumbar radiculopathy.

The utility, or lack thereof, of various physical examination findings has been studied. Defining positivity as radiating pain in the symptomatic leg, wide variability has been reported for the sensitivity (53% to 98%) and specificity (11% to 89%) of the SLR for radiculopathy in patients with sciatica, with a positive LR of only 1.5 and a modest negative LR of 0.4.[15] The best predictors of S1 radiculopathy are S1 distribution sensory loss (LR 2.4), ipsilateral calf wasting (LR 2.4) and a decreased ankle jerk (LR 2.7).[15]

Straight thumb sign: See **OK sign**.

Stransky's sign: See **minor extensor toe signs** (see Table M.3).

Stretch reflex: See **deep tendon reflex**.

Striatal toe: See **dystonic foot**.

Stroop test: An assessment of the patient's ability to inhibit automatic responses. In some disease processes, especially those with frontal lobe involvement, the patient may display **defective response inhibition, environmental dependency** and **stimulus bound behavior**. In the Stroop "little-big" test, the words little and big are printed on separate cards in both upper- and lowercase letters. The patient is required to answer "big" aloud if the print is uppercase, even in response to the word little, or vice versa. A variation is to write several color names in nonmatching colors, e.g., write the word blue with a red marker, then ask the patient to read the cards by stating the color of the print, not the written name of the color. Patients with frontal lobe dysfunction have trouble inhibiting the tendency to read the color name or don't answer "little" when "big" is written in lowercase.

Strümpell's phenomenon: A **minor extensor toe sign** (see Table M.3).

Strümpell's pronator sign: One of several **pronator signs**. An abnormal **associated movement** seen in **hemiparesis**; active flexion of a paretic forearm is followed by pronation and flexion of the hand; if patient can bring the hand to the shoulder, the dorsum of hand strikes the shoulder with palm forward. If the supinated forearm is actively flexed or the forearm is passively flexed and supinated by examiner, it immediately assumes a position of pronation (the same as the **pronation sign of Neri**). See Table P.3.

Strümpell's signs: See **anterior tibial sign, radialis sign of Strümpell**, and **Strümpell's pronator sign**.

Stuttering: Faulty, spasmodic, interrupted speech characterized by involuntary hesitations in which the speaker is unable to produce the next expected sound. The flow of speech is broken by pauses during which articulation is entirely arrested. Speech is faltering and characterized by difficulty in enunciating syllables and joining them together. Stuttering speech is stumbling and hesitant in character, with habitual and spasmodic repetitions of consonants or syllables, alternating with pauses. There may be localized cramps, spasms, and tic-like contractions of the muscles essential to articulation, sometimes accompanied by grimaces, spasms and contractions of the muscles of the head and extremities, and spasm and incoordination of the respiratory muscles. The individual may be unable to pronounce certain consonants, with particular difficulty in using dentals and labials. Often the first syllable or consonant of a word is repeated many times. The individual may remain with his mouth open until the articulatory spasm relaxes, then the words explode out until the breath is gone. He then takes another breath, and the process is repeated. In spite of difficulty in speaking, the individual may be able to sing without hesitation. There have been accomplished professional singers who stuttered severely in ordinary speech **(Video Links S.8 and S.9)**.

    Stuttering is markedly influenced by emotional excitement and by the presence of strangers. Interference with communication may be profound and the social consequences severe. Britain's King George VI stuttered severely, as memorably depicted in the motion picture *The King's Speech*. Many theories have been offered regarding the etiology of stuttering. New onset stuttering, or the re-emergence of childhood stuttering, may occur as an early manifestation of PD.

Subcortical (extrasylvian) aphasia: Language disorders that arise not from damage to the perisylvian language areas, but from lesions—usually vascular—involving the thalamus, caudate, putamen, periventricular white matter or internal capsule of the language dominant hemisphere **(Fig. S.20)**.[34]

    Two types have been described: an anterior and a posterior syndrome. The anterior syndrome (caudate or striatocapsular aphasia) is characterized by slow

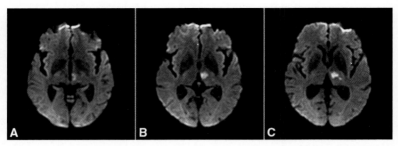

Figure S.20. MRI of the brain shows acute ischemic stroke involving the left thalamus. Axial diffusion-weighted images at different levels show restricted diffusion in the left thalamus. Affected thalamic nuclei include dorsomedial nucleus **(A)**, anterior nuclear group **(B)**, ventral nuclear group, and reticular nuclei **(C)**. (From Afzal U, Farooq MU. Teaching neuroimages: thalamic aphasia syndrome. *Neurology.* 2013;81:e177, with permission.)

dysarthric speech with preserved phrase length, i.e., not telegraphic, preserved comprehension and poor naming. In the posterior syndrome (thalamic aphasia), there is fluent speech without dysarthria, poor comprehension and poor naming. In both forms, repetition is relatively preserved, and the patients usually have an accompanying **hemiparesis**. The anterior syndrome resembles a transcortical motor aphasia, and the posterior syndrome resembles **Wernicke's aphasia** or transcortical sensory aphasia but accompanied by a hemiparesis (see **transcortical aphasia**). The relative preservation of repetition suggests a link between the subcortical and transcortical syndromes. The anterior syndrome shows more clinical variability than the posterior. Some include a third type associated with white matter paraventricular lesions.[35]

The mechanism by which subcortical lesions cause aphasia remains conjectural, but it may involve secondary dysfunction of the perisylvian language areas due to interruption of fibers that communicate between cortical and subcortical structures. Imaging has shown that cortical hypoperfusion is common in subcortical aphasia. In a SPECT study, left cerebral cortical hypoperfusion was observed in all patients with striatocapsular infarction.[36]

Subhyaloid (preretinal) hemorrhage: See **Terson's syndrome.**

Subjective visual vertical (SVV): The capacity to determine the vertical alignment of objects in the absence of any visual reference. An abnormality of SVV is a sensitive clinical brain stem sign and is very common in acute brain stem infarctions. The deviation is typically ipsiversive with pontomedullary lesions and contraversive with pontomesencephalic lesions. More than 90% of patients with acute vestibulopathy show ipsilateral deviation of SVV. Simple bedside testing has been described using the "bucket method."[37] Patients look into a plastic bucket so that the rim of the bucket obscures visual references, and then rotate a line on the bottom to their perception of vertical. The deviation from true vertical is read off on an outside scale by the examiner.

Subtle signs of hemiparesis: Clinical signs indicative of CST dysfunction in the absence of gross, overt weakness (see Video F.4). The importance of such subtle signs is inversely proportional to the adequacy of the formal motor examination.

These relatively subtle signs become most apparent with side-to-side comparison but frequently occur in some form in patients with paraparesis and quadriparesis as well. These signs occur primarily because of preferential innervation of certain muscle groups by the CST. There is heavy CST input to distal extremity muscles, especially the hand, as reflected by the huge amount of motor cortex devoted to hand function. The CST also preferentially innervates the extensors, supinators and external rotators in the upper extremity and the flexors (hip, knee and ankle dorsi-flexors) in the lower extremity.

Impaired distal upper extremity function produces abnormal **forearm rolling,** or posting, which may also involve the forefinger or thumb, decreased **fine motor control** and loss of dexterity when performing **rapid alternating movements** (see **finger tapping test**). The relatively preserved strength in the pronators and flexors as compared to the extensors and supinators leads to **pronator drift** and other **pronator signs** (see Table P.3).

Abnormalities of **associated movements** may also occur relatively early. These may include the absence of a normal associated movement, such as a decreased arm swing while walking, or the presence of an abnormal associated movement, such as Wartenberg's thumb adduction sign (see **Wartenberg's signs**).

Subtle signs are more difficult to detect in the lower extremity, but **leg drift** and impaired **foot tapping** may also occur. The **anterior tibial sign** is an abnormal associated movement.

See also **digiti quinti sign, finger escape sign, myelopathy hand, and Babinski trunk–thigh sign.**

Sucking (suck) reflex: A **primitive reflex** or **frontal release sign**, normal in infants; stimulation of the perioral region is followed by sucking movements of the lips, tongue, and jaw. The response may be elicited by lightly touching, striking, or tapping the lips, stroking the tongue, or stimulating the palate. See **pathologic reflexes, rooting reflex, snout reflex.**

Sugiura's sign: Perilimbal depigmentation of the iris that occurs in Vogt-Koyanagi-Harada disease.[38]

Sulcus sign: A step-off that appears between the humeral head and acromion when pulling downward on the relaxed arm in the presence of inferior instability of the shoulder.

Sunglasses sign: An indication that a patient may have nonorganic visual loss (NOVL). Patients with visual loss who wear sunglasses in clinic have an increased likelihood of having NOVL. In a series of 34 patients who wore sunglasses, only 7 (20.6%) had organic visual loss.[39] The sensitivity of wearing sunglasses for NOVL was 0.46 (95% CI 0.33–0.59) and the specificity was 0.995 (95% CI 0.989–0.998). Either a highly positive review of systems, workers' compensation claim, disability, or lawsuit was found in 96.3% of NOVL patients wearing sunglasses and in none of the sunglasses patients with organic neuro-ophthalmic disorders. The "sunglasses sign" in a patient without an obvious ophthalmic reason to wear sunglasses is highly suggestive of NOVL.

Sunset glow fundus: Atrophy of the retinal pigment epithelium due to Vogt-Koyanagi-Harada disease. The choroid takes on a yellowish orange appearance.

Superficial anal reflex: See **anal reflex.**

Superficial reflexes: Responses to stimulation of either the skin or mucous membrane. Cutaneous reflexes are elicited by a superficial skin stimulus, such as a light touch or scratch. The response occurs in the same general area where the stimulus is applied (local sign). Superficial reflexes are polysynaptic, in contrast to the stretch reflexes, which are monosynaptic. The superficial reflexes respond more slowly to the stimulus than do the stretch reflexes, their latency is longer, they fatigue more easily, and are not as consistently present as tendon reflexes. The primary utility of superficial reflexes is related to the changes that occur with CST lesions, which characteristically produce the combination of increased **deep tendon reflexes** and decreased or absent superficial reflexes. The superficial reflexes obtained most often are the superficial **abdominal reflexes** and the **cremasteric reflex**. Many of the superficial reflexes are arcane, of minor clinical significance, and primarily of historical interest. See **palmar reflex, interscapular reflex, gluteal reflex, plantar reflex, anal reflex,** and **bulbocavernosus reflex.**

Supinator reflex: See **brachioradialis reflex.**

Suprapatellar reflex: An alternative method for eliciting the **knee reflex** and one of the occasionally useful DTRs (see Table D.1, Video B.4). Tapping over the suprapatellar tendon elicits the knee reflex **(Fig. S.21).** The response is minimal normally. When the reflexes are exaggerated, the response may be obtained more easily. With reflex spread, hip adduction, sometimes bilaterally, may accompany knee extension, or bilateral knee extension may occur. The suprapatellar reflex is often useful is determining whether there is knee reflex asymmetry. Presence of the response on the side of the suspiciously hyperactive knee reflex and not on

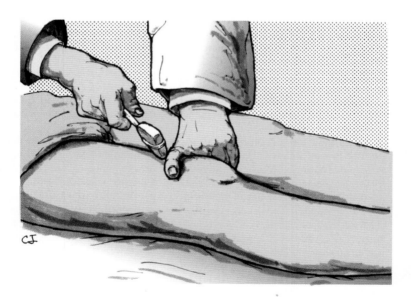

Figure S.21. Method of obtaining the suprapatellar reflex. (From Campbell WW. *DeJong's the Neurologic Examination.* 7th ed. Philadelphia, PA: Wolters Kluwer Health/ Lippincott Williams & Wilkins; 2013, with permission.)

the opposite side helps confirm asymmetry. The tendon can be tapped directly, or, with the patient recumbent, the examiner can place her index finger on the upper border of the patella and tap the finger to push down the patella. Contraction of the quadriceps causes a brisk upward movement of the tendon, together with knee extension.

Superior oblique myokymia: A rare ocular motility disorder characterized by brief episodes of pendular ocular oscillation due to spasmodic contraction of the superior oblique. Superior oblique myokymia presents as episodes of diplopia or oscillopsia lasting several seconds to several minutes. Patients often complain of "dizziness." It is similar to **ocular neuromyotonia**, which can involve any muscle. Injury, inflammation or microvascular compression of CN IV is thought to cause spontaneous discharges. Myokymia has also been reported to involve the inferior oblique[40] **(Video Link S.10).**

The condition has also been referred to as an intermittent uniocular rotatory microtremor. It was originally described by Duane in 1906, who called it "unilateral rotatory nystagmus," then rediscovered by Hoyt and Keane in 1970, who coined the present terminology.[41] Contraction of the superior oblique by looking down, then returning gaze to primary position, will sometimes initiate the spasmodic contractions. The rapid, low-amplitude microtremor is difficult to see with the naked eye and is better visualized with a direct ophthalmoscope or Frenzel lenses.

Suspended sensory loss: A pattern of sensory loss most commonly seen in syringomyelia. Syrinxes usually occur in the cervical region and more or less centrally within the cord substance. The syrinx interferes with the function of the pain and temperature sensory fibers crossing in the anterior commissure just ventral to the central canal. Sensory fibers ascending from the lower extremities are running in the posterior columns and lateral spinothalamic tracts located on the periphery of the cord. Head and neck sensory fibers coursing above the level of the syrinx are not affected. The sensory loss therefore only involves the upper extremities, leaving normal sensation in the lower extremities, head, and neck (Fig. S.22D). The sensory loss is therefore described as "suspended" or in a cape or shawl pattern. The sensory loss caused by a cervical syrinx is also "dissociated" because only pain and temperature fibers are affected with preservation of light touch and other sensory functions (see **dissociated sensory loss**). Figure S.23 shows the sensory loss pattern in a patient who had a cervical syrinx.

Swinging flashlight test: See **afferent pupillary defect.**

Sympathetic apraxia: The inability of a patient to perform a complex motor act with the nonparetic limb in the presence of a unilateral dominant hemisphere lesion. For instance, a patient with a left hemisphere lesion causing **Broca's aphasia** may be unable to show how to wave goodbye using the left hand. Sympathetic apraxia occurs because the fibers connecting the language areas of the left hemisphere with the motor areas of the right hemisphere are disrupted. The patient understands the request, has no weakness of the left hand, but is unable to execute because the right hemisphere never receives the command.

Symphysis pubis reflex: Tapping over the symphysis pubis elicits contraction of the abdominal muscles and a downward movement of the umbilicus. The patient should be recumbent, with the abdominal muscles relaxed and the thigh in slight abduction and internal rotation. If a unilateral stimulus is applied by tapping 1.5 to

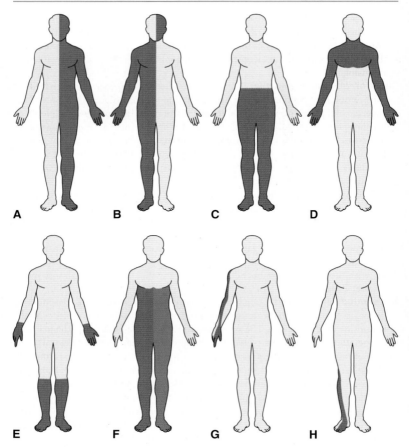

Figure S.22. Some common patterns of sensory loss. **A:** Hemisensory loss due to a hemispheric lesion. **B:** Crossed sensory loss to pain and temperature due to a lateral medullary lesion. **C:** Midthoracic spinal cord level. **D:** Suspended, dissociated sensory loss to pain and temperature due to syringomyelia. **E:** Distal, symmetric sensory loss due to peripheral neuropathy. **F:** Crossed spinothalamic loss on one side with posterior column loss on the opposite side due to Brown-Sequard syndrome. **G:** Dermatomal sensory loss due to cervical radiculopathy. **H:** Dermatomal sensory loss due to lumbosacral radiculopathy. (From Campbell WW. *DeJong's the Neurologic Examination*. 7th ed. Philadelphia, PA: Wolters Kluwer Health/Lippincott Williams & Wilkins; 2013, with permission.)

2 cm from the midline, there is not only the "upper response" just described, but also a "lower response," or puboadductor reflex, with contraction of the ipsilateral adductor muscles of the thigh and some flexion of the hip. The latter response is also seen if the reflex is exaggerated. The symphysis pubis reflex is innervated by the lower intercostal, ilioinguinal, and iliohypogastric nerves (T11–T12 and upper lumbar segments). With spasticity, percussion over the symphysis may cause

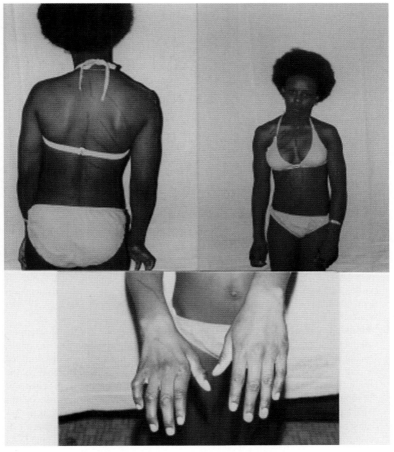

Figure S.23. Suspended, dissociated syrinx (hatched areas) and clawing of the hand due to a syrinx.

S

adduction of both legs. The symphysis pubis reflex may be considered a variation of the deep **abdominal reflexes** in which the stimulus is directed toward the site of insertion.

Syndactyly: Fusion of two or more digits (Fig. S.24). In simple syndactyly, soft tissue joins the digits; in complex syndactyly, the bones are also fused. With complete syndactyly, the webbing extends to the tips of the digits; with incomplete syndactyly, the fusion is partial. Simple syndactyly is a common congenital anomaly. Polydactyly, the most common anomaly of the hand, is more than the normal number of fingers and toes. These anomalies are a feature of many congenital dysmorphic syndromes. Syndactyly or polydactyly occur in **acrocephalosyndactyly**, such as Carpenter's and Apert's syndromes, and other forms of **craniosynostosis**. Other notable conditions with digital fusion as a feature include: Möebius syndrome, Prader-Willi

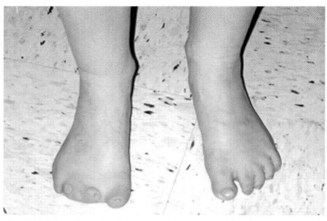

Figure S.24. Syndactyly in a patient with Andersen-Tawil syndrome. (From Donaldson MR, Jensen JL, Tristani-Firouzi M, et al. PIP2 binding residues of Kir2.1 are common targets of mutations causing Andersen syndrome. *Neurology.* 2003;60:1811–1816, with permission.)

syndrome, David anomaly, craniodigital syndrome, HSP with syndactyly, fetal anticonvulsant syndrome, hereditary brachial plexopathy, Klippel-Trenaunay-Weber syndrome, and de Lange syndrome.

Synkinesis (synkinesias): Abnormal muscle contractions due to anomalous innervation or **aberrant reinnervation**. **Facial synkinesis** is the most common example. During recovery from a facial nerve lesion, most often Bell's palsy, axons destined for one muscle regrow to innervate another, resulting in abnormal twitching of the face outside the area of intended movement. On blinking or winking, the corner of the mouth may twitch. On smiling or opening the jaw, the eye may close (Marin Amat sign, see **inverse jaw winking**). These movements are prominent in some patients; more often synkinesis is subtle, such as a slight twitch of the orbicularis oris synchronous with blinking of the eye. When misdirection is conspicuous, the main effect of smiling on the involved side of the face may be eye closure.

Swinging flashlight test: See **afferent pupillary defect**.

Szapiro's sign: A **minor extensor toe sign** (see Table M.3).

Video Links

S.1. Opsoclonus. (From Zaganas I, Prinianakis G, Xirouchaki N, et al. Opsoclonus-myoclonus syndrome associated with cytomegalovirus encephalitis. *Neurology.* 2007;68:1636.) Available at: http://www.neurology.org/content/suppl/2007/05/01/68.19.1636.DC1/Video.mpg

S.2. Opsoclonus due to diphenhydramine poisoning. (From Carstairs SD, Schneir AB. Images in clinical medicine. Opsoclonus due to diphenhydramine poisoning. *N Engl J Med.* 2010;363:e40.) Available at: http://www.nejm.org/doi/pdf/10.1056/NEJMicm1002035

S.3. Slowly progressive ataxia, neuropathy, and oculomotor dysfunction. (From Jordan JT, Samuel G, Vernino S, et al. Slowly progressive ataxia, neuropathy, and oculomotor dysfunction. *Arch Neurol.* 2012;69:1366–1371.) Available at: http://archneur.jamanetwork.com/multimediaPlayer.aspx?mediaid=4268300

S.4. Scapular winging. Available at: http://www.youtube.com/watch?v=dfTe0nPclDE

S.5. A demonstration of the SIC test. (From LaFrance WC Jr. Video neuroimage: diagnosing conversion weakness with the Spinal Injuries Center test: when Hoover doesn't help. *Neurology.* 2008;71:e57.) Available at: http://www.neurology.org/content/71/19/e57/suppl/DC1

S.6. A discussion of strabismus and the cover tests. (From Root T. Ophthobook.) Available at: http://www.ophthobook.com/videos/tropias-and-phorias-video

S.7. Findings in various types of paralytic strabismus. (From The University of California, Davis: The Neurological Eye Simulator.) Available at: at cim.ucdavis.edu/eyes

S.8. Stuttering. Available at: https://www.youtube.com/watch?v=5aweaoakyK8

S.9. Stuttering. Available at: https://www.youtube.com/watch?v=U7XPh481E9A

S.10. Inferior oblique myokymia. (From Chinskey ND, Cornblath WT. Inferior oblique myokymia: a unique ocular motility disorder. *JAMA Ophthalmol.* 2013;131(3):404–405.) Available at: http://archopht.jamanetwork.com/multimediaPlayer.aspx?mediaid=5414740

References

1. Thurtell MJ, Leigh RJ. Nystagmus and saccadic intrusions. *Handb Clin Neurol.* 2011;102:333–378.

2. Lemos J, Eggenberger E. Saccadic intrusions: review and update. *Curr Opin Neurol.* 2013;26:59–66.

3. Zaganas I, Prinianakis G, Xirouchaki N, et al. Opsoclonus-myoclonus syndrome associated with cytomegalovirus encephalitis. *Neurology.* 2007;68:1636.

4. Carstairs SD, Schneir AB. Images in clinical medicine. Opsoclonus due to diphenhydramine poisoning. *N Engl J Med.* 2010;363:e40.

5. Tilikete C, Koene A, Nighoghossian N, et al. Saccadic lateropulsion in Wallenberg syndrome: a window to access cerebellar control of saccades? *Exp Brain Res.* 2006;174:555–565.

6. Frohman EM, Frohman TC, Fleckenstein J, et al. Ocular contrapulsion in multiple sclerosis: clinical features and pathophysiological mechanisms. *J Neurol Neurosurg Psychiatry.* 2001;70:688–692.

7. Jordan JT, Samuel G, Vernino S, et al. Slowly progressive ataxia, neuropathy, and oculomotor dysfunction. *Arch Neurol.* 2012;69:1366–1371.

8. Schwarzer AC, Aprill CN, Bogduk N. The sacroiliac joint in chronic low back pain. *Spine (Phila Pa 1976).* 1995;20:31–37.

9. Laslett M, Williams M. The reliability of selected pain provocation tests for sacroiliac joint pathology. *Spine (Phila Pa 1976).* 1994;19:1243–1249.

10. Broadhurst NA, Bond MJ. Pain provocation tests for the assessment of sacroiliac joint dysfunction. *J Spinal Disord.* 1998;11:341–345.

11. Fortin JD, Falco FJ. The Fortin finger test: an indicator of sacroiliac pain. *Am J Orthop (Belle Mead NJ).* 1997;26:477–480.

12. Murakami E, Aizawa T, Noguchi K, et al. Diagram specific to sacroiliac joint pain site indicated by one-finger test. *J Orthop Sci.* 2008;13:492–497.

13. Makanji HS, Becker SJ, Mudgal CS, et al. Evaluation of the scratch collapse test for the diagnosis of carpal tunnel syndrome. *J Hand Surg Eur Vol.* 2014;39:181–186.

14. Blok RD, Becker SJ, Ring DC. Diagnosis of carpal tunnel syndrome: interobserver reliability of the blinded scratch-collapse test. *J Hand Microsurg.* 2014;6:5–7.

15. McGee S. *Evidence Based Physical Diagnosis.* 3rd ed. Philadelphia, PA: Elsevier/Saunders; 2012.

16. Ghosh SK, Bandyopadhyay D, Chatterjee G, et al. Mucocutaneous changes in tuberous sclerosis complex: a clinical profile of 27 Indian patients. *Indian J Dermatol.* 2009;54:255–257.

17. Sackellares JC, Swift TR. Shoulder enlargement as the presenting sign in syringomyelia. *JAMA.* 1976;236:2878.

18. Dennis M, Bowen WT, Cho L. *Mechanisms of Clinical Signs.* Sydney, Australia: Churchill Livingstone; 2012.

19. MacDonald PB, Clark P, Sutherland K. An analysis of the diagnostic accuracy of the Hawkins and Neer subacromial impingement signs. *J Shoulder Elbow Surg.* 2000;9:299–301.

20. McFarland EG, Garzon-Muvdi J, Jia X, et al. Clinical and diagnostic tests for shoulder disorders: a critical review. *Br J Sports Med.* 2010;44:328–332.

21. Colsant B, Sams R, Paden S. Clinical inquiries. Which history and physical findings are most useful in identifying rotator cuff tears? *J Fam Pract.* 2010;59:179–181.

22. Simkin PA. Simian stance: a sign of spinal stenosis. *Lancet.* 1982;2:652–653.

23. Brodsky MC, Donahue SP, Vaphiades M, et al. Skew deviation revisited. *Surv Ophthalmol.* 2006;51:105–128.

24. Sullivan HC, Kaminski HJ, Maas EF, et al. Lateral deviation of the eyes on forced lid closure in patients with cerebral lesions. *Arch Neurol.* 1991;48:310–311.

25. Weber KP, Thurtell MJ, Halmagyi GM. Teaching neuroimage: convergence spasm associated with midbrain compression by cerebral aneurysm. *Neurology.* 2008;70:e49–e50.

26. Mayer NH. Clinicophysiologic concepts of spasticity and motor dysfunction in adults with an upper motoneuron lesion. *Muscle Nerve Suppl.* 1997;6:S1–13.

27. Fleuren JF, Voerman GE, Erren-Wolters CV, et al. Stop using the Ashworth Scale for the assessment of spasticity. *J Neurol Neurosurg Psychiatry.* 2010;81:46–52.

28. Yugue I, Shiba K, Ueta T, et al. A new clinical evaluation for hysterical paralysis. *Spine (Phila Pa 1976).* 2004;29:1910–1913.

29. LaFrance WC Jr. Video neuroimage: diagnosing conversion weakness with the Spinal Injuries Center test: when Hoover doesn't help. *Neurology.* 2008;71:e57.

30. Eisen A, Kuwabara S. The split hand syndrome in amyotrophic lateral sclerosis. *J Neurol Neurosurg Psychiatry.* 2012;83:399–403.

31. Ho BK, Morgan JC, Sethi KD. "Starfish" hand. *Neurology.* 2007;69:115.

32. van der Windt DA, Simons E, Riphagen II, et al. Physical examination for lumbar radiculopathy due to disc herniation in patients with low-back pain. *Cochrane Database Syst Rev.* 2010;(2):CD007431.

33. De Luigi AJ, Fitzpatrick KF. Physical examination in radiculopathy. *Phys Med Rehabil Clin N Am.* 2011;22:7–40.

34. Afzal U, Farooq MU. Teaching neuroimages: thalamic aphasia syndrome. *Neurology.* 2013;81:e177.

35. Kuljic-Obradovic DC. Subcortical aphasia: three different language disorder syndromes? *Eur J Neurol.* 2003;10:445–448.

36. Choi JY, Lee KH, Na DL, et al. Subcortical aphasia after striatocapsular infarction: quantitative analysis of brain perfusion SPECT using statistical parametric mapping and a statistical probabilistic anatomic map. *J Nucl Med.* 2007;48:194–200.

37. Zwergal A, Rettinger N, Frenzel C, et al. A bucket of static vestibular function. *Neurology.* 2009;72:1689–1692.

38. Friedman AH, Deutsch-Sokol RH. Sugiura's sign. Perilimbal vitiligo in the Vogt-Koyanagi-Harada syndrome. *Ophthalmology.* 1981;88:1159–1165.

39. Bengtzen R, Woodward M, Lynn MJ, et al. The "sunglasses sign" predicts nonorganic visual loss in neuro-ophthalmologic practice. *Neurology.* 2008;70:218–221.

40. Chinskey ND, Cornblath WT. Inferior oblique myokymia: a unique ocular motility disorder. *JAMA Ophthalmol.* 2013;131:404–405.

41. Hoyt WF, Keane JR. Superior oblique myokymia. Report and discussion on five cases of benign intermittent uniocular microtremor. *Arch Ophthalmol.* 1970;84:461–467.

Tachylalia (tachyphemia): Rapid, jumbled speech that may occur due to anxiety and agitation. The speech is broken, tremulous, high-pitched, uneven, and breathless. Stuttering and stammering are common.

Tactile agnosia: See **agnosia.**

Tactile perception of direction: See **direction of scratch test.**

Tactile perseveration: A sensation of the continuing presence of a sensory stimulus after the stimulus has been removed; an occasional feature of parietal lobe lesions.

Tadpole pupil: See Table P.1.

Talipes equinovarus: See **pes cavus.**

Tandem gait test: See **gait disorders.**

Tandem Romberg: See **Romberg sign.**

Task specific tremor: A tremor that appears during or is exacerbated by a specific movement or activity, e.g., **primary writing tremor.**

Tardive akathisia: An inner restlessness and urge to move associated with neuroleptic therapy. The sensation is unpleasant and often accompanied by repetitive, purposeless **stereotypies**, such as pacing (see **akathisia**). Tardive movement disorders are those associated with long-term use of neuroleptic agents that are dopamine receptor antagonists (DRA), particularly with the discontinuation or decrease in dose of a neuroleptic, as in **tardive dyskinesias**, the most common tardive syndrome.[1] Akathisia can occur as a tardive phenomenon, following a decrease in dose or discontinuation of a DRA or a decrease in the dose of medication used to control akathisia, such as benztropine. Risk factors for the development of tardive akathisia include female gender, advanced age, iron deficiency, cognitive dysfunction, and affective disorders. In contrast to acute akathisia, which tends to respond to anticholinergics, propranolol, or clonazepam, tardive akathisia may improve with monoamine depleting agents, such as reserpine.

Tardive dyskinesias (TD): Involuntary movements that usually develop in patients who have received dopamine receptor antagonists or related compounds, usually as treatment for major psychosis, for prolonged periods (see Table A.2).[2] The movements typically involve primarily the mouth, tongue, and jaw with incessant chewing, smacking, licking, and tongue-thrusting movements that are difficult to eradicate (see **orofacial dyskinesias**). Some patients are unaware they have these movements. Tardive dyskinesias are more prone to develop in older patients, especially women. Unfortunately, the term TD is often used for all involuntary orofacial movements, even those that develop with no drug exposure, especially in older or edentulous patients. Anti-emetic agents that block the dopamine receptor, such as metoclopramide, can cause tardive syndromes. The atypical antipsychotics, such as quetiapine, and olanzapine are less likely to cause tardive syndromes, but the risk is not eliminated. See **dyskinesias, rabbit syndrome, bon bon sign.** Involuntary movements of the upper face or an abnormal gait suggest an alternate diagnosis, such as HD.

Tardive dystonia: A movement disorder related to the use of dopamine-blocking agents, such as neuroleptics (see Table A.2).[3] These agents most often cause acute dystonic reactions, such as **oculogyric crisis**, but may also produce **dystonia** in the setting of chronic use, particularly a decrease in dose or discontinuation of a neuroleptic. Drug-induced dystonia is an important cause of secondary dystonia.

Tardive dystonia is distinct from **tardive dyskinesias**, and there are important reasons to differentiate between these two disorders. Tardive dyskinesias are most common in elderly women; tardive dystonia occurs in younger patients and has no gender predilection. Anticholinergic medications tend to worsen tardive dyskinesias but are helpful in tardive dystonia. In one large series, only 39% had received DRAs for schizophrenia and 9.5% of patients had been treated for nonpsychiatric disorders.[4] Tardive dystonia may develop after a relatively short exposure to neuroleptics. The dystonic movements in tardive dystonia are identical to those that occur with idiopathic dystonia, but in tardive dystonia other abnormal involuntary movements, such as **orofacial dyskinesias**, may coexist. The presence of multiple movement disorders in the same patient should raise suspicion of a drug-induced disorder. Tardive dystonia usually begins focally but may progress to a segmental or even a generalized disorder. Neck involvement typically causes retrocollis or anterocollis. **Pisa syndrome** occurs more commonly with tardive dystonia than with idiopathic dystonia.

Tay's sign: See **cherry red spot.**

Tectal pupils: The large pupils with light near dissociation sometimes seen when lesions affect the upper midbrain. Such pupils may accompany the **upgaze palsy** and **convergence retraction nystagmus** of Parinaud's syndrome. Tectal pupils have a poor, rarely absent, light response and much better near response. The pupils tend to be large, but this may be in part due to the fact that young people have larger pupils and lesions in this region tend to occur in younger patients. Sometimes, upgaze paresis is severe enough that the eyes are forced into sustained downgaze with retracted eyelids: the "**setting sun sign**," seen in children with obstructive hydrocephalus ballooning the posterior third ventricle and rostral aqueduct.

Telangiectasias: Dilated dermal blood vessels that occur in a number of conditions. Telangiectasias appear as red or purple spidery or punctate lesions; because the lesions are vascular, they blanch when pressure is applied.

From a neurologic perspective, important conditions associated with telangiectasias include DM, SLE, Cushing's syndrome, sickle cell disease, carcinoid syndrome, alcoholism, scleroderma, and CREST (calcinosis, Raynaud's phenomenon, esophageal dysmotility, sclerodactyly, and telangiectasias), a limited, cutaneous form of scleroderma. In ataxia-telangiectasia, the lesions occur in the conjunctiva (Fig. T.1). In hereditary hemorrhagic telangiectasia (Osler-Weber-Rendu syndrome), the telangiectasias are actually tiny, cutaneous AVMs (Fig. T.2). Capillary telangiectasias may also occur in the brain but are rarely symptomatic.

Telecanthus: See **hypertelorism.**

Telegraphic speech: See **agrammatism.**

Temperature reversal: An unusual and dramatic sensory disturbance that occurs in ciguatera intoxication. The disorder causes a primarily sensory neurologic syndrome with paresthesias and bizarre sensations. With temperature reversals, cold feels hot and vice versa. A cold tuning fork applied to the skin is perceived as warm or hot. Temperature reversal has also been reported with neurotoxic shellfish poisoning.

Temporal crescent: A rare finding on visual field examination. Fibers that carry visual impulses from the peripheral portions of the retina terminate on the anterior

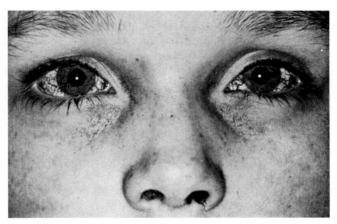

Figure T.1. Telangiectasias in the bulbar conjunctiva in ataxia telangiectasia. (From Rowland LP, Pedley TA, eds. *Merritt's Neurology*. 12th ed. Philadelphia, PA: Wolters Kluwer Health/Lippincott Williams & Wilkins; 2009, with permission.)

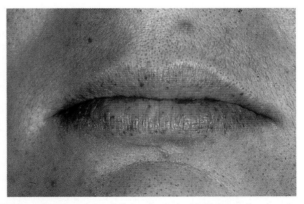

Figure T.2. Hereditary hemorrhagic telangiectasia. Multiple small red spots on the lips strongly suggest hereditary hemorrhagic telangiectasia. Spots may also be visible on the face and hands and in the mouth. The spots are dilated capillaries and may bleed when traumatized. The most common neurological complication is brain abscess. (From Langlais RP, Miller CS. *Color Atlas of Common Oral Diseases*. Philadelphia, PA: Lea & Febiger; 1992, with permission.)

third or half of the visual cortex of the occipital lobe in concentric zones, with macular fibers terminating most posteriorly. The most peripheral parts of the retina are represented most anteriorly in the calcarine cortex; the closer a retinal point lies to the macula, the more posterior its calcarine representation. The nasal hemiretina representation extends farther forward than the temporal (the temporal field is more extensive than the nasal), creating a portion of retina for which no homology exits in the opposite eye. This unpaired nasal retina is represented in the most anterior portion of the calcarine cortex, near the area of the tentorium, just outside the binocular visual field, which creates an isolated temporal crescent in each field. Sparing or selective involvement of this monocular temporal crescent has localizing value.[5] Occipital lobe lesions may spare the monocular temporal crescent if the damage does not involve the anterior part of the cortex.[6] Conversely, small, far anteriorly placed lesions may involve only the temporal crescent in the contralateral eye (half [quarter might be more appropriate] moon or temporal crescent syndrome).[7] Preservation of the temporal crescent results in strikingly incongruous fields. Preservation of the temporal crescent has been called an "endangered" finding because detecting it requires the now seldom used kinetic (Goldmann) perimetry; the currently used static perimetric techniques that concentrate on the central 30 degrees of the visual field tend to miss this phenomenon.[8]

Temporal pallor: Pallor of the temporal portion of the disc. Temporal pallor is a classical finding in MS and may precede definite **optic atrophy**, but normal physiologic temporal pallor makes this finding often equivocal (Fig. T.3; see Fig. O.4).

Terson's syndrome: An ophthalmoscopic picture that may occur after SAH or other intracranial bleeding. There are bilateral multiple posterior segment hemorrhages that may be subhyaloid, intraretinal, or intravitreal in location (Figs. T.4 and T.5). Intraocular hemorrhage occurs in approximately 20% of patients with acute intracranial bleeding, most often subarachnoid but occasionally subdural or intracerebral. The most common cause is spontaneous aneurysmal SAH. Intraocular hemorrhages are thought to occur because of the sudden increase in ICP that may complicate intracranial hemorrhage. The precise mechanism remains unclear, but the extent of intraocular hemorrhage correlates with the rapidity and degree of ICP elevation. The increased ICP is thought to obstruct retinal venous outflow and

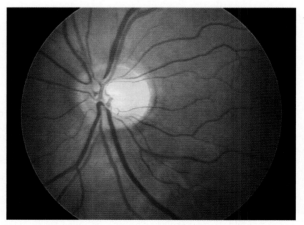

Figure T.3. Temporal optic disc pallor with decreased vision and central scotomas in a patient with presumed nutritional deficiency optic neuropathy. (From Savino PJ, Danesh-Meyer HV; Wills Eye Hospital (Philadelphia Pa). *Neuro-ophthalmology.* 2nd ed. Philadelphia, PA: Wolters Kluwer Health/Lippincott Williams & Wilkins; 2012, with permission.)

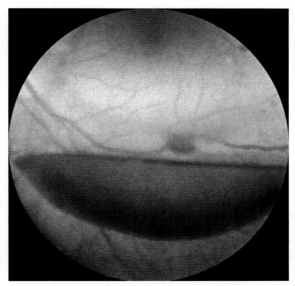

Figure T.4. Subhyaloid hemorrhage in a patient with subarachnoid hemorrhage (Terson's syndrome). The hemorrhage occurs between the posterior layer of the vitreous and the retina, are globular and often form a meniscus if the patient is examined upright, if supine the hemorrhage appears globular. (From Campbell WW. *DeJong's the Neurologic Examination*. 7th ed. Philadelphia, PA: Wolters Kluwer Health/Lippincott Williams & Wilkins; 2013, with permission.)

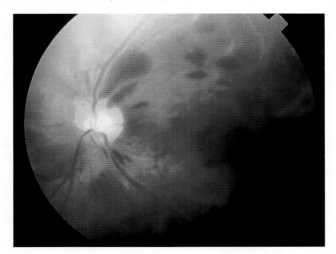

Figure T.5. Terson's syndrome. Multiple superficial retinal hemorrhages are present in the posterior pole. (From Tasman W, Jaeger E. *The Wills Eye Hospital Atlas of Clinical Ophthalmology*. 2nd ed. Philadelphia, PA: Wolters Kluwer Health/Lippincott Williams & Wilkins; 2001, with permission.)

cause the rupture of superficial retinal blood vessels. The presence of intraocular hemorrhages is associated with higher mortality.

Tetany: Hyperexcitability of the entire peripheral nervous system, as well as the musculature, to even minimal stimuli that most often occurs with alkalosis, typically due to hyperventilation, or with hypocalcemia or hypomagnesemia.[9] A normocalcemic variation occurs as a familial disorder. The clinical manifestations of tetany include spasm and tonic contractions of the skeletal muscles, principally the distal muscles of the extremities. Signs of tetany are more easily obtained if the patient first hyperventilates for a few minutes (latent tetany). Severe tetany may cause seizures, laryngospasm, stridor, and respiratory arrest.

Common manifestations of tetany include **carpopedal spasm**, with tonic contraction of the muscles of the wrists, hands, fingers, feet, and toes, **Chvostek's sign** and **Trousseau's sign**. The **Lust phenomenon** may also occur. Patients often have a very active **Tinel's sign** over multiple peripheral nerves. Both Chvostek's sign and the Lust peroneal phenomenon are essentially examples of a **motor Tinel's sign**. Other signs of tetany are summarized in **Table T.1**.

Thalamic aphasia: See **subcortical aphasia**.

Thalamic astasia: An inability to stand or sit out of proportion to weakness or sensory loss, with a tendency to fall backward or to the side contralateral to a thalamic lesion. This postural difficulty has been attributed to dysfunction of thalamic area X, a cerebellar relay nucleus in the ventral lateral complex.

Table T.1. Other Signs of Tetany

Sign	Technique	Finding
Pool-Schlesinger's	Forceful abduction and elevation of the arm to produce tension on the brachial plexus; or forceful flexion of the thigh on the trunk while the leg is extended to stretch the sciatic nerve	Tetanic spasm of the muscles of the forearm, hand, and fingers; or spasm of the muscles of the leg and foot
Schultze's	Mechanical stimulation of protruded tongue (e.g., by tapping with a percussion hammer)	Transient depression or dimpling at the site of stimulation (similar response may occur in myotonia or myotonic dystrophy)
Kashida's thermic	Application of either hot or cold irritants	Hyperesthesias and spasms
Escherich's	Percussion of the inner surface of the lips or percussion of the tongue	Contractions of the lips, masseters, and tongue
Hochsinger's	Pressure on the inner aspect of biceps muscle	Spasm and contraction of the hand (may be a variation of Trousseau sign)
Peroneal (Lust phenomenon)	Tapping over the common peroneal nerve as it winds around the neck of the fibula	Dorsiflexion and eversion of the foot

From Campbell WW. *DeJong's the neurologic examination.* 7th ed. Philadelphia, PA: Wolters Kluwer Health/Lippincott Williams & Wilkins; 2013.

Thalamic ataxia: Incoordination that develops due to a lesion involving the mid to posterior thalamus, particularly the ventrolateral and ventral posterior nuclei, probably because of involvement of the dentatorubrothalamic tract and ascending sensory pathways as they enter the thalamus. Thalamic ataxia usually occurs after ischemic lesions, primarily infarction involving the distribution of the thalamogeniculate artery, occasionally after hemorrhage. **Hemiparesis** may occur, but only transiently. Patients develop "cerebellar" findings, but these are associated with sensory loss (hemiataxia–hypesthesia syndrome) and sometimes pain. Findings may include **ataxia, dysmetria, dysdiadochokinesia,** and **loss of rebound**. The thalamic ataxia syndrome has distinct localizing value. The findings are distinguishable from ataxic hemiparesis, in which hemiparesis is more prominent but sensory loss does not occur. When the immediately adjacent posterior limb of the internal capsule is also involved, hemiparesis may be more prominent. In addition to ataxia and tremor, posterior thalamic infarction may cause dystonia, myoclonus and chorea: "the jerky dystonic unsteady hand."[10] When these involve the hand, the condition is referred to as thalamic hand.

Thalamic esotropia: Loss of abduction of the contralateral eye in acute thalamic lesions, either ischemic infarction or, more often, hemorrhage.[11] Esotropia of the ipsilateral eye occurs less commonly and is usually less severe. **Upgaze palsy** often occurs in association. When severe, thalamic hemorrhage may produce bilateral acute esotropia with tonic downward deviation of the eyes so that the patient seems to peer at the tip of the nose.[12] Thalamic esotropia may be mistaken for CN VI palsy.

Thalamic hand: See **thalamic ataxia.**

Thalamic neglect: See **attentional deficits.**

Thalamic sensory loss: A pattern of sensory loss that occurs with thalamic lesions and has some unusual characteristics not typically seen with hemisensory deficits caused by lesions in other locations. Thalamic sensory loss tends to involve all modalities, including vibration, which is never lost with a lesion of the cortex. Marked loss of appreciation of heavy contact, posture, passive movement, and deep pressure perception occurs, and the thresholds for light touch, pain, and temperature sensations are raised. Small lesions limited to the ventral posterior lateral nucleus may cause paresthesias without demonstrable sensory loss. The sensory loss may cause **midline splitting,** especially on the face. The sensory loss may be bilateral around the umbilicus and intraorally. The bilateral, intraoral involvement is characteristic of ventral posterior medial lesions. The sensory impairment tends to involve the distal extremities maximally. It may involve the tips of all the fingers; this pattern is diagnostic of involvement of the ventral posterior inferior nucleus. Thalamic lesions are often associated with sensory perversions, such as paresthesias and hyperesthesias, or painful hyperpathia or **allodynia**. Some thalamic lesions may blunt cold but not heat sensation.[13] Many patients have active paresthesias with a burning quality, and a thalamic pain (Dejerine-Roussy) syndrome may ensue. In addition to the sensory changes, hemiparesis and hemianopia usually occur and, less frequently, hemiataxia, choreoathetosis, and unmotivated emotional responses (see **thalamic ataxia**).

In a series of 25 patients with thalamic stroke, nine had a loss of all modalities of sensation with faciobrachiocrural distribution, five suffered dissociated sensory loss with faciobrachiocrural distribution, 11 showed a dissociated involvement of sensation with a partial distribution pattern, 18 had contralateral paresthesias, six complained of pain and/or dysesthesias during the stroke, and four developed delayed pain and/or dysesthesias.

Thalamic tremor: See **tremor.**

Thenar hypoplasia: See **muscle aplasia.**

Thermanesthesia: Loss of thermal sensibility.

Thoracic outlet syndrome provocative tests: Maneuvers used in the diagnosis of thoracic outlet syndrome (TOS). TOS is a very controversial clinical entity.[14,15] Among proponents, the diagnosis is frequently based on physical examination findings. There is no confirmatory test, and a frequent statement in the surgical literature is that the diagnosis is based on "careful clinical evaluation" or words to that effect. In fact, careful studies have shown that the clinical tests on which the diagnosis is usually based are themselves quite unreliable.

As with the **carpal tunnel syndrome provocative tests**, the physical examination in TOS employs various maneuvers seeking to reproduce symptoms. The examination techniques most often used include Adson's test, the **elevated arm stress test** (EAST), Wright's hyperabduction maneuver and the costoclavicular maneuver. For Adson's test, the patient sits upright with the hands resting on the knees with the neck extended and the chin up, then takes a deep breath and turns the head toward the affected side. A positive test is diminution of the radial pulse or blood pressure in the symptomatic arm. In Wright's test, the radial pulse decreases when the arm is held overhead at a 90-degree angle with the elbow flexed. The EAST attempts to reproduce symptoms by having the patient hold the arms at shoulder level with the elbows flexed to 90 degrees and repetitively clench the fists for 3 minutes. The costoclavicular test assesses the radial pulse as the shoulders are braced downward and backward with the chest protruded in an exaggerated military attention posture. Other signs may include pain or paresthesias with firm supraclavicular pressure, **Tinel's sign** over the plexus or a bruit over the supraclavicular fossa or in the axilla. The Cyriax release test seeks to relieve symptoms by holding up the elbows, the same maneuver described for droopy shoulder syndrome. The **upper limb tension test** is a complex maneuver not considered very reliable by evidence-based assessment, but touted as one of the very best tests for TOS.

There have been few studies on the validity of any of these signs.[16,17] The available information indicates that the sensitivity, specificity, and LRs of the various physical examination maneuvers are singularly unimpressive. These provocative maneuvers result in a high false-positive rate in normal subjects and an even higher false-positive rate in CTS patients. One of the main criteria for the diagnosis, a positive Adson maneuver, is positive in many normal asymptomatic individuals. In an investigation of TOS provocative maneuvers, 94% of patients with CTS and 56% of normals had at least one positive TOS diagnostic maneuver.[18] The EAST was positive in 77% of patients with CTS and in 47% of normal controls. A study of 200 upper extremities in 100 normal volunteers found that 7.5% of the extremities had a Tinel sign. Pulse obliteration was present in 13.5% with the Adson maneuver, 47% with the costoclavicular maneuver, and 57% with Wright's hyperabduction maneuver.[19] Similar results were obtained in a study of 64 normal subjects.[20]

Even the surgeons now admit that Adson's, Wright's, and related maneuvers are useless. Sanders et al.[21] stated, "The Adson test has been shown to be of no clinical value . . . The test is normal in most patients with true neurogenic TOS and at the same time can be positive in many control volunteers." Roos,[22] a leading TOS proponent, when describing the EAST, stated "pulse obliteration with the arms and head in various positions is a normal finding in the majority of asymptomatic people and therefore has no relation to the etiology or presence of symptoms" and that studies have shown "no correlation with impairment of circulation or positional radial pulse changes in almost all patients with true TOS." Advocates claim greater sensitivity comes with multiple positive tests, but this approach ignores the statistical issues involved with multiple tests and the increasing likelihood of a false positive as more tests are performed. In one study, 12% of normal subjects had two or more positive tests.[20]

Thorburn sign: See **Jolly sign.**

Three-clap test: See **applause sign.**

Three-paper test: See **Marie's paper test.**

Three-step test for vertical diplopia: See **Bielschowsky's head tilt test.**

Throckmorton's sign: See Table M.3.

Thumb rolling: See **finger rolling, forearm rolling,** and **subtle signs of hemiparesis.**

Thumb–chin reflex: See **palmomental reflex.**

Tibialis anterior reflex: See **peroneal reflex.**

Tibialis posterior reflex: Inversion of the foot with tapping the tendon of the tibialis posterior just above and behind the medial malleolus (see Table D.1). This reflex is best examined with the patient prone and the foot in a neutral position or slight eversion, extended beyond the edge of the bed. It may be absent in L5 or S1 radiculopathy but is difficult to obtain even in normal subjects.

Tibialis sign of Strumpell: See **anterior tibial sign.**

Tic (habit spasms): Quick, irregular but repetitive movements that are more often seen in children than in adults. A tic may be defined as a coordinated, repetitive, seemingly purposeful act involving a group of muscles in their normal synergistic relationships. Tics are stereotyped, recurrent movements that may seem purposeful but are relatively involuntary, consisting of brief contractions of whole muscles or groups of muscles, always accompanied by motion of the affected part. Patients are able to suppress the movements temporarily with concentration, but they quickly return when attention is diverted to some other task. Voluntary suppression causes a sense of intolerable mounting tension and an urge to move that is temporarily relieved by indulgence in a tic. Tics are exaggerated by emotional strain and tension; they cease during sleep.

Tics may involve any portion of the body. Common examples of simple motor tics include repetitive blinking, facial contortions, or shoulder shrugging. More complicated tics can occur, and tics can also involve the vocal tract (phonic or vocal tic), producing throat-clearing as well as bizarre vocalizations, such as barking and grunting or sounds resembling a hiccup.

Patients affected with Gilles de la Tourette syndrome (maladie des tics) have multifocal tics, compulsive behavior, imitative gestures, stereotyped movements, grunts and groans, and evidence of regressive behavior. Tics are very common and usually benign; patients with Tourette syndrome have exaggerated, complex tics, which together with the other features of the disease can be very disabling. The large repertoire of tics and the combination of motor and vocal tics distinguish Tourette's syndrome from ordinary tics.

Tic convulsif: The rare combination of both **hemifacial spasm** and trigeminal neuralgia, with lancinating pain accompanying the facial spasms.

Tilted discs: An optic disc anomaly that may produce a constellation of findings occasionally confused with pituitary tumor. Tilted disks occur in 1% to 2% of the population and the condition is bilateral in 75% of cases.[23] The disc does not lie flat against the retina because the optic nerve enters the globe at an angle superiorly, causing the superior margin of the disc to protrude slightly and the disc to slant from above to below (Fig. T.6). Confusion with **papilledema** may arise because the protrusion and obscuration of the superior aspect of the disc can simulate disc edema. In addition, there is usually accompanying ectasia of the inferior nasal part of the retina that can cause a superior temporal **visual field defect**. The combination of superior temporal field defects and the appearance of disc edema have led to the misdiagnosis of pituitary tumor. The field defect may not respect the vertical meridian, as would be expected with a chiasmal lesion. Associated findings include an anomalous pattern of retinal vessels, astigmatism, **strabismus**, and inferonasal pigmentary accumulation. See **pseudopapilledema**.

Time agnosia: See agnosia.

Tinel's (Hoffman-Tinel) sign: Paresthesias produced by percussion over a peripheral nerve that may indicate focal nerve pathology, aka neuroma sign **(Video T.1)**. Originally described in traumatic nerve injury, an advancing Tinel sign along the course of a nerve is used as a marker of regeneration.[24] Mechanical sensitivity often accompanies neural regeneration and following a peripheral nerve injury the region of mechanical sensitivity will advance down the nerve along with axonal sprouting. Failure of the Tinel sign to advance is a poor prognostic sign. The Tinel sign is often used as a one of the **carpal tunnel syndrome provocative tests** and in other suspected nerve compressions, where eliciting a Tinel sign can be useful. Bear in mind that many normal patients "Tinel" over all their nerves; only the presence of a disproportionately active Tinel sign over the clinically suspect nerve has any localizing value (see Video T.1).

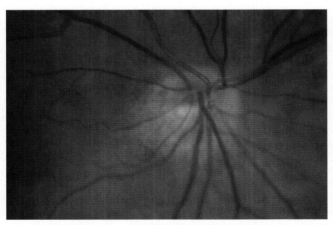

Figure T.6. The congenital tilted optic disk is apparent as the oval of nerve tissue superiorly. There is no apparent optic cup. (From Chern KC, Saidel MA. *Ophthalmology Review Manual.* 2nd ed. Philadelphia, PA: Wolters Kluwer Health/Lippincott Williams & Wilkins; 2012, with permission.)

Rarely, percussion over a nerve may elicit paresthesias radiating proximally, referred to as a reverse Tinel or Valleix sign.

Titubation: The rhythmic head and trunk oscillations seen in severe truncal **ataxia** due to midline cerebellar lesions. The head movements in titubation are primarily anteroposterior (yes–yes) at 3 to 4 Hz.

Toe-to-finger test: See **finger-to-nose** and **heel-to-shin tests.**

Toe walking: An abnormal gait pattern in which the patient tends to walk on tiptoe. Toe walking is not considered abnormal unless it persists past age 2 years. When the walking pattern continues into later childhood and adolescence without any other demonstrable abnormalities, the condition is referred to as idiopathic toe walking. However, toe walking may occur in a number of disorders, and may be the presenting or primary manifestation of such conditions as muscular dystrophy, hereditary neuropathy, cerebral palsy, and autism.

In myopathy, toe walking occurs because the pelvis is thrust forward to compensate for hyperlordosis, and the patient bears weight on the forefoot to adapt and maintain balance. Toe walking also requires less knee extensor strength than normal walking and may help compensate for quadriceps weakness.[25] Toe walking also requires less ankle plantar flexor and dorsiflexor strength, and may occur as a manifestation of peripheral nerve disease. In a series of 18 patients with toe walking, six had muscular dystrophy, five CMT disease, and four had other neuropathies.[26] Evidence of early involvement with conditions such as Becker muscular dystrophy and CMT disease may not be obvious, and some patients with these conditions have been thought to have idiopathic toe walking. Eight of 16 patients with Becker muscular dystrophy and 13 of 44 with CMT disease presented either entirely or predominantly because of toe walking.[26]

Toe walking also occurs with upper motor neuron disease; it may be a feature of cerebral palsy, particularly mild spastic diplegia, and may be an early manifestation of HSP. Toe walking is also associated with autism and may be the first sign of a global developmental disorder. Before accepting toe walking as idiopathic, look for evidence of muscle weakness or pseudo-hypertrophy, pes cavus, bladder dysfunction, hyperreflexia or hyporeflexia, as well as learning and behavior difficulties.

Tongue deviation: Failure of the tongue to protrude in the midline. Unilateral tongue weakness causes the tongue to deviate toward the weak side on protrusion because of the unopposed action of the normal genioglossus—the principal protractor of the tongue—which protrudes the tip of the tongue by drawing the root forward. Because the tip of the tongue is pulled out of the mouth it deviates toward the paretic side. There is impairment of the ability to deviate the protruded tongue toward the opposite side. There is impairment of the ability to push the tongue against the cheek on the sound side, but not on the paralyzed side. Lateral movements of the tip of the nonprotruded tongue, controlled by the intrinsic tongue muscles, may be preserved.

Facial muscle weakness or jaw deviation makes it difficult to evaluate deviation of the tongue. Patients with significant lower facial weakness often have distortion of the normal facial appearance that can produce the appearance of tongue deviation when none is present. The lack of mobility of the corner of the mouth may simulate tongue deviation. Manually pulling up the weak side of the face eliminates the "deviation." It may also be helpful to gauge tongue position in relation to the tip of the nose or the notch between the upper incisors. See **glossoplegia.**

Tongue weakness may be due to a supranuclear, nuclear, or infranuclear lesion. Supranuclear lesions cause weakness but no atrophy, and the weakness is rarely severe. Since the genioglossus has mainly crossed supranuclear innervation, the tongue protrudes toward the weak side, but to the side opposite the supranuclear lesion. Supranuclear tongue weakness may occur with a destructive lesion of the cerebral cortex or the corticobulbar tract in the internal capsule, cerebral peduncle, or pons.

In addition to weakness, nuclear and infranuclear lesions cause atrophy of the involved side. The tongue protrudes toward the weak side, which is also the side of the lesion. Progressive nuclear lesions, such as motor neuron disease, often cause **fasciculations** in addition to weakness **(Video Link T.1)**. Common disorders that may involve the hypoglossal nucleus include neoplasms, vascular lesions, and motor neuron disease. Nuclear lesions and infranuclear, intramedullary lesions may exhibit involvement of the contiguous ascending sensory or descending motor pathways, as in the medial medullary syndrome causing tongue weakness and contralateral hemiparesis. Processes involving the extramedullary, intracranial course of the nerve include disorders involving the meninges, such as infectious and neoplastic meningitis, neoplasms and other mass lesions (e.g., schwannoma), inflammation, and trauma.

Processes involving the skull base—such as basal skull fractures, basilar impression, platybasia, or Chiari malformation may affect the nerve before it leaves the skull. Lesions along the clivus may cause bilateral hypoglossal palsies or involve other cranial nerves. Processes involving the extracranial course of the nerve include trauma of various types, especially penetrating wounds, carotid aneurysms (especially dissections) and tumors involving the neck, tongue base, or salivary glands. Hypoglossal nerve palsy can also occur as an idiopathic, benign syndrome that resolves spontaneously. Rarely, primary neural tumors involve CN XII extracranially. CN XII may be involved with other lower cranial nerves in a multiple cranial neuropathy syndrome. In a series of 100 cases of hypoglossal palsy, the nerve was involved bilaterally in one-third; tumor and trauma accounted for the majority.[27]

Tonic plantar response: A slow, tonic flexion of the toes and distal part of the foot produced by rubbing the sole; reputedly a sign of extrapyramidal disease.

Tonic pupil: See **Adie's tonic pupil.**

Topagnosia: See **agnosia.**

Touch-me-not sign: See **Waddell signs.**

Tournay pupillary phenomenon: The pupil of the abducting eye dilates and the pupil of the adducting eye constricts with extreme lateral gaze, causing transient physiologic anisocoria; a normal finding.

Torsional nystagmus: See **nystagmus.**

Torticollis: See **cervical dystonia.**

Tottering gait: See **gait disorders.**

Tourniquet test: A procedure described for the diagnosis of CTS. Studies have shown low sensitivity and specificity. See **carpal tunnel syndrome provocative tests.** The test has also been used for tarsal tunnel syndrome, with even less in the way of reliability data.

Tower skull: See **craniosynostosis.**

Trail-making tests: A **mental status examination** test in which the patient is required to connect in sequence either letters or numbers scattered around a page (Trails A), or to alternate connecting letters and numbers, e.g., A-1-B-2-C-3 (Trails B).

Transcortical aphasia: Types of **aphasia** in which the perisylvian language area is preserved but disconnected from the rest of the brain. The usual etiology is a border-zone infarction. Because the posterior inferior frontal and the posterior superior temporal language areas and the connecting arcuate fasciculus are intact, patients with transcortical aphasia (TCA) are aphasic but have a paradoxical preservation of the ability to repeat. Repetition can be so well preserved that the patients display **echolalia**. When the condition is severe and the entire perisylvian language complex is separated from the rest of the brain, the patients are not fluent in spontaneous speech and are unable to comprehend. This syndrome has been termed isolation of the speech area, or mixed TCA. When the lesion is primarily anterior, the syndrome resembles **Broca's aphasia** with nonfluency in spontaneous speech but intact comprehension. Repetition is better than spontaneous speech. This is the syndrome of transcortical motor aphasia (anterior isolation syndrome). The supplementary motor area and dorsolateral prefrontal cortex, which are responsible for the planning and initiation of speech, are isolated from the posterior inferior frontal region. In transcortical sensory aphasia (posterior isolation syndrome), there is greater involvement of the posterior language areas. The posterior superior temporal region is isolated from the surrounding parietal, occipital, and temporal cortex that store word associations. The patients are fluent but have difficulty with comprehension; repetition is better than spontaneous speech. The TCAs are more common than is often appreciated.

Trapezius hump: A sign of shoulder girdle weakness, which occurs particularly in FSH and is most notable from the front during arm abduction (Fig. T.7). The hump is due to prominence of the midportion of the trapezius. In patients with mild shoulder girdle weakness, the hump is due to trapezius contraction as it tries to stabilize the scapula. With more severe weakness, much of the hump may be the scapula as it rides up.

Traquair scotoma: See **scotoma.**

Tremblement affirmative/negatif: See **essential tremor.**

Tremor: Involuntary, relatively rhythmic, purposeless, oscillatory movements of a body part. The excursion may be small or large, and may involve one or more parts of the body. A simple tremor involves only a single muscle group; a compound tremor involves several muscle groups and may have several elements in combination, resulting in a series of complex movements (e.g., alternating flexion and extension together with alternating pronation and supination). Not only the agonist and antagonist, but muscles of fixation and synergists may play a part in the movements. A tremor may be present at rest or with activity. Some tremors are accentuated by having the patient hold the fingers extended and separated with the arms outstretched. Slow movements, writing, and drawing circles or spirals may bring tremor out.

Tremors are classified in various ways: by location, rate, amplitude, rhythmicity, relationship to rest and movement, etiology, and underlying pathology. Amplitude and frequency typically exhibit an inverse relationship, with the coarser tremors having a lower frequency and the finer tremor a higher frequency. Other important

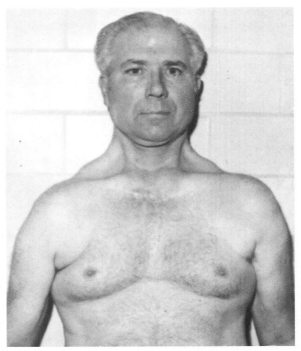

Figure T.7. Shoulder girdle weakness with "trapezius hump," "step-sign" with prominent down-sloping clavicles, and an oblique anterior axillary crease in a patient with LGMD. (From Weiner W. *Neurology for the Non-Neurologist.* 6th ed. Philadelphia, PA: Wolters Kluwer Health/Lippincott Williams & Wilkins; 2010, with permission.)

factors include the relationship to fatigue, emotion, and the use of medications, alcohol, or street drugs. Tremor may be unilateral or bilateral; and most commonly involves distal parts of the extremities—the fingers or hands—but may also affect the arms, feet, legs, tongue, eyelids, jaw, and head. The rate classification includes slow, medium, or fast. Oscillations of 3 to 5 Hz are considered slow, 10 to 20 Hz rapid; amplitude may be fine, coarse, or medium. Tremor may be constant or intermittent, rhythmic or relatively nonrhythmic, although a certain amount of rhythmicity is implied in the term tremor.

The relationship to rest or activity is the basis for classification into two primary tremor types: rest and action. A **rest tremor** is present mainly during relaxation when voluntary muscle activity is absent and the part completely supported against gravity (e.g., with the hands in the lap), and attenuate when the part is used. Rest tremor is seen primarily in PD and other forms of **parkinsonism**. An **action tremor** appears with voluntary movement, such as when performing some activity. Action tremors are divided into postural and kinetic subtypes. Postural tremors become evident when the limbs are maintained in an antigravity position (e.g., arms outstretched, fingers pointed at each other, heel perched on opposite knee).

Common types of postural tremor are **enhanced physiologic tremor** and **essential tremor** (ET). A kinetic tremor, such as **intention tremor** and **task-specific tremor,** appears when making a voluntary movement. An isometric tremor is one that appears during contraction of a muscle against resistance without actual movement of the body part, as in **orthostatic tremor**. Some tremors fall into more than one potential classification. ET has both postural and kinetic components. The real severity of a kinetic tremor is often best appreciated during activities such as writing and drinking from a cup.

Coarse tremors occur in a variety of disease states, and are usually slow. **Parkinsonian tremor** is one of the most characteristic. Coarse tremor also occurs in Wilson's disease and other extrapyramidal syndromes. The tremors of general paresis and alcoholism are typically coarse, especially if the movements are diffuse, as in delirium tremens. **Psychogenic tremor** and the tremors associated with midbrain and cerebellar disease are also usually coarse and slow. A unilateral, postural and kinetic tremor of the upper limb associated with a single focal thalamic lesion has rarely been reported (thalamic tremor).[28] Thalamic tremor may result from the interruption of the cerebellar outflow tract to the ventral intermediate nucleus within the thalamus.

Trendelenburg's sign (gait, test): Abnormalities of station and gait related to weakness of the hip abductor muscles, primarily the gluteus medius **(Video T.2).** The hip abductors are very important in walking. With each step, the abductors of the stance leg must generate enough force to balance all the weight of the rest of the body in order to keep the pelvis level. Without contraction of the hip abductors, the hip would slide laterally toward the stance leg as the weight bearing leg was forced into adduction and the pelvis tilted. Normally, when standing on one leg the pelvis remains level or slants slightly upward away from the stance leg and toward the unsupported leg. With unilateral hip abductor weakness, standing on the affected leg causes the pelvis to slant downward away from the stance leg. The hip moves laterally and up on the weak side and the pelvis sags toward the normal, unsupported leg (the "sound side sags"). This is Trendelenburg's sign and having the patient stand on one leg is the Trendelenburg test. It may be confusing because the sag is toward the normal and away from the weak side.

To compensate for the pelvic tilt the patient may shift weight so that the trunk sways as the shoulder moves down on the weight-bearing side, the compensated Trendelenburg sign or Trendelenburg lurch. Neurologic causes of a unilateral Trendelenburg sign include L5 radiculopathy and superior gluteal neuropathy, both of which cause gluteus medius weakness.

When walking, hip abductor weakness causes the weight-bearing leg to adduct and the hip to jut laterally on the affected side, causing an exaggerated pelvic swing during the stance phase as the pelvis on the side of the swing leg drops downward. This is the Trendelenburg gait or gluteus medius lurch. When hip abductor weakness is bilateral, the result is a gait pattern referred to as a pelvic waddle, which resembles the exaggerated hip swing of a fashion model. The waddling gait is particularly common in myopathies that weaken the pelvic girdle musculature. The Trendelenburg sign or gait may also occur with musculoskeletal disease, such as hip dislocation, fracture of the femoral head, slipped capital femoral epiphysis, coxa vara or avulsion of the abductor muscle tendon, which may occur after hip surgery.

To understand the Trendelenburg phenomenon, stand on one leg and note how the pelvis remains fairly level. Then execute an exaggerated adduction movement by shifting the body weight ipsilaterally and note how the pelvis sags downward on the opposite side, away from the weight-bearing leg ("pelvic ptosis"). Then abduct the leg and the pelvis will return to level. Weakness of hip abduction results in abnormal adduction of the stance leg: the Trendelenburg stance and gait. A biomechanical study using superior gluteal nerve blocks showed that the Trendelenburg compensations only occur after about a 50% reduction in hip abductor strength.[29] The static Trendelenburg test has only limited use as a measure of hip abductor function and cannot substitute for direct strength examination.

The patient with a myopathic gait due to bilateral hip abductor weakness has abnormal hip adduction with each step (see **gait disorders**). He walks with a broad base, with an exaggerated rotation of the pelvis, rolling or throwing the hips from side to side with every step to shift the weight of the body. There is an abnormal drop of the pelvis on the side of the swing leg and the shoulders tilt in compensation, causing the hips and shoulders to slant in opposite directions each time the gait enters stance phase. In the extreme forms, this gait pattern has a bizarre appearance. The patient walks with a pronounced waddle, shoulders thrown back and pelvis thrust forward. This form of gait is particularly common in FSH dystrophy (**Video Link T.2**).

Patients with hip pain may also lurch toward the painful side, the coxalgic gait, but there is no drop of the pelvis as in a Trendelenburg gait.

Triceps reflex: The DTR elicited by percussion of the triceps tendon, causing contraction of the triceps muscle and extension of the elbow (C7,8). (**Fig. T.8**, see Video B.4) The most common cause of reflex depression is cervical radiculopathy.

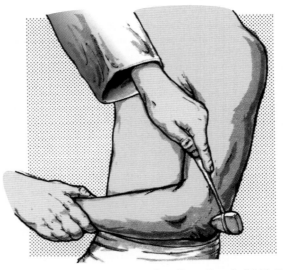

Figure T.8. Method of obtaining the triceps reflex. (From Campbell WW. *DeJong's the Neurologic Examination*. 7th ed. Philadelphia, PA: Wolters Kluwer Health/Lippincott Williams & Wilkins; 2013, with permission.)

A decreased triceps jerk has an LR of 3.0 for the diagnosis of C7 radiculopathy.[30] How to elicit the triceps reflex is nicely demonstrated in **Video Link T.3**. Occasionally, the reflex is inverted or paradoxical and percussion of the tendon causes the elbow to flex; see **inverted reflexes, olecranon reflex**.

Trident (triple furrowed) tongue: An appearance of three parallel longitudinal grooves in the tongue characteristic of MG **(Fig. T.9)**. Although muscle atrophy is rare in MG, patients with long-standing disease may develop a characteristic pattern of tongue atrophy with grooves on either side of the genioglossus paralleling the central fissure.

Trigeminal-mediated reflexes: Reflexes that depend on the motor or sensory functions of the trigeminal nerve; these reflexes include **head retraction, zygomatic reflex, oculopupillary reflex, corneomandibular, nasal reflex, trigeminobrachial,** and the **trigeminocervical**.

Trigeminobrachial reflex: Contralateral flexion and supination of the forearm after stimulation in the distribution of CN V.

Trigeminocervical reflex: Contralateral head turn after stimulation in the distribution of CN V.

Trigonocephaly: See **craniosynostosis**.

Triple flexion reflex: A variation of the withdrawal reflex, a primitive flexion response that is a spinal defense reflex mechanism (the reflex of spinal automatism, the pathologic shortening reflex). **Babinski's plantar sign** and related extensor plantar responses are fragments of the withdrawal reflex that occur with damage to the descending motor pathways. More fully developed is the triple flexion response, in which extension of the great toe is accompanied by dorsiflexion of the foot and

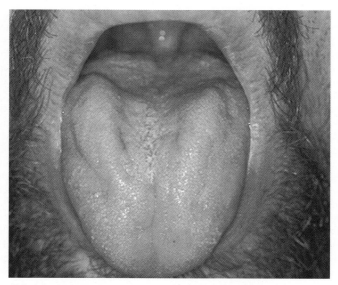

Figure T.9. A triple furrowed atrophic tongue in MUSK antibody positive myasthenia gravis. (From Selcen D, Fukuda T, Shen XM, Engel AG. Are MuSK antibodies the primary cause of myasthenic symptoms? *Neurology.* 2004;62:1945–1950, with permission.)

flexion of the knee and hip. The triple flexion reflex is seen with more severe and extensive disease of the corticospinal pathways. In addition, there is often contraction of the tensor fascia lata causing slight internal rotation at the hip and more rarely abduction of the hip (see **Brissaud's reflex**).

Triple furrowed tongue: See **trident tongue**.

Tripod (Amoss's, Hoyne's) sign: A sign of meningeal irritation. To avoid spinal flexion, the patient may sit in bed with the hands placed far behind, the head thrown back, the hips and knees flexed, and the back arched. See **meningeal signs**.

Trismus (lockjaw): Marked spasm of the muscles of mastication: The teeth are tightly clenched, the muscles hard and firm, and the patient is unable to open his jaw. Trismus is a classical manifestation of tetanus, and sometimes occurs in encephalitis, rabies, acute dystonic reactions due to neuroleptic medications, malignant hyperthermia, NMS, and **tetany**. Trismus may occur in Foix-Chavany-Marie syndrome.[31] Some myopathies, especially polymyositis, may result in fibrosis of the masseters, which causes painless trismus.[32] Psychogenic trismus does occur.

Trombone tongue: A sign of motor impersistence, characteristic of chorea. Patients are unable to maintain tongue protrusion, and the tongue moves back and forth like the slide on a trombone, aka flycatcher, snake or darting tongue (see Video C.5).

Trömner sign: See Hoffman sign.

Trousseau's sign: A sign of **tetany**. Ischemia of the peripheral nerve trunks increases nerve excitability and causes spontaneous discharges that produce **carpopedal spasm**. Compression of the arm by manual pressure, a tourniquet, or a sphygmomanometer cuff for 3 minutes is followed first by distal paresthesias that progress centripetally, then twitching of the fingers, and finally by cramping and contraction of the muscles of the fingers and hand with the thumb strongly adducted and the fingers stiffened, slightly flexed at the MCP joints, and forming a cone clustered about the thumb (obstetrician's or accoucheur's hand, main d' accoucheur) **(Fig. T.10)**. There may be a latent period of 0.5 to 4 minutes. Similar pressure around the leg or thigh will cause pedal spasm. A modification is to keep a moderately inflated sphygmomanometer cuff on one arm for about 10 minutes, then remove it and have the patient hyperventilate; typical tetanic spasm occurs earlier in the previously ischemic arm.

Truncal ataxia: Inability to maintain an upright position, with swaying and unsteadiness when standing, typically due to midline cerebellar disease. When severe, patients may lose the ability to remain erect even when seated, or to hold the neck and head steady and upright, leading to constant, to-and-fro swaying, nodding and weaving movements of the head and trunk when the patient is upright known as **titubation**. Lesions of the flocculonodular lobe (vestibulocerebellum) may cause severe truncal ataxia and make standing, or even sitting, very difficult without producing appendicular ataxia.

Trunk–thigh sign: See **Babinski trunk–thigh sign**.

Tubular visual fields: Concentric constriction of the visual fields (VF); the fields fail to enlarge as expected with testing at increasing distance. Normally, the field of vision widens progressively as the test objects are held farther away from the eye, but in nonorganic visual loss this normal widening is not seen, and the entire width of the field is as great at 1 foot from the eye as it is at 2, 5, 10, or 15 feet. The normal VF is a funnel, the nonorganic VF is a tunnel. The tubular field can be demonstrated either by testing the extent of the VF at varying distances from the patient, or it

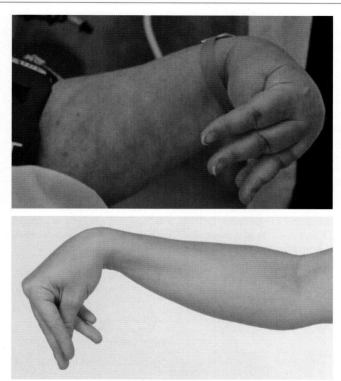

Figure T.10. Trousseau's sign in hypocalcemia. The wrist and metacarpophalangeal joints are flexed, the interphalangeal joints are hyperextended, and the thumb opposed. (From Campbell WW. *DeJong's the Neurologic Examination.*7th ed. Wolters Kluwer Health/Lippincott Williams & Wilkins; 2013, with permission.)

can be shown by using test objects of different sizes at a constant distance. The VF should be wider with larger test objects. Deficits at the same isopter with all size test objects suggest nonorganicity.

Tucked lid sign: See **eyelid retraction.**

Turricephaly: See **craniosynostosis.**

Two-point discrimination: The ability to differentiate, eyes closed, cutaneous stimulation by one point from stimulation by two points. The best instrument for testing is a two-point discriminator designed for the purpose. Commonly used substitutes are electrocardiogram calipers, a compass, or a paper clip bent into a "V," adjusting the two points to different distances. There are two types of two-point discrimination: static and moving. To test static two-point, the test instrument is held in place for a few seconds on the site to be tested. To test moving two-point on a finger pad, the discriminator would be pulled from the crease of the distal interphalangeal joint toward the tip of the finger over several seconds. The findings on the two sides of the body, or between involved and uninvolved regions, are compared.

Either one-point or two-point stimuli are delivered randomly, and the minimal distance that can be discerned as two points is determined. This distance varies considerably in different parts of the body. Normal two-point discrimination is about 1 mm on the tip of the tongue, 2 to 3 mm on the lips, 2 to 4 mm on the fingertips, 4 to 6 mm on the dorsum of the fingers, 8 to 12 mm on the palm, 20 to 30 mm on the back of the hand, and 30 to 40 mm on the dorsum of the foot. For moving two-point, the technique is the same except that the instrument is drawn slowly across the test area. Discrimination for two moving points is slightly better than for two stationary points. Moving two-point tests the rapidly adapting mechanoreceptors, and may have some advantages in the management of patients with peripheral nerve injuries.

Two-point discrimination requires keen tactile sensibility. The pathway is mainly through the posterior columns and medial lemniscus. Loss of two-point discrimination with preservation of other discriminatory tactile and proprioceptive sensation occurs as a subtle sign of a lesion of the opposite parietal lobe. Loss of two-point discrimination limited to the distribution of a peripheral nerve or root is helpful in diagnosis and management. Two-point discrimination may also be used to demonstrate a sensory level on the trunk in myelopathy.

Video Links

T.1. Unilateral tongue atrophy and fasciculations due to a cervicomedullary junction mass lesion. Available at: http://www.youtube.com/watch?v=-LvlVqhPfNE

T.2. A patient with a myopathic gait with waddling, toe walking, and hyperlordosis. (From Paul D. Larsen, MD, University of Nebraska Medical Center and Suzanne S. Stensaas, PhD, University of Utah School of Medicine, http://library.med.utah.edu/neurologicexam/html/gait_abnormal.html.) Available at: http://library.med.utah.edu/neurologicexam/html/video_window.html?vidurl=../movies/gait_ab_11.mov&vidwidth=320&vidheight=240

T.3. How to elicit the triceps reflex. (From Stanford Medicine 25, An Initiative to Revive the Culture of Bedside Medicine.) Available at: http://stanfordmedicine25.stanford.edu/the25/tendon.html

References

1. Fernandez HH, Friedman JH. Classification and treatment of tardive syndromes. *Neurologist.* 2003;9:16–27.
2. Aquino CC, Lang AE. Tardive dyskinesia syndromes: current concepts. *Parkinsonism Relat Disord.* 2014;20(suppl 1):S113–S117.
3. Skidmore F, Reich SG. Tardive dystonia. *Curr Treat Options Neurol.* 2005;7:231–236.
4. Kiriakakis V, Bhatia KP, Quinn NP, et al. The natural history of tardive dystonia. A long-term follow-up study of 107 cases. *Brain.* 1998;121:2053–2066.
5. Landau K, Wichmann W, Valavanis A. The missing temporal crescent. *Am J Ophthalmol.* 1995;119:345–349.
6. Benton S, Levy I, Swash M. Vision in the temporal crescent in occipital infarction. *Brain.* 1980;103:83–97.
7. Chavis PS, al-Hazmi A, Clunie D, et al. Temporal crescent syndrome with magnetic resonance correlation. *J Neuroophthalmol.* 1997;17:151–155.
8. Lepore FE. The preserved temporal crescent: the clinical implications of an "endangered" finding. *Neurology.* 2001;57:1918–1921.
9. Cooper MS, Gittoes NJ. Diagnosis and management of hypocalcaemia. *BMJ.* 2008;336:1298–1302.
10. Ghika J, Bogousslavsky J, Henderson J, et al. The "jerky dystonic unsteady hand": a delayed motor syndrome in posterior thalamic infarctions. *J Neurol.* 1994;241:537–542.
11. Gomez CR, Gomez SM, Selhorst JB. Acute thalamic esotropia. *Neurology.* 1988;38:1759–1762.
12. Choi KD, Jung DS, Kim JS. Specificity of "peering at the tip of the nose" for a diagnosis of thalamic hemorrhage. *Arch Neurol.* 2004;61:417–422.
13. Kim JH, Greenspan JD, Coghill RC, et al. Lesions limited to the human thalamic principal somatosensory nucleus (ventral caudal) are associated with loss of cold sensations and central pain. *J Neurosci.* 2007;27:4995–5004.

14. Campbell WW, Landau ME. Controversial entrapment neuropathies. *Neurosurg Clin N Am.* 2008;19:597–608, vi–vii.
15. Stewart JD. *Focal Peripheral Neuropathies.* 4th ed. West Vancouver, Canada: JBJ Publishing; 2010.
16. Marx RG, Bombardier C, Wright JG. What do we know about the reliability and validity of physical examination tests used to examine the upper extremity? *J Hand Surg Am.* 1999;24:185–193.
17. Malanga GA, Nadler S. *Musculoskeletal Physical Examination.* Philadelphia, PA: Elsevier Mosby; 2006.
18. Nord KM, Kapoor P, Fisher J, et al. False positive rate of thoracic outlet syndrome diagnostic maneuvers. *Electromyogr Clin Neurophysiol.* 2008;48:67–74.
19. Rayan GM, Jensen C. Thoracic outlet syndrome: provocative examination maneuvers in a typical population. *J Shoulder Elbow Surg.* 1995;4:113–117.
20. Warrens AN, Heaton JM. Thoracic outlet compression syndrome: the lack of reliability of its clinical assessment. *Ann R Coll Surg Engl.* 1987;69:203–204.
21. Sanders RJ, Hammond SL, Rao NM. Diagnosis of thoracic outlet syndrome. *J Vasc Surg.* 2007;46:601–604.
22. Roos DB. Congenital anomalies associated with thoracic outlet syndrome. Anatomy, symptoms, diagnosis, and treatment. *Am J Surg.* 1976;132:771–778.
23. Vongphanit J, Mitchell P, Wang JJ. Population prevalence of tilted optic disks and the relationship of this sign to refractive error. *Am J Ophthalmol.* 2002;133:679–685.
24. Davis EN, Chung KC. The Tinel sign: a historical perspective. *Plast Reconstr Surg.* 2004;114:494–499.
25. Kerrigan DC, Riley PO, Rogan S, et al. Compensatory advantages of toe walking. *Arch Phys Med Rehabil.* 2000;81:38–44.
26. Shield LK. Toe walking and neuromuscular disease. *Arch Dis Child.* 1984;59:1003–1004.
27. Keane JR. Twelfth-nerve palsy. Analysis of 100 cases. *Arch Neurol.* 1996;53:561–566.
28. Krystkowiak P, Martinat P, Cassim F, et al. Thalamic tremor: correlations with three-dimensional magnetic resonance imaging data and pathophysiological mechanisms. *Mov Disord.* 2000;15:911–918.
29. Kendall KD, Patel C, Wiley JP, et al. Steps toward the validation of the Trendelenburg test: the effect of experimentally reduced hip abductor muscle function on frontal plane mechanics. *Clin J Sport Med.* 2013;23:45–51.
30. McGee S. *Evidence Based Physical Diagnosis.* 3rd ed. Philadelphia, PA: Elsevier/Saunders; 2012.
31. Frontera JA, Palestrant D. Acute trismus associated with Foix-Marie-Chavany syndrome. *Neurology.* 2006;66:454–455.
32. Singer PA, Chikarmane A, Festoff BW, et al. Trismus. An unusual sign in polymyositis. *Arch Neurol.* 1985;42:1116–1118.

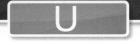

Ulnar flexion maneuver: See **elbow flexion test.**

Ulnar griffe: See **claw hand.**

Uncrossed diplopia: See **crossed diplopia.**

Unterberger-Fukuda stepping test: A test for vestibular imbalance (see Video P.3). With eyes closed, the patient steps in place for 1 minute and the degree of rotation noted. Normally there is none. With vestibular imbalance, the patient slowly pivots in the direction of the less active labyrinth. In most instances, the less active labyrinth is the diseased one. The pathophysiology is the same as for **past pointing, saccadic lateropulsion,** and **star walking.** The stepping test was first described by Unterberger in 1939 and modified by Fukuda in 1959.[1] It is referred to as the Fukuda test in the United States and Asia and the Unterberger test in Europe. The term *Unterberger-Fukuda* has been suggested **(Video Link U.1).**[2] See **head impulse test.**

Upbeat nystagmus: See **nystagmus.**

Upgaze palsy: Difficulty looking up with preservation of other eye movements **(Fig. U.1).** The pathways controlling upgaze and downgaze course in the region of the rostral midbrain, pretectum, and posterior commissure. The vertical gaze equivalent of the PPRF is the rostral interstitial nucleus of the MLF (riMLF), which lies in the midbrain near the red nucleus. The lateral portion of the riMLF is concerned with upgaze and the medial portion with downgaze. Connections via the posterior commissure coordinate the activity on the two sides. Upgaze and downgaze pathways occupy different positions, and abnormalities may affect one without the other. Conversely, in some instances both upgaze and downgaze are affected; see **combined vertical gaze palsy.**

Impaired upgaze is the core feature of Parinaud's (dorsal midbrain, periaqueductal) syndrome. Patients are unable to look up, and when they attempt it the eyes may spasmodically converge and retract backward into the orbits (see **convergence retraction nystagmus**). Upgaze palsy due to a structural lesion is frequently accompanied by **tectal pupils** and **eyelid retraction** (see **Collier's sign**). PSP is another common cause of upgaze palsy.

In some conditions, upgaze palsy is so severe there is tonic downgaze. Forced downgaze may occur in thalamic hemorrhage, obstructive hydrocephalus (see **setting sun sign**), severe metabolic encephalopathy, and massive SAH. Occasionally there is also tonic convergence, so that the patient seems to peer at the tip of the nose (see **thalamic esotropia**).

Upper limb tension test: See **cervical radiculopathy signs, Bakody's sign, cervical distraction test, Naffziger's sign, Viets' sign.**

Upper motor neuron signs: Clinical signs due to dysfunction of the upper motor neuron. UMN signs include **weakness** in the pattern characteristic of CST pathology, hyperactive **deep tendon reflexes,** depressed **superficial reflexes, spasticity, pathologic reflexes,** and changes in **associated movements** (see Table L.3). With bilateral UMN pathology, other signs may emerge depending on the level of involvement, such as pseudobulbar palsy and sphincter dysfunction.

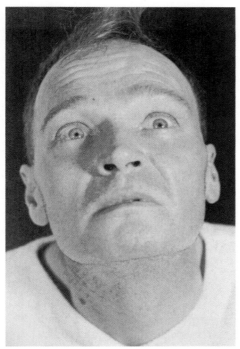

Figure U.1. Paresis of upward gaze in a patient with a neoplasm of the posterior third ventricle. (From Campbell WW. *DeJong's the Neurologic Examination.* 7th ed. Wolters Kluwer Health/Lippincott Williams & Wilkins; 2013, with permission.)

Upside-down ptosis: See **Horner's syndrome.**

Useless hand (of Oppenheim): A classical but rare manifestation of MS. There is loss of function of one hand with relatively normal strength but severe deafferentation with a marked proprioceptive deficit out of proportion to the impairment of other sensory modalities. The responsible lesion involves the posterior columns of the spinal cord ipsilateral to the affected hand.[3,4]

Utilization behavior: A type of **defective response inhibition** first described by Lhermitte in patients with frontal lobe damage. Patients with utilization behavior will automatically reach out and use objects in the environment and are not able to inhibit this response, a phenomenon referred to as **environmental dependency** or **stimulus-bound behavior.**[5] See **imitation behavior.**

Uveitis: See **iritis/uveitis.**

Video Link

U.1. Abnormal Unterberger-Fukuda stepping test in a patient with vestibular neuritis. (From Bassani R. Teaching video neuroimages: vestibular neuritis: basic elements for clinical and instrumental diagnosis. *Neurology.* 2011;76:e71.) Available at: http://www.neurology.org/content/suppl/2011/04/03/76.14.e71.DC1/Video_1.mov

References

1. Grommes C, Conway D. The stepping test: a step back in history. *J Hist Neurosci.* 2011;20:29–33.
2. Bassani R. Teaching video neuroimages: vestibular neuritis: basic elements for clinical and instrumental diagnosis. *Neurology.* 2011;76:e71.
3. Coleman RJ, Russon L, Blanshard K, et al. Useless hand of Oppenheim—magnetic resonance imaging findings. *Postgrad Med J.* 1993;69:149–150.
4. Rae-Grant AD. Unusual symptoms and syndromes in multiple sclerosis. *Continuum (Minneap Minn).* 2013;19:992–1006.
5. Besnard J, Allain P, Aubin G, et al. Utilization behavior: clinical and theoretical approaches. *J Int Neuropsychol Soc.* 2010;16:453–462.

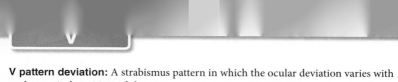

V pattern deviation: A strabismus pattern in which the ocular deviation varies with the vertical position of the eyes, causing **exotropia** on upgaze and **esotropia** on downgaze. See **A pattern deviation.**

V sign: See **dermatomyositis skin changes.**

Valgus deviation: A deformity with displacement of part of an extremity away from the midline. A cubitus valgus deviation of the elbow is associated with ulnar neuropathy at the elbow.

Valleix's sign: (1) Paresthesias radiating proximally on percussion over an entrapped nerve (see **Tinel's sign**); (2) tenderness on palpation of the sciatic nerve in the buttock or posterior thigh in S1 radiculopathy.

Valsalva test: See **cervical radiculopathy signs, Spurling's sign, straight leg-raising test.**

Varus deviation: A deformity with displacement of part of an extremity toward the midline, as in genus varus (knock knees). In talipes (pes) equinovarus the foot deviates medially; see **pes cavus.**

Venous hum: See **bruit.**

Verbal paraphasia: See **paraphasia.**

Verbigeration: See **monophasia.**

Vergences: See **ductions.**

Vernet rideau phenomenon: A pharyngeal movement seen with unilateral weakness of the superior pharyngeal constrictor; with phonation or gagging there is a "**curtain sign**" with motion of the pharyngeal wall toward the nonparalyzed side.

Versions: See **ductions.**

Vertical nystagmus: See **nystagmus.**

Vertical smile: See **mysasthenic snarl.**

Vestibular nystagmus: See **nystagmus.**

Vestibulo-ocular reflex (VOR): An oculomotor control system linked to the vestibular system. The VOR serves to move the eyes at an equal velocity but in the direction opposite a head movement; this keeps the eyes still in space and maintains visual fixation while the head is in motion. There are several ways to examine the VOR, including the **oculocephalic response** (doll's eye test), **head impulse test**, **dynamic visual acuity**, and **caloric tests.**

Vestibulopupillary reflex: Constriction of the pupil following stimulation of the vestibular system.

Vibration-induced nystagmus: Induction of nystagmus by vibration of approximately 100 Hz applied to the mastoids, vertex, or forehead. Although it may occur to a slight degree in normals, in the patient with dizziness vibration-induced nystagmus (VIN) usually indicates unilateral peripheral vestibular dysfunction.[1] It is a marker for superior canal dehiscence, where a horizontal or torsional component beating toward the side of the lesion usually results.[2] VIN may also occur in otosclerosis, but is typically sparse, low amplitude, and not systematically lateralized to a specific side. When VIN is present, it only appears while the vibrating stimulus is applied and stops immediately when the vibration ceases.

Viets' sign: See **Naffziger's sign, Bakody's sign, cervical distraction test, upper limb tension test**.

Violaceous discoloration: See **heliotrope rash.**

Visual acuity: A measure of the eye's ability to resolve details. Visual acuity (VA) depends on several functions. Visual acuity charts, the Snellen chart for distance and the near card for near, consist of letters, numbers, or figures that get progressively smaller and can be read at varying distances by normal individuals (Fig. V.1).

The difference between near and distance vision and between vision with and without correction are points of primarily ophthalmological interest. For neurologic purposes, only the patient's best-corrected visual acuity is pertinent. Refractive errors, media opacities, and similar optometric problems are irrelevant. Acuity is always measured using the patient's accustomed correction. Ophthalmologists and neuro-ophthalmologists often employ more detailed methods to clarify the refractive component of a patient's visual impairment.

For distance vision measurement in the United States, a Snellen chart is placed 20 ft from the patient; at that distance there is relaxation of accommodation, and the light rays are nearly parallel. The eyes are tested separately. In countries using the metric system, the distance is usually given as 6 m. The ability to resolve test characters (optotypes) approximately 1-in high at 20 ft is normal (20/20 or 6/6) visual acuity. These characters subtend 5 minutes of visual arc at the eye; the components of the characters (e.g., the crossbar on the letter "A") subtend 1 minute of arc. The acuity is the line where more than half of the characters are accurately read. If the patient can read the 20/30 line and two characters on the 20/25 line, the notation is 20/30 + 2. By conventional notation, the distance from the test chart, 20 or 6, is the numerator, and the distance at which the smallest type read by the patient should be seen by a person with normal acuity is the denominator. The patient is the numerator; a normal person is the denominator. An acuity of 20/40 (6/12) means the individual must move in to 20 ft to read letters a normal person can read at 40 ft. This does not mean the patient's acuity is one half of normal. In fact, an individual with a distance acuity of 20/40 has only a 16.4% loss of vision.

Since few neurology clinics, offices, or hospital rooms have 20-ft eye lanes, neurologists usually assess near vision. Near vision is tested with a near card, such as the Rosenbaum pocket vision screening card, held at the near point (14 in. or 35.5 cm). Good lighting is essential. A penlight shone directly on the line being read is useful for bedside testing. Various electronic devices have acuity-measuring capability (Neuro Toolkit, Pocket Eye Exam, and others). In some circumstances, a device designed for assessment at an intermediate distance is useful. The Maxwell card is designed for testing at 6 ft, a convenient distance that lessens the need for presbyopic correction. The eye chart in the Neuro Toolkit is used at 1 m on a smartphone and 2 m on an iPad or equivalent. The Pocket Eye Exam chart is used at 6 ft.

If the patient cannot read the 20/200 line at 20 ft, the distance may be shortened and the fraction adjusted. Ability to read the line at 5 ft is vision of 5/200, equivalent to 20/800 (5 × 4/200 × 4 = 20/800). Vision worse than the measurable 20/800 is described as counts fingers (CF), hand motion (HM), light perception (LP), or no light perception (NLP). The average finger is approximately the same size as the 20/200 character, so ability to count fingers at 5 ft is equivalent to an acuity of 20/800.

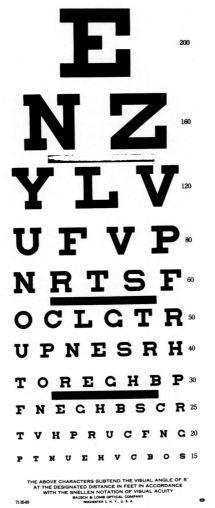

Figure V.1. The Snellen test chart. (From Campbell WW. *DeJong's the Neurologic Examination.* 7th ed. Wolters Kluwer Lippincott Williams & Wilkins; 2013, with permission.)

When a patient has impaired vision, an attempt should be made to exclude refractive error by any available means. If the patient has corrective lenses, they should be worn. In the absence of correction, improvement of vision with the **pinhole test** suggests impairment related to a refractive error.

Suspected NOVL is best evaluated by an ophthalmologist, who has the proper tools to answer the question. Clever and determined patients with functional visual loss present a major challenge. There may be certain clues. The **sunglasses sign** is often an indication of NOVL. A truly blind person can sign his name without difficulty. A functionally blind patient often cannot. A truly blind person asked to look at his hand will look wherever proprioception tells him his hand should be; a person with NOVL may gaze in any direction and perhaps never where the hand actually is. A truly blind person can touch his forefingers together without difficulty; a functionally blind person may make half-hearted inaccurate thrusts. The presence of normal visual reflexes excludes organic blindness. A patient with NOVL ignorant of the laws of reflection may have much improved vision reading the image of an acuity chart held to his chest in a mirror 10 ft away compared with reading the actual chart at 20 ft; the acuity in fact should be the same. Some patients with NOVL can suppress the OKN response. An excellent test is to have the patient look into a large mirror that can be held and moved. Tilting and moving the mirror will elicit OKN responses because the entire visual environment is moving. The patient cannot suppress or "blur out" by willfully failing to fixate on a single target, as he may be able to do with the usual methods of OKN testing.

Visual agnosia: See **agnosia.**

Visual field defects: A deficit of visual function causing an impairment of the ability to see in certain portions of the visual field (VF). For neurologic purposes, VF abnormalities can be divided into **scotomas**, hemianopias, **altitudinal visual field defects**, and concentric constriction or contraction of the fields. Figure S.5 depicts examples of different types of field defects. Because of the anatomy and organization of the visual system, neurologic disorders tend to produce straight-edged defects that respect either the horizontal or vertical meridian or have a characteristic shape because of the arrangement of the nerve fiber layer (NFL). Respect of the horizontal meridian may occur because of the horizontal temporal raphe and the arching sweep of NFL axons above and below the macula. This pattern is characteristic of optic nerve, optic disc, and NFL lesions. The vascular supply of the retina consists of superior and inferior branches of the central retinal artery, which supply the upper and lower retina, respectively. Vascular disease characteristically causes altitudinal field defects that are sharply demarcated horizontally. The calcarine cortex is organized into a superior and an inferior bank, and lesions involving only one bank may produce VF defects that respect the horizontal meridian. The vertical meridian is respected because of the division into nasal and temporal hemiretinas that occurs at the chiasmal decussation and is maintained through the retrochiasmal visual pathways.

Hemianopia is impaired vision in half the visual field of each eye; hemianopic defects do not cross the vertical meridian. Hemianopias may be homonymous or heteronymous. A homonymous hemianopia causes impaired vision in corresponding halves of each eye (e.g., a right homonymous hemianopia is a defect in the right half of each eye). Homonymous hemianopias are caused by lesions posterior to the optic chiasm, with interruption of the fibers from the temporal half of the ipsilateral retina and the nasal half of the contralateral retina. Vision is lost in the ipsilateral nasal field and the contralateral temporal field. A heteronymous hemianopia is impaired vision in opposite halves of each eye (e.g., the right half in one eye and the left half in the other). Unilateral homonymous hemianopias, even those with macular splitting, do not affect visual acuity. Patients can read normally with the preserved half of the macula, but those with left-sided hemianopias may have trouble finding the line to be read. Occasionally patients with homonymous hemianopia will read only half of the line on the acuity chart.

A homonymous hemianopia may be complete or incomplete. If incomplete, it may be congruous or incongruous. A congruous hemianopia shows similarly shaped defects in each eye (see Fig. S.5 H). The closer the optic radiations get to the occipital lobe, the closer lie corresponding visual fibers from the two eyes. The more congruous the field defect, the more posterior the lesion is likely to be. An incongruous hemianopia is differently shaped defects in the two eyes (see Fig. S.5 I). The more incongruous the defect, the more anterior the lesion. The most incongruous hemianopias occur with optic tract and lateral geniculate lesions. With a complete hemianopia, congruity cannot be assessed; the only localization possible is to identify the lesion as contralateral and retrochiasmal. A superior quadrantopia implies a lesion in the temporal lobe affecting Meyer's loop (inferior retinal fibers): "pie in the sky" (see Fig. S.5 J). Such a defect may occur after temporal lobe epilepsy surgery because of damage to the anteriorly looping fibers. An inferior quadrantopia ("pie on the floor") implies a parietal lobe lesion affecting superior retinal fibers (see Fig. S.5 K). A macular-sparing hemianopia is one that spares the area immediately around fixation; it implies an occipital lobe lesion (see Fig. S.5 L).

Incomplete homonymous VF defects are common. These include partial or irregular defects in one or both of the hemifields, relative rather than absolute loss of vision, an inability to localize the visual stimulus, and hemianopia only for objects of a certain color (see **hemiachromatopsia**). Extinction, a visual **attentional deficit**, is hemianopic suppression of the visual stimulus in the involved hemifield when bilateral simultaneous stimuli are delivered. Visual extinction is most characteristic of lesions involving the nondominant parieto-occipital region. **Riddoch's phenomenon** is a dissociation between the perception of static and kinetic stimuli.

Heteronymous hemianopias are usually bitemporal; only rarely are they binasal. A bitemporal hemianopia is usually due to chiasmatic disease, such as a pituitary tumor growing up out of the sella tursica and pressing on the underside of the chiasm (Fig. V.2). Bitemporal field defects can usually be detected earliest by demonstrating bitemporal **color desaturation**, particularly to red. Because of the anterior inferior position of decussating inferior nasal fibers, lesions impinging from below produce upper temporal field defects, which evolve into a bitemporal hemianopia. Lesions encroaching from above tend to cause inferior temporal defects initially. The defect will be first and worst in the upper quadrants with infrachiasmatic masses (e.g., pituitary adenoma), and it will be first and worst in the lower quadrants with suprachiasmatic masses (e.g., craniopharyngioma). Patients with postfixed chiasms and pituitary tumors may present with optic nerve defects, and those with prefixed chiasms may have optic tract defects.

The most common cause of bitemporal hemianopia is a pituitary adenoma; occasionally, it results from other parasellar or suprasellar lesions such as meningioma and craniopharyngioma, as well as glioma of the optic chiasm, aneurysms, trauma, and hydrocephalus. Other VF defects that may simulate bitemporal hemianopia include **tilted discs**, bilateral cecocentral **scotomas**, and bilaterally enlarged **blind spots**. Binasal hemianopias may occur from disease impinging on the lateral

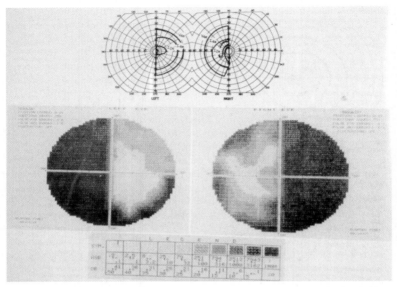

Figure V.2. Visual field performed on a Goldmann perimeter in a patient with a chiasmal lesion **(Top)**. Humphrey perimeter field in the same patient **(Bottom)**. (From Beck RW, Bergstrom TJ, Lichter PR. A clinical comparison of visual field testing with a new automated perimeter, the Humphrey Field Analyzer, and the Goldmann perimeter. *Ophthalmology.* 1985;92:77–82, with permission.)

aspect of the chiasm bilaterally (e.g., bilateral intracavernous carotid aneurysms), but they are more likely to be due to bilateral optic neuropathy.

An **altitudinal visual field defect** is one involving the upper or lower half of vision, usually in one eye. Constriction of the VFs is characterized by a narrowing of the range of vision, which may affect one or all parts of the periphery. Constriction may be regular or irregular, concentric or eccentric, temporal or nasal, and upper or lower. Symmetric concentric contraction is most frequent and is characterized by a more or less even, progressive reduction in field diameter through all meridians. Such constriction is referred to as funnel vision, as opposed to tunnel vision (see below). Concentric constriction of the VFs may occur with optic atrophy, especially secondary to papilledema or late glaucoma, or with retinal disease, especially **retinitis pigmentosa**. Narrowing of the fields due to fatigue, poor attention, or inadequate illumination must be excluded, as must spurious contraction due to decreased visual acuity or delayed reaction time. Diffuse depression is the static perimeter equivalent of constriction on kinetic perimetry. Concentric constriction of the fields is sometimes seen in NOVL. A suspicious finding is when the fields fail to enlarge as expected with testing at increasing distance (see **tubular visual fields**).

Visual grasp reflex: See **antisaccade task.**
Visual neglect: See **attentional deficits.**
Visual-palpebral reflex: Blinking in response to light.
Visual perseveration: See **palinopsia.**

Visuospatial agnosia: See **agnosia.**
Visuospatial neglect: See **attentional deficits, line bisection test.**
Vocal agnosia: See **auditory agnosia.**
Vocal tics: See **motor tics.**
Volitional facial palsy: See **facial weakness.**
Voluntary nystagmus: An ability in some normal individuals to saccade very rapidly back and forth horizontally, producing a high-frequency, low-amplitude, pendular eye movement that is startling but of no consequence. It has been described as **ocular flutter** under voluntary control. Voluntary nystagmus may alarm the physician who has not previously seen these impressive oscillations. The movements cannot be sustained for long, generally lasting <30 seconds **(Video Link V.1)**.[3]
Von Bechterew reflex: See **carpometacarpal reflex.**
Von Graefe sign: See **lid lag.**
Von Monakow sign (reflex): A lower extremity **pathologic reflex**, seen with CST lesions. Stroking the lateral margin of foot causes foot eversion and abduction.
Von Stein test: See **Romberg sign.**
Vulpian's sign: See **gaze palsy.**

Video Link

V.1. Voluntary nystagmus. (From Bassani R. Images in clinical medicine. Voluntary nystagmus. *N Engl J Med.* 2012;367:e13.) Available at: http://www.nejm.org/doi/full/10.1056/NEJMicm1104924

References

1. Perez N. Vibration induced nystagmus in normal subjects and in patients with dizziness. A video-nystagmography study. *Rev Laryngol Otol Rhinol (Bord).* 2003;124:85–90.
2. Dumas G, Lion A, Karkas A, et al. Skull vibration-induced nystagmus test in unilateral superior canal dehiscence and otosclerosis: a vestibular Weber test. *Acta Otolaryngol.* 2014;134:588–600.
3. Bassani R. Images in clinical medicine. Voluntary nystagmus. *N Engl J Med.* 2012;367:e13.

V

Waddell (touch-me-not) signs: A set of tests for nonorganicity in low back pain (see Video B.2).[1] An evidence-based review of 61 studies addressing the concept of nonorganic findings challenged this orthodoxy.[2] The study concluded that the Waddell signs are associated with decreased functional performance, poorer treatment outcomes, and greater levels of pain but no evidence of an association with psychological distress, abnormal illness behavior, or secondary gain and no evidence they can discriminate organic from nonorganic disease.

The Waddell signs include a discrepancy between the positivity of **straight leg raising** in the supine and seated position; pain in the back on pressing down on top of the head; widespread and excessive tenderness (the "touch me not" sign); general overreaction during testing; pain during simulated spinal rotation, pinning the patients hands to the sides while rotating the hips (no spine rotation occurs as shoulders and hips remain in a constant relationship); and nondermatomal/nonmyotomal neurologic signs.

In the skin roll test, the loose skin over the lower back or neck is gently rolled. Pain produced by skin rolling in the patient with low back pain or headache suggests an exaggerated pain response and is analogous to the Waddell "touch me not" sign.

Waddling gait: See **gait disorders.**

Waiter's (porter's, policeman's) tip position: The posture of the upper extremity in the patient with Erb's palsy (Fig. W.1). Because of weakness of muscles innervated by the upper plexus, the arm is held in a position of adduction and internal rotation, with the elbow extended and the forearm pronated. The hand rests with the palm facing out and backward, with the wrist and fingers flexed; the appearance is as if the patient were reaching behind to receive a gratuity.

Walker effect: See **Mary Walker test.**

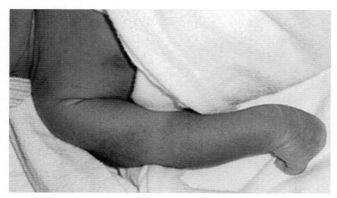

Figure W.1. Waiter's tip posture in a newborn with Erb's palsy. (From Hemady N, Noble C. Newborn with abnormal arm posture. *Am Fam Physician.* 2006;73:2015–2016, with permission).

Wall-eyed bilateral INO: See **internuclear ophthalmoplegia.**
Warm pack test: See **ice pack test.**
Warm-up effect: Improvement of **myotonia** with repeated contractions.
Wartenberg's reflex (winking jaw phenomenon): See **corneomandibular reflex.**
Wartenberg's pendulum test: See **pendulum test.**
Wartenberg signs: (1) Adduction, flexion, and opposition of the thumb following active flexion of the terminal phalanges of the four fingers of a paretic hand about a firm object, or against resistance offered by the examiner's fingers similarly flexed (Wartenberg's thumb adduction sign; **Fig. W.2**). Normally, the thumb remains in abduction and extension. A variation is for patient and examiner to hook and pull with only the index fingers; the response is the same. (2) the **finger flexor reflex;** (3) the **Bergara-Wartenberg sign;** (4) inability to adduct the small finger with a tendency for it to drift into abduction in ulnar neuropathy **(Fig. W.3)**. See **pathologic reflexes, associated movements.**

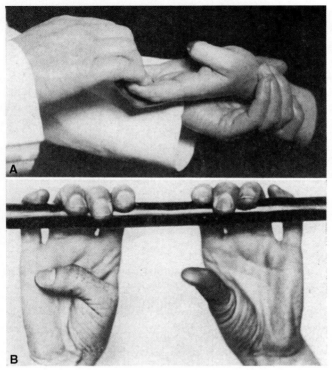

Figure W.2. Associated movement of the thumb (Wartenberg's sign). **A:** The patient bends his last four fingers against resistance of four hooked fingers of the examiner. Thumb moves toward palm. Mild spastic paralysis of hand. **B:** With his fingers hooked over a horizontally fastened rod, the patient is asked to pull it down. Right thumb performs an associated movement toward the palm. Right-sided spastic hemiplegia. (From Wartenberg R. *Diagnostic Tests in Neurology.* Chicago, IL: Year Book Medical Publishers; 1953, with permission.)

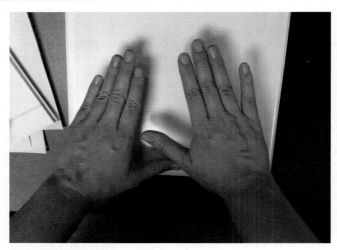

Figure W.3. Small finger abduction in ulnar neuropathy.

Weakness: Loss of muscle strength, a cardinal sign of CST lesions and neuromuscular disorders. The suffix *paresis* means decreased strength; *plegia* is paralysis, an absence of muscle contraction. *Paresis* is used to describe many grades of motor impairment up to complete paralysis, with qualifiers such as mild, moderate, or severe, as well as distribution descriptors (hemi-, para-, quadri-). Associated features provide additional useful information, such as flaccid or spastic. The acuity of the problem is also relevant. The patient with an acute, flaccid hemiparesis is a far different clinical problem than one with a long-standing spastic quadraparesis. When paralysis is complete, the term *plegia* is preferred, but these distinctions are frequently disregarded.

Weakness of a muscle must be distinguished from loss of range of motion for other reasons and from **contracture** of antagonists. Passive movements to assess range of motion are sometimes necessary to help distinguish whether limitation of movement is due to weakness, pain, muscle spasm, or contracture.

In manual muscle testing, the strength of individual muscles is tested and graded quantitatively using some scale, most commonly the 5-level **MRC scale**. The muscle strength scale used by physical therapists grades muscles on a six-point scale from zero (no motion) through trace, poor, fair, and good to normal. The Mayo clinic grades muscle strength on a five-point scale that is more linear. Normal is designated as zero, mild weakness is 1, and total paralysis is 4.

There are common patterns of weakness. Recognition of a pattern may help greatly in lesion localization and differential diagnosis. Identification of the process causing weakness is further aided by accompanying signs, such as reflex alterations and sensory loss. **Table W.1** reviews the features of upper motor neuron versus lower motor neuron weakness. **Table W.2** summarizes some common patterns of weakness and their localization.

Table W.1. Features of Upper Motor Neuron versus Lower Motor Neuron Weakness

Feature	Upper Motor Neuron	Lower Motor Neuron
Weakness distribution	Corticospinal distribution; hemiparesis, quadriparesis, paraparesis, monoparesis, faciobrachial	Generalized, predominantly proximal, predominantly distal or focal. No preferential involvement of corticospinal innervated muscles
Sensory loss distribution	Central pattern	None, stocking glove or peripheral nerve or root distribution
Deep tendon reflexes	Increased unless very acute	Normal or decreased
Superficial reflexes	Decreased	Normal
Pathologic reflexes	Yes	No
Sphincter function	Sometimes impaired	Normal (except for cauda equina lesion)
Muscle tone	Increased unless very acute	Normal or decreased
Pain	No	Sometimes
Other CNS signs	Possibly	No

CNS, central nervous system.
From Campbell WW. *DeJong's the Neurologic Examination.* 7th ed. Wolters Kluwer Health/Lippincott Williams & Wilkins; 2013, with permission.

Weakness may be focal or generalized. When focal, it may follow the distribution of some structure in the peripheral nervous system, such as a peripheral nerve or spinal root. It may affect one side of the body in a "hemi" distribution. A hemi distribution may affect the arm, leg, and face equally on one side of the body, or one or more areas may be more involved than others. The CST preferentially innervates certain muscle groups, and these are often selectively impaired in weakness due to a lesion of the CST (see Video F.2). The CST preferentially innervates distal muscles, and impaired **fine motor control** detected by testing **rapid alternating movements** with the **finger tapping test, forearm rolling, foot tapping test,** or similar is often an early sign (see Video F.2). In the upper extremity, the muscles preferentially innervated by the CST tract, are the extensors, supinators, and external rotators. Weakness of these muscles is responsible for **pronator drift** and other **pronator signs** (see **subtle signs of hemiparesis**). In the lower extremity, the CST distribution includes the hip and knee flexors and the foot dorsiflexors. **Facial weakness** is limited to the lower face, and voluntary facial movements are affected more than emotional ones (dissociated facial palsy). Bulbar functions, movements of the trunk, and other functions with bilateral supranuclear innervation are little affected.

When weakness is nonfocal, it may be generalized, predominantly proximal, or predominantly distal. The term *generalized weakness* implies that the weakness involves both sides of the body, more or less symmetrically. When a patient has truly generalized weakness, bulbar motor functions—such as facial movements, speech, chewing, and swallowing—are involved as well. Weakness of both arms

Table W.2. Common Patterns of Weakness with Lesions at Different Locations in the Neuraxis

Location of Lesion	Distribution of Weakness	Sensory Loss	DTRs*	Possible Accompanying Signs
Middle cerebral artery	Contralateral arm and face > leg**	Y	Incr	Aphasia, apraxia, visual field deficit, gaze palsy
Anterior cerebral artery	Contralateral leg > arm and face**	Y	Incr	Cortical sensory loss in contralateral leg, frontal lobe signs, sometimes incontinence
Internal capsule	Contralateral face = arm = leg**	N	Incr	None ("pure motor stroke")
Brainstem	Ipsilateral cranial nerve and contralateral body**	Y	Incr	Variable, depending on level
Cervical cord (transverse)	Both arms and both legs**	Y	Incr	Bowel, bladder, or sexual dysfunction common
Thoracic cord (transverse)	Both legs**	Y	Incr	Bowel, bladder, or sexual dysfunction common
Cauda equina	Both legs, asymmetric, multiple root pattern	Y	Decr	Occasional bowel, bladder, or sexual dysfunction; sometimes pain
Anterior horn cell	Focal early, generalized late	N	Incr	Atrophy, fasciculations, bulbar weakness
Single nerve root	Muscles of the affected myotome	Y	Decr	Pain
Plexus	Plexus pattern, complete or partial	Usually	Decr	Pain is common, especially with brachial "plexitis"
Mononeuropathy	Muscles of the affected nerve	Usually	Decr	Variable atrophy, variable pain
Polyneuropathy	Distal > proximal (usually)	Usually	Decr	Variable pain, atrophy late
Neuromuscular junction	Bulbar, proximal extremities	N	Normal	Ptosis, ophthalmoparesis, fatigable weakness, fluctuating weakness
Muscle	Proximal > distal (usually)	N	Normal	Pain uncommon, many potential patterns (limb girdle, facioscapulohumeral, etc.), pseudohypertrophy, myotonia

*With corticospinal lesions, DTRs acutely may be normal or decreased (neural shock).
**Extremity weakness in a corticospinal tract distribution.
DTR, deep tendon reflex; Y, yes; N, no; Incr, increased; Decr, decreased.
From Campbell WW. *DeJong's the Neurologic Examination.* 7th ed. Wolters Kluwer Health/Lippincott Williams & Wilkins; 2013, with permission.

and both legs with normal bulbar function is **quadraparesis** or tetraparesis. Weakness of both legs is **paraparesis**. When weakness affects all four extremities, the likely causes include spinal cord disease, peripheral neuropathy, a neuromuscular junction disorder, or a myopathy. When spinal cord disease is the culprit and the deficit is incomplete, more severe involvement of those muscles preferentially innervated by the CST can frequently be discerned. **Deep tendon reflexes** are usually increased (though in the acute stages they may be decreased or absent); there is usually some alteration of sensation, sometimes a discrete spinal "level"; **superficial reflexes** disappear; and there may be bowel and bladder dysfunction. Generalized peripheral nerve disease tends to predominantly involve distal muscles, although there are exceptions. There is no preferential involvement of CST-innervated muscles, reflexes are usually decreased, sensory loss is frequently present, and bowel and bladder function are not disturbed. With a neuromuscular junction disorder, the weakness is likely to be worse proximally, sensation is spared, reflexes are normal, and there is usually involvement of bulbar muscles, especially with ptosis and ophthalmoplegia. When the problem is a primary muscle disorder, weakness is usually more severe proximally, reflexes are normal, sensation is normal, and, with only a few exceptions, bulbar function is spared except for occasional dysphagia.

Focal weakness may occur in many different patterns. Weakness of the arm and leg on one side of the body is hemiparesis. Monoparesis is weakness limited to one extremity. **Diplegia** is weakness of like parts on the two sides of the body. Weakness of one arm and the opposite leg is referred to as **cruciate weakness**.

Certain patterns of muscle weakness point to a peripheral nerve, plexus, or root lesion. With a peripheral nerve lesion, all muscles below the level of the lesion are at risk, although not all are necessarily equally affected. When multiple muscles of an extremity are weak, localization depends on recognizing the common innervating structure. In cervical radiculopathy, the muscles involved are innervated by different peripheral nerves and different brachial plexus components, but all by the same root. For instance, lesions of the middle trunk of the brachial plexus are exceedingly rare, so weakness of the triceps (radial nerve) and the pronator teres (median nerve) always means a lesion of the C7 root.

A focal neuropathy, such as a radial nerve palsy, or a spinal root lesion—such as from a herniated disc—causes weakness limited to the distribution of the involved nerve or root. A complete plexopathy, such as a traumatic brachial plexopathy, may cause weakness of the entire limb. Partial lesions may cause weakness only in the distribution of certain plexus components. With such lower motor neuron pathology, reflexes are typically decreased, and there is often accompanying sensory loss. Localization of focal weakness due to root, plexus, and peripheral nerve pathology requires intimate familiarity with peripheral neuroanatomy. Anterior horn cell disease often begins with focal weakness that may simulate mononeuropathy, but it evolves into a more widespread pattern as the disease progresses, culminating in generalized weakness. Except for extraocular muscle involvement in myasthenia gravis, it is rare for a myopathy or neuromuscular junction disorder to cause focal weakness.

Functional weakness, or nonorganic weakness, is a pattern of weakness seen in patients whose motor deficit is not the result of neurologic disease.

Weber test: A vibrating tuning fork is placed in the midline on the vertex of the skull. It may be placed anywhere in the midline: over the nasal bridge, forehead, or maxilla, but works best over the vertex. Normally, the sound is heard equally in both ears or seems to resonate somewhere in the center of the head; it is "not lateralized." In **conductive hearing loss**, the sound is heard better ("lateralized") to the involved side. In **sensorineural hearing loss**, the sound is heard better in the normal ear (see Table C.5). Lateralization to the side with poorer hearing suggests conductive hearing loss in that ear. Lateralization to the side with better hearing suggests sensorineural hearing loss in the opposite ear.

WEBINO/WEMINO: See **internuclear ophthalmoplegia.**

Wernicke's (fluent, receptive, sensory, posterior, postrolandic) aphasia: Aphasia due to a lesion in the posterior superior temporal region that involves the auditory association cortex and the angular and supramarginal gyri. Patients are unable to understand speech (see **word deafness**) or read (see **word blindness**). They are relatively fluent, with a normal or even increased word output (see **logorrhea**), but there is loss of the ability to comprehend the significance of spoken words or recall their meaning. Speech production is effortless; phrase and sentence length and prosody are normal. Although speech is abundant, it is devoid of meaningful content. The patient can still hear and can recognize voices, but not the words they utter. **Paraphasias** are frequent, resulting in incorrect or unintelligible words, unconventional and gibberish sounds, and senseless combinations. The speech abounds in **neologisms**. There may be **circumlocution** and an excess of small filler words. In its mildest form, there are mild paraphasias and minimal difficulty understanding grammatically complex material (mini-Wernicke's).

Speech may be fluent, but the patient cannot understand his own speech; he is not aware of, and does not correct, his errors in speaking. The frequent paraphasias and neologisms, combined with **agrammatism**, along with the high word output, may lead to completely unintelligible gibberish, termed **jargon aphasia**. Hughlings Jackson described this type of aphasia as "plentiful words wrongly used." Naming and repetition deficits arise from poor comprehension. There is usually an accompanying proportional **alexia**. Often the patient lacks awareness of the deficit and may actually appear euphoric. Patients with Wernicke's aphasia often have a **visual field defect** but no **hemiparesis**. When due to vascular disease, the ischemia is usually in the distribution of the inferior division of the MCA. With large, acute lesions Wernicke's aphasia may evolve from a state of **mutism**. As with **Broca's aphasia**, lesions causing Wernicke's aphasia usually extend beyond the superior temporal gyrus. Patients with acute Wernicke's aphasia may become agitated because of their comprehension difficulty. The agitated patient, speaking gibberish and with no gross neurologic deficit, is frequently thought to be psychotic **(Video Link W.1).**

Wernicke's hemianopic pupil: A decreased pupillary light reflex when light is shone on the affected hemiretina in an optic tract lesion. The phenomenon is near impossible to appreciate at the bedside because of intraocular light scatter but may be seen with infrared pupillography.

Westphal's sign: Absence of the **knee reflex**, initially described in tabes dorsalis but which may occur in a variety of conditions.

Wheelchair sign: The use of a wheelchair early in the course of a patient with **parkinsonism**. Because **postural instability** severe enough to cause frequent falls and require the use of a wheelchair is unusual in idiopathic PD, the wheelchair sign is considered suggestive of one of the atypical parkinsonian syndromes.

Whispering dysphonia: See **dysphonia.**

Whistle-smile (Hanes) sign: An efficient way to bring out the **masked facies** in PD, described by FM Hanes[3] in 1943. His description is as follows: When the normal individual is asked to whistle, he does so and then smiles, probably as a response to the apparent absurdity of the request. The patient suffering from parkinsonism does not smile after whistling because of bradykinesia affecting the facial muscles.

White rabbit sign: See **orthostatic tremor.**

Wide-based gait: See **gait disorders.**

Wilson's sign: (1) See **eccentric pupil;** (2) see **pronator sign;** (3) persistence of the glabellar tap response in PD.

Wing-beating (bat wing) tremor: The proximal tremor of the upper extremity characteristic of Wilson's disease; may also be seen in MS, dystonia, essential tremor, and PD **(Video Link W.2)**.

Wink reflex: See **anal reflex.**

Winking jaw: See **corneomandibular reflex.**

Withdrawal reflex: See **flexion reflex.**

Witzelsucht: Inappropriate joking and punning, due to disinhibition, seen in patients with orbitofrontal lesions. See **moria.**

Woltman's sign: See **hung-up reflex.**

Word blindness: See **alexia.**

Word deafness: See **auditory agnosia.**

Working memory: See **memory.**

Wright's hyperabduction maneuver: See **thoracic outlet syndrome provocative tests.**

Wrist drop: Weakness of wrist extension; the most common cause is radial neuropathy **(Fig. W.4)**. Acute radial neuropathy usually results from sustained compression in the spiral groove over a period of several hours during sleep or a drug- or alcohol-induced stupor ("Saturday night" or "bridegroom's" palsy). The radial nerve is also particularly prone to involvement in systemic vasculitis. Weakness involves all radial innervated muscles distal to the triceps and **finger drop** is present as well. Confusion commonly arises on two points: (a) because of mechanical factors, the interossei cannot exert normal power in the face of finger drop and may seem weak—the patient is thought to also have ulnar neuropathy; and (b) weakness of thumb abduction occurs due to dysfunction of the radial innervated abductor pollicis longus—the patient is thought to also have median neuropathy. Pseudoradial nerve palsy is weakness in an apparently radial distribution due to a cerebral hemispheric lesion.[4]

Writing tremor: See **primary writing tremor.**

Wrong-way eyes: See **gaze palsy.**

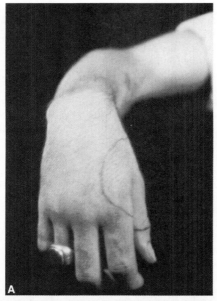

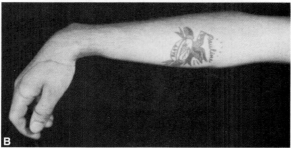

Figure W.4. A: Wrist drop secondary to radial nerve palsy. **B:** Sensory deficit in this instance involved the shaded area only. (From Campbell WW. *DeJong's the Neurologic Examination.* 7th ed. Wolters Kluwer Health/Lippincott Williams & Wilkins; 2013, with permission.)

Video Links

W.1. Wernicke's aphasia. Available at: http://www.youtube.com/watch?v=aVhYN7NTIKU&feature=related
W.2. Wing-beating (bat wing) tremor. Available at: http://www.doctorshangout.com/video/video/show?id=2002836%3AVideo%3A109321

References

1. Waddell G, McCulloch JA, Kummel E, et al. Nonorganic physical signs in low-back pain. *Spine (Phila Pa 1976).* 1980;5:117–125.
2. Fishbain DA, Cole B, Cutler RB, et al. A structured evidence-based review on the meaning of nonorganic physical signs: Waddell signs. *Pain Med.* 2003;4:141–181.
3. Hanes FM. Two clinically useful signs. *J Am Med Assoc.* 1943;121:1152–1153.
4. Celebisoy M, Ozdemirkiran T, Tokucoglu F, et al. Isolated hand palsy due to cortical infarction: localization of the motor hand area. *Neurologist.* 2007;13:376–379.

Xanthoma: A collection of lipid. There are various subtypes of xanthoma. Xanthelasma are yellowish plaques or nodules deposited around the eyelids (Fig. X.1). The deposits are particularly prone to occur on the medial upper eyelid and in patients with hyperlipidemia, but often there is no underlying lipid abnormality. The prevalence of atherosclerosis among patients with xanthelasma is 15% to 69%.[1] Patients with hyperlipidemia who have xanthelasma are at an increased risk of cardiovascular disease. Eyelid xanthomas occur in primary biliary cirrhosis, a cause of peripheral neuropathy.

Tendon xanthomas may occur in hyperlipidemia but are also a feature of cerebrotendinous xanthomatosis, an inborn metabolic error that causes the accumulation of cholestanol, a cholesterol metabolite, in tendons and in the CNS (Fig. X.2). In this rare, autosomal recessive lipid storage disease, cholestanol replaces cholesterol in myelin, leading to the neurological manifestations.

Xerophthalmia: Dryness of the eyes (keratoconjunctivitis sicca). Xerophthalmia may be an important clue to the presence of sicca syndrome. Sicca syndrome produces dryness of the eyes and mouth (xerostomia), and the term is sometimes used synonymously with Sjögren's syndrome. However, sicca symptoms are often due to medication side effects, particularly from drugs with anticholinergic properties, such as antidepressants and antihistamines, and may occur as a manifestation of vitamin A deficiency. Autoimmune sicca syndrome, or Sjögren's syndrome, occurs in primary and secondary forms. In primary Sjögren's syndrome, there is an autoimmune attack on exocrine glands, particularly the lacrimal and salivary glands. Primary Sjögren's syndrome has a host of neurological manifestations. Neurological

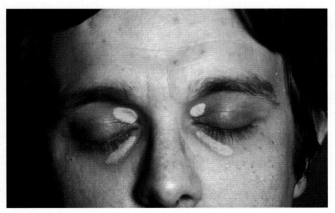

Figure X.1. Dramatic palpebral xanthelasma in a patient with familial hypercholesterolemia. (From Schaaf CP, Zschocke J, Potocki L. *Human Genetics: From Molecules to Medicine.* Philadelphia, PA: Wolters Kluwer Health/Lippincott Williams & Wilkins; 2012, with permission.)

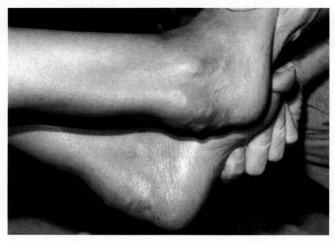

Figure X.2. Xanthomas involving the Achilles tendons in an adult patient with cerebro-tendinous xanthomatosis who presented with cerebellar ataxia.

involvement occurs in 20% of patients with Sjögren's syndrome, and in 81% the neurological manifestations precede the diagnosis.[2] The disease may mimic MS and often causes a polyneuropathy. Headache, particularly chronic tension-type head-ache, is common.[3] The diagnosis is often challenging. Anti-Ro/SSA or anti-La/SSB antibodies are detectable in only about 20% of patients initially. Documentation of xerophthalmia with the **Schirmer test** is helpful.

In secondary Sjögren's syndrome, exocrine gland involvement occurs due to an underlying connective tissue disease, most commonly rheumatoid arthritis, in which case the neurological complications are those of the underlying disease. Other causes of sicca syndrome include conditions such as sarcoidosis, amyloido-sis, primary biliary cirrhosis, and hyperthyroidism, which also have neurological manifestations. Botulism, autonomic neuropathy, and LEMS may cause prominent dry mouth.

Xerostomia: See **xerophthalmia.**

References

1. Dennis M, Bowen WT, Cho L. *Mechanisms of Clinical Signs.* Sydney, Australia: Churchill Livingstone; 2012.
2. Delalande S, de Seze J, Fauchais AL, et al. Neurologic manifestations in primary Sjogren syndrome: a study of 82 patients. *Medicine (Baltimore).* 2004;83:280–291.
3. Tjensvoll AB, Harboe E, Goransson LG, et al. Headache in primary Sjogren's syndrome: a population-based retrospective cohort study. *Eur J Neurol.* 2013;20:558–563.

Yawning: A complex respiratory reflex with deep, prolonged inspiration, usually involuntary, through open mouth. It typically occurs during sleepiness and fatigue but may also be brought on by suggestion or boredom. Yawning can occur in neurologic disease as well. It may occur with brainstem lesions and has been reported as the presenting symptom of brainstem stroke.[1] When yawning occurs in anterior circulation stroke, the paretic limbs may move, supporting the idea that yawning is mediated primarily by extrapyramidal pathways.[2]

Yeoman's sign: See **sacroiliac joint signs**.

Yergason's test (sign): A test primarily for bicipital tendonitis; see **shoulder examination tests**.

Yoshimura's sign: See **Chaddock's sign**.

References

1. Cattaneo L, Cucurachi L, Chierici E, et al. Pathological yawning as a presenting symptom of brain stem ischaemia in two patients. *J Neurol Neurosurg Psychiatry.* 2006;77:98–100.
2. Krestel H, Weisstanner C, Hess CW, et al. Insular and caudate lesions release abnormal yawning in stroke patients. *Brain Struct Funct.* 2015;220(2):803–812.

Y

Z

Zygomatic reflex: A modification of the jaw jerk. Percussion over the zygoma produces ipsilateral deviation of the mandible. Seen only with supranuclear lesions.

List of Signs by Conditions

This section is an index of sorts. It lists major neurologic disorders, conditions, and syndromes and the physical signs associated with them that are discussed in this book. It is not a comprehensive list of all the physical signs that might be seen in any particular condition. The subheadings refer to entries in the text.

Note: Page locators followed by "*f*" and "*t*" indicate figures and tables, respectively.

A

Aberrant regeneration (reinnervation), 2
  aberrant reinnervation of CN III, 2–3, 25
  Adie's pupil, 8
  arm–diaphragm synkinesia, 25
  breathing arm/hand, 50
  crocodile tears, 85
  facial synkinesis, 2, 123
  gustatory sweating, 161
  inverse jaw winking, 194
  jaw winking, 200
  lacrimal sweating, 206
  lid lag, 210
  pseudo-Argyll Robertson pupil, 287
  pseudo-Graefe sign, 3, 210, 288
  pupillary light near dissociation, 212*t*
Acid maltase deficiency (adult)
  bent spine syndrome, 43
  calf enlargement, 56
  dropped head, 104
  macroglossia, 216
  myotonia, 237
  respiratory failure, 301, 301*t*
Acromegaly, 5–6, 5*f*
  angioid streaks, 17
  clubbing, 76
  frontal bossing, 6, 139
  galactorrhea, 154
  hypertrichosis, 185
  macroglossia, 6, 216
  prognathism, 6, 283
Adie's pupil/syndrome, 6–8, 7*f*, 8*f*, 18, 25, 227, 278, 362
  aberrant regeneration, 8
  anisocoria, 8, 8*f*
  light-near dissociation, 6, 25
Alcoholism
  alcoholism, signs of, 13
  pupillary light near dissociation, 212*t*
  telangiectasias, 13, 352
  tremor, 364, 365
Alzheimer's disease
  anosmia, 19
  autoprosopagnosia, 31
  clock drawing test, 75
  cognitive screening instruments, 76–77, 76*t*
  executive functions, impaired, 118

  head turning sign, 166
  mental status examination, abnormal, 224
  myoclonus, 235
  orthostatic myoclonus, 258
Amyloidosis
  lymphadenopathy, 215
  macroglossia, 216
  organomegaly, 257
  proptosis, 286
  pseudohypertrophy, 232, 288
  pupillary light near dissociation, 212*t*
  raccoon eyes, 298
  retinal vascular sheathing, 305*t*
  scalloped pupils, 111*t*, 265*t*
  xerophthalmia, 392
Amyotrophic lateral sclerosis, 16
  bent spine syndrome, 43
  corneomandibular reflex, 83
  dropped head, 103
  dysarthria, 105, 106
  fasciculations, 127
  flail arm(s), 134, 135*f*
  flail leg(s), 134
  gag reflex, 147
  glossoplegia, 157
  jaw reflex, 200
  nasal speech, 240
  paradoxical respiration, 302
  Rust's sign, 311
  split hand, 334
Ankylosing spondylitis
  bent spine syndrome, 43
  iritis/uveitis, 196
  kyphosis, 205
Antiphospholipid syndrome
  livedo reticularis, 214
  retinal artery occlusion, 303
Ataxia-telangiectasia
  gray hair, 160
  hyperpigmentation, 183
  hypertrichosis, 185
  telangiectasias, 352
Autonomic neuropathy
  hyperhidrosis, 180
  pupillary light near dissociation, 212*t*
  xerophthalmia, 392

B

Basilar invagination
  downbeat nystagmus, 101–102, 244*t*, 247
  facial myokymia, 122
  short neck, 324
Basilar skull fracture
  Battle's sign, 41
  hemotympanum, 169, 169*f*
  raccoon eyes, 298
  tongue deviation, 362